The American

Occupational Structure

The American Occupational Structure

Peter M. Blau and Otis Dudley Duncan

WITH THE COLLABORATION OF ANDREA TYREE

THE FREE PRESS
A Division of Macmillan Publishing Co., Inc.
NEW YORK

Collier Macmillan Publishers
LONDON

The Free Press
A Division of Macmillan Publishing Co., Inc.
866 Third Avenue, New York, N.Y. 10022

Collier Macmillan Canada, Ltd.

First Free Press Edition 1978

Library of Congress Catalog Card Number: 78-50657

Printed in the United States of America

printing number

1 2 3 4 5 6 7 8 9 10

Library of Congress Cataloging in Publication Data

Blau, Peter Michael.
  The American occupational structure.

  Reprint of the ed. published by Wiley, New York.
  Includes bibliographical references.
  1. Occupational mobility--United States. 2. Social
mobility--United States. 3. United States--Occupations
--Social aspects. I. Duncan, Otis Dudley, joint author.
II. Title.
[HN90.S65B53 1978]   301.44'044'0973   78-50657
ISBN 0-02-903670-4

TO

Theodor I. Blau and Otis Durant Duncan
whose occupational achievements greatly
facilitated those of their sons

Preface

We may assume, then, that in contemporary life we have to do with a society in which the constitution of classes, so far as we have them, is partly determined by inheritance and partly by a more or less open competition, which is, again, more or less effective in placing men where they rightly belong. . . .

Where classes do not mean separate currents of thought, as in the case of caste, but are merely differentiations in a common mental whole, there are likely to be several kinds of classes overlapping one another, so that men who fall in the same class from one point of view are separated in another. The groups are like circles which, instead of standing apart, interlace with one another so that several of them may pass through the same individual. . . .

In modern life, then, and in a country without formal privilege, the question of classes is practically one of wealth, and of occupation considered in relation to wealth. . . .

Charles Horton Cooley, Social Organization

. . . There is a certain opposition between the ideal of equal opportunity and that of family responsibility. Responsibility involves autonomy, which will produce divergence among families, which, in turn, will mean divergent conditions for the children; that is, unequal opportunities. . . .

I think that equal opportunity, though not wholly practicable, is one of our best working ideals. We are not likely to go too far in this direction. There is a natural current of privilege, arising from the tendency of advantages to flow in the family line, and any feasible diversion into broader channels will probably be beneficial.

Charles Horton Cooley, Social Process

Men's careers occupy a dominant place in their lives today, and the occupational structure is the foundation of the stratification system of contemporary industrial society. In the absence of hereditary castes or feudal estates, class differences come to rest primarily on occupational positions and the economic advantages and powers associated with them. A knowledge of the occupational structure and of the conditions that govern men's chances of achieving economic success by moving up in the occupational hierarchy is, therefore, essential for understanding modern society and, particularly, its stratified character. In a democratic country where equality of opportunity, though never perfectly realized, is an important ideal, the question of the extent to which the class or ethnic group into which an individual is born furthers or hinders his career chances is of special theoretical as well as political significance. The present monograph provides an analysis of the American occupational structure and the factors that influence social mobility in it on the basis of a large-scale empirical survey of the working lives of men in the United States.

This book is the result of a collaborative effort extending over seven years. We have tried hard to make the book a genuine joint product to which each of us made the contributions he is best qualified to make. There is no senior author; the sequence of name is simply alphabetical, and we have reversed it in signing the pref. ce and elsewhere to emphasize this fact. Our collaboration was motivated by our shared interest in social stratification, our common concern with advancing scientific social theory on the basis of systematic research, and the conviction that the inquiry would benefit from the different qualifications and viewpoints the two of us represent. There can be no doubt that our interests in and approaches to sociological problems differ to a considerable degree. Although we agree that refining research methods and advancing social theory are both important, for example, it is only fair to state that Duncan puts priority on developing rigorous methods and Blau lays more stress on deriving theoretical generalizations.

Joining forces in this research endeavor posed the challenge for us of whether we could reconcile the disagreements resulting from our divergent perspectives sufficiently to take advantage of our complementary skills. It is not for us to say how successful we were in meeting this challenge. We do realize, however, that the problems created by our collaboration are reflected in certain limitations of the book. It is unquestionably not as well integrated—either in style or in continuity of thought—as it would be had it not been written by two social scientists with rather different orientations. One conclusion our experience has impressed upon us is that reasonable men (if we may so describe ourselves) may reasonably differ when jointly exploring a rough terrain. We have not only differed concerning the best interpretation of a set of empirical findings, which is to be expected, but sometimes even disagreed as to what the findings themselves show. Confronted by the same set of quantitative data, two men do not necessarily arrive at the same conclusion regarding the empirical "facts" of the case, let alone regarding the inferences to be drawn from them. A configuration clearly apparent in a number of complex tables to one may be seen by the other as conforming to a different pattern, dependent on initial assumptions and problem focus. Orders of significance and priority of emphasis may fail to coincide, and what looks like an interesting discovery from one point of view seems trivial from another. Moreover, there can hardly be full consensus on what demands to place on the reader—whether to let him draw his own conclusions or present what possibly only one of us considers to be the most plausible interpretation of the findings. We have reconciled these differences as best we could and in various ways. Sometimes, we have carried out additional empirical analysis to clarify a problem to our joint satisfaction (for instance, in Chapter 2); at other times, we reached a compromise conclusion after discussion; at still others, we agreed to differ and presented alternative perspectives (for instance, in Chapter 11). We have also given preference to the inclination of the author of a given chapter in respect to how far to go beyond the data in suggesting interpretations for them. If we have often erred in both directions, offering insufficient interpretations on some occasions and engaging in excessive speculations on others, and if this has produced some unevenness in the book, we must ask the reader's indulgence in sharing with us the vicissitudes of a collaborative effort of this kind.

Given the differences in our skills and concerns, it appears appropriate to outline the division of labor that produced this book, if only to help the reader understand any inconsistencies that have remained in the volume despite our awareness of the problem and our efforts to achieve coherence. The study as a whole was initiated by Blau, having been originally conceived over 12 years ago in discussions with Nelson N. Foote and with Clyde W. Hart, then director of the National Opinion Research Center. The involvement of Duncan occurred at the time when it was determined that the project could best be carried out in cooperation with the U. S. Bureau of the Census. Early planning was carried out in close collaboration through the stages of questionnaire design and the first round of tabulation specifications. Generally, however, Blau was more concerned with conceptual issues and hypothesis formulation, and Duncan with problems of measurement and hypothesis testing. A second round of tabulation specifications was primarily the work of Duncan, in connection with the separately funded study of fertility in relation to social mobility (this material is presented mainly in Chapter 11 and, to some extent, in Chapter 10).

The development of statistical methods and models and the supervision of the bulk of the calculations fell on Duncan. Results of this work were allocated between the two authors, each taking primary responsibility for drafting certain chapters. Subsequently, intensive mutual criticism and exchange of ideas led to extensive revisions. The primary responsibility for the final as well as the preliminary versions of Chapters 3, 4, 5, 8, 10, and 11 was Duncan's, and that for Chapters 2, 6, 7, 9, and 12 was Blau's. But most chapters include not only many ideas and suggestions but also entire passages contributed by the author not primarily responsible for them. Andrea Tyree was Blau's research assistant while these chapters were prepared and helped him in the over-all organization of the volume, and her designation as collaborative author is in acknowledgment of her substantial contributions to the book.

The analysis of empirical findings is presented in ten chapters, preceded by a general introduction to the study of occupational structure and mobility and followed by a concluding chapter dealing with some broader theoretical issues raised by the research findings. The organization of the material in the volume is discussed at the end of the introductory chapter, but a few preliminary remarks on the tabulations and the appendices are in order. Unless otherwise indicated all tables refer to all men between the ages of 20 and 64 in the civilian noninstitutional population of the United States in March 1962. The numbers are population estimates, in thousands, derived from our representative national sample. Whenever a table pertains to a narrower age range, such as 25 to 64, or a subgroup or a different sample, the population base is explicitly specified in the table heading. We have devoted considerable time and energy to the analysis of differences between age cohorts. Most relationships between variables were observable in all age groups (with the partial exception of the youngest group, the men less than 25 years, many of whom are still in preparatory stages of their careers). We have combined age cohorts in these instances in the interest of preserving larger case bases for refined analysis, considering it unnecessary to present separate data for different cohorts merely to demonstrate the parallel patterns. The noteworthy differences between age cohorts are, of course, discussed at various appropriate points in the text, and Chapter 3 deals extensively with age differences and their implications.

Some basic descriptive information on the variables used in the study and their relationships as well as on a variety of methodological points is presented in ten appendices. The first of these is a bibliography of Census publications containing material relevant for this study. The last appendix consists of supplementary tables. Most of the other appendices deal with methodological questions. For example, two reliability checks on our data are discussed. Of special interest is Appendix H. It contains not only a specification of every variable used, but it also shows how much of the variance in occupational status and in education is explained by each independent variable singly and by a large number of combinations of independent variables. These data disclose much information about the conditions that influence success in our society.

OTIS DUDLEY DUNCAN
PETER M. BLAU

Ann Arbor and Chicago,
February 1967

Acknowledgments

This study would not have been possible, of course, without the cordial cooperation of the Bureau of the Census and the conscientious exercise of its wide array of skills. Most of the people who carried out the exacting operational tasks—interviewing, data processing, and tabulating —were not known to us, but we appreciate their excellent work nonetheless. Several members of the professional staff of the Bureau were directly involved with the research at various points. We should particularly like to mention that Conrad Taeuber, as Assistant Director, was the person with whom our initial discussions of feasibility took place, and he has maintained a friendly interest in the study. Robert B. Pearl, Chief of the Demographic Surveys Division (the unit responsible for the Current Population Survey), provided sound counsel on the many perplexing details of research design. Three members of the Economic Statistics Branch of the Population Division served as Project Coordinator of our study of Occupational Changes in a Generation: Stuart Garfinkle during the period when the questionnaire was designed and pretested, William J. Milligan during the period of the field work, and Stanley Greene during the period of data processing and tabulation. It was a great advantage to have the guidance of these experts in the field of occupational statistics. We should like, finally, to express our thanks for the several useful suggestions made by members of the staff of the Population Division: Howard G. Brunsman, Henry S. Shryock, Jr., Paul C. Glick, Charles B. Nam, and Robert Parke, Jr. It should only be added that the conclusions drawn in this book are the sole responsibility of its authors, as are any errors in the analysis and interpretation of the data provided by the Bureau of the Census.

We gratefully acknowledge financial support by three research grants: from the National Science Foundation to the University of Chicago (G-16233); from the National Institutes of Health to the University of Chicago (RG-8386) and to the University of Michigan (GM-10386). We want to thank particularly Henry W. Riecken of the National Science Foundation, who gave us much encouragement when we initially approached him with our proposal, and Robert L. Hall, then at the National Science Foundation and now at the University of Illinois, whose cooperative attitude and helpful counsel were of great assistance in formulating the research proposal.

A number of students at the University of Chicago and the University of Michigan served as associates and assistants in this study. Robert W. Hodge worked with us at the beginning of the study, preparing an illuminating review of the literature and contributing significant observations to the evaluation of the pretest. The execution of the statistical analysis would not have been possible without the expertise of J. Michael Coble in programming and data handling. Bruce L. Warren lived with the data for several years and made substantive as well as technical contributions to the analysis. Their labors were augmented by the faithful services of Ruthe C. Sweet and Sally Frisbie. More than ordinary skill and diligence went into the work of Beulah El Dareer and Alice Y. Sano in typing tables and manuscript.

The colleagues with whom we discussed one problem or another of our research in the long period of its gestation are too numerous to mention, and we can only express our appreciation to them collectively. We were particularly fortunate, however, to be able to benefit from the insightful suggestions and penetrating criticisms of two colleagues throughout these many years, two colleagues on whose perceptive understanding of social research and our own work we had come to rely long before this project had been started. We are greatly indebted for their supportive assistance to Beverly Duncan and Zena Smith Blau.

Table of Contents

The American
Occupational Structure

CHAPTER 1

Occupational Structure and Mobility Process

The objective of this book is to present a systematic analysis of the American occupational structure, and thus of the major foundation of the stratification system in our society. Processes of social mobility from one generation to the next and from career beginnings to occupational destinations are considered to reflect the dynamics of the occupational structure. By analyzing the patterns of these occupational movements, the conditions that affect them, and some of their consequences, we attempt to explain part of the dynamics of the stratification system in the United States. The inquiry is based on a considerable amount of empirical data collected from a representative sample of over 20,000 American men between the ages of 20 and 64.

Many of the research findings and conclusions we report have significant implications for social policy and action programs. For example, we repeatedly indicate whether the inferior occupational chances of some groups compared to those of others are primarily due to the former's inferior educational attainments or to other factors. These differences reveal whether educational programs would suffice or other social actions are necessary to effect improvements in the occupational opportunities of the groups under consideration. We hope that the documented generalizations presented will be helpful to policy makers and the interested public in formulating appropriate action programs and clarifying partisan controversy, but we have not seen it as our task to spell out the practical implications of our findings in detail.

Neither have we set ourselves the objective of formulating a theory of stratification on the basis of the results of our empirical investiga-

1

tion. This does not mean that we have restricted our responsibility to reporting "the facts" and letting them speak for themselves, or that we favor an artificial separation of scientific research and theory. On the contrary, we seek to place our research findings into a theoretical framework and suggest theoretical interpretations for them. To bring theoretical considerations to bear upon our empirical data on occupational achievement and mobility, however, is a much more modest undertaking than to construct a theory of stratification. The latter is not the aim of this book, although we shall speculate in the concluding chapter about some of the broader implications of our results for such a theory.

STRATIFICATION THEORY AND MOBILITY RESEARCH

In a classical presentation of social mobility as an important problem for sociological inquiry, completed four short decades ago, the author lamented,

> Within our societies vertical circulation of individuals is going on permanently. But how is it taking place? . . . what are the characteristics of this process of which very little is known? Individuals have been speculating too much and studying the facts too little. It is high time to abandon speculation for the somewhat saner method of collecting the facts and studying them patiently.[1]

It was only after World War II that Sorokin's challenge began to be met in any substantial way. To be sure, many of the great social thinkers of the last century, stimulated by the great impact of industrialization on society and the resulting concern with social change in general and the role of class differentiation for change in particular, developed theories of stratification or differentiation. The classical example is Marx's theory of class conflict as the prime force generating historical change, which has dominated much of social thought in the nineteenth century and much of political life in the twentieth.[2] Marx would probably not be displeased to see that his theory today is much more influential in actual political life than in the social sciences, since he held that the action implications of a social theory, not its objective scientific merits, are what justifies it. Durkheim's theory of the division of labor focuses more specifically on occupational differentiation, its roots in social density, and its implications

---

[1] Pitirim A. Sorokin, *Social Mobility*, New York: Harper, 1927, p. 414.
[2] For a concise summary of Marx's class theory, see Reinhard Bendix and Seymour M. Lipset (eds.), *Class, Status, and Power*, Glencoe: Free Press, 1953, pp. 26-35.

for lessening consensus and altering the nature of social solidarity.[3] But neither these two nor any of the many other broad theories of social class and differentiation had much influence on the systematic research on social mobility that has been carried out in the last two decades. Indeed, most empirical studies of occupational mobility never refer to these theories. Thus even investigators known to be conversant with and sympathetic to Marx's theory do not make reference to it in their mobility research.

The reason for this neglect of stratification theory in mobility research is not simply the often-voiced complaint that the grand theories developed in the last century are not formulated in terms that make them easily amenable to empirical investigation. It is more specific than that. Stratification theories seek to explain the features of social differentiation in a society by reference to the historical conditions that have produced them, which implies a comparative framework in which differences in institutional conditions between historical periods or societies are related to consequent differences in the stratification systems. To explain the conditions that have produced the distinctive features of a stratification system it is necessary to contrast it with other systems or, at the very least, with one other, whether the comparison is based on systematic data or relies on impressionistic observation. Empirical studies of social status and mobility in one society cannot make the relevant comparisons to formulate or refine the propositions of stratification theories, because each society constitutes merely a single case from the perspective of these theories, regardless of the volume of quantitative data collected. Moreover, stratification theories generally are concerned with other institutional conditions in a society that produce the characteristic class structure, or with other conditions that have been produced by this class structure. Empirical studies typically have no information on these other variables. Thus both Marx and Durkheim consider extensive social interaction an essential condition for the development of social differentiation—specifically, for the development of the class consciousness that crystallizes class differences in Marx's case, and for the development of the division of labor in Durkheim's. But mobility research rarely if ever collects information on the extent of social interaction. The design of mobility research is not suited for the study of the problems posed by stratification theory, for it centers attention not on the institutional differences between societies but on the differ-

[3] Émile Durkheim, *On the Division of Labor in Society*, New York: Macmillan, 1933.

ential conditions that affect occupational achievements and mobility within any one.

Although no single empirical study of social status and mobility in one society can advance stratification theory—which is the reason we have stressed that doing so is not the aim of our book—this does not mean that such research is irrelevant for the theory. Far from it; the cumulative results of empirical studies of stratification in different societies are essential for testing and refining stratification theory. Sorokin called for this kind of cumulative research effort in the passage quoted, and he attempted in his own work to derive theoretical generalizations about stratification from the limited bodies of empirical data then available.[4]

A number of local studies of occupational mobility in one community were pioneering endeavors that provided important insights into the problem,[5] but the tendency to use their results—as the only ones available—to draw inferences about social mobility in the society at large soon called attention to their evident limitations for such a purpose. It became increasingly apparent that nationwide studies based on representative samples are needed to clarify the process of social mobility, particularly in modern society where occupational mobility is often accompanied by geographical moves that take individuals from one local community to another. A number of such national mobility surveys in different countries were initiated shortly after the end of World War II by a group of scholars who formed an international committee on social stratification and mobility under the auspices of the International Sociological Association. Outstanding illustrations are the studies of mobility in Britain by Glass and his colleagues, in Denmark by Svalastoga, and in Sweden by Carlsson.[6] National studies in numerous other countries have also been carried out, but there is no need to review them here since a comprehensive bibliography of these and a few local studies, together with some comparative analysis of their results, has been presented by Miller.[7]

---

[4] Sorokin, loc. cit. For a critique, see Gösta Carlsson, "Sorokin's Theory of Social Mobility," in Philip J. Allen (ed.), Pitirim A. Sorokin in Review, Durham: Duke Univer. Press, 1963, pp. 123-139.

[5] For two American studies, see H. Dewey Anderson and Percy E. Davidson, Occupational Mobility in an American Community, Stanford: Stanford Univer. Press, 1937; and Natalie Rogoff, Recent Trends in Occupational Mobility, Glencoe: Free Press, 1953.

[6] D. V. Glass (ed.), Social Mobility in Britain, London: Routledge and Kegan Paul, 1954; Kaare Svalastoga, Prestige, Class and Mobility, Copenhagen: Gyldendal, 1959; and Gösta Carlsson, Social Mobility and Class Structure, Lund: CWK Gleerup, 1958.

[7] S. M. Miller, "Comparative Social Mobility," Current Sociology, Vol. 9, No. 1, 1960. A recent Italian study not included in Miller's review is presented in Joseph

Our research on the American occupational structure is in the tradition of these national surveys of occupational mobility. It shares with them the assumption that the understanding of social stratification in modern society is best promoted by the systematic investigation of occupational status and mobility. In short, the focus is on the stratified hierarchy of occupations rather than on some other aspects of social differentiation. The limitation of this approach as well as the justification for it should be pointed out. The major limitation is that it does not make it possible to analyze the various dimensions of stratification.

Max Weber's famous distinction between class, status, and political party calls attention to different dimensions of social stratification.[8] He granted the importance of economic classes that is stressed in Marx's theory. These classes are differentiated on the basis of the position of men in relation to the economy, particularly the possession of property in the form of capital, and they determine the life chances of individuals and their economic interests. But Weber emphasized that this economic differentiation is not the only dimension along which society is stratified. Men are also differentiated into social strata in terms of the social honor or prestige accorded to them, and the members of a status group, as Weber called prestige strata, share a distinctive style of life, accept each others as equals, and restrict noninstrumental social intercourse to the ingroup. Moreover, the roles individuals play in the struggle among parties for political power refer to still another aspect of stratification, which must be distinguished from both class position and prestige status. The difference between the latter two can be summarized by saying "that 'classes' are stratified according to their relations to the *production* and *acquisition* of goods; whereas 'status groups' are stratified according to the principles of their *consumption* of goods as represented by special 'styles of life.' "[9]

Although Warner did not utilize Weber's conceptual scheme, and was apparently not even aware of it, his community studies led him to the same conclusion: other criteria than strictly economic ones govern the differentiation of men into various prestige strata.[10] The

Lopreato, "Social Mobility in Italy," *American Journal of Sociology*, 71(1965), 311-314.

[8] Max Weber, *Essays in Sociology*, New York: Oxford Univer. Press, 1946, pp. 180-195.

[9] *Ibid.*, p. 193 (italics in original).

[10] See especially W. Lloyd Warner and Paul S. Lunt, *The Social Life of a Modern Community*, New Haven: Yale Univer. Press, 1941, pp. 81-126. This is the first volume of the *Yankee City Series*. There is no reference to Max Weber in the entire series.

prestige status of individuals is not directly determined by their economic affluence or personal attributes but by the social stratum in which their families have found social acceptance. Social strata rather than individuals are ranked by the community into a prestige hierarchy. The family's possessions and characteristics affect its prestige status only indirectly, by influencing the stratum in which members are accepted, as indicated by their patterns of social participation and association. Important as these prestige strata studied by Warner may be in the social life of a community, however, economic rather than prestige criteria are undoubtedly the crucial ones in the stratification system of the entire society, particularly the industrial society.

Occupational position is not identical either with economic class or with prestige status, but it is closely connected with both, particularly with the former. Class may be defined in terms of economic resources and interests, and the primary determinant of these for the large majority of men is their occupational position. To be sure, Marx stressed that the criterion of class is not a man's occupation but whether he is an employer who has the capital to buy the labor of others or an employee who sells his labor. This criterion, however, is no longer adequate for differentiating, as Marx intended it to do, men in control of the large capitalistic enterprises from those subject to their control, because the controlling managers of the largest concerns today are themselves employees of corporations. If class refers to the role persons occupy in the economy and their managerial influence on economic concerns, it is more accurately reflected in a man's specific occupation than in his employment status in contemporary society, where the economy is dominated by corporations rather than individual proprietors. Occupational position does not encompass all aspects of the concept of class, but it is probably the best single indicator of it (although more refined measures should take economic influence directly into account). Conceptually, there is a closer relationship between economic class and occupational position than there is between occupational position and prestige status. But there is also some relationship between the latter two because many occupational pursuits (notably those involving physical labor) are incompatible with the "honor" of belonging to the higher prestige strata. In addition, the maintenance of the "proper" style of life of these higher strata requires considerable economic resources.

The occupational structure in modern industrial society not only constitutes an important foundation for the main dimensions of social stratification but also serves as the connecting link between different institutions and spheres of social life, and therein lies its great significance. The hierarchy of prestige strata and the hierarchy of economic classes have their roots in the occupational structure; so does the hierarchy of political power and authority, for political authority in modern society is largely exercised as a full-time occupation. It is the occupational structure that manifests the allocation of manpower to various institutional spheres, and it is the flow of movements among occupational groups that reflects the adjustment of the demand for diverse services and the supply of qualified manpower. The occupational structure also is the link between the economy and the family, through which the economy affects the family's status and the family supplies manpower to the economy.[11] The hierarchy of occupational strata reveals the relationship between the social contributions men make by furnishing various services and the rewards they receive in return, whether or not this relationship expresses some equitable functional adjustment, as assumed by the functional theory of stratification.[12] Indeed, there is good reason to suspect that such adjustment is often disturbed, because the occupational hierarchy is not only an incentive system for eliciting services in demand but also a power structure that enables men in controlling positions, such as corporation managers, to influence the distribution of rewards.

The variegated role of the occupational structure in connecting different elements of social organization makes an understanding of it essential for the student of modern society. The study of social stratification, in particular, presupposes a thorough knowledge of the occupational hierarchy, which is a major source of the various aspects of social stratification in industrial society. Many problems of stratification cannot be investigated on the basis of research on the occupational structure, however, because such research does not provide information on the various manifestations of stratification and their interrelations—the extent to which class, status, and power differences overlap or diverge—but only deals with the underlying dimension common to them all. Hence inquiries into the occupational structure are merely a first step, albeit an important one, in the analysis of social stratification.

Our study builds on the tradition that has developed in national surveys of occupational mobility but departs from this tradition both methodologically and substantively. Previous studies of occupational mobility have devoted much attention to methodological problems of

[11] See Talcott Parsons and Neil J. Smelser, *Economy and Society*, Glencoe: Free Press, 1956, pp. 51-55, 70-72.
[12] See Kingsley Davis and Wilbert Moore, "Some Principles of Stratification," *American Sociological Review*, 10(1945), 242-249.

measurement, notably, how to rank occupations and how to measure the extent of mobility between social origins and occupational destinations. In addition to the use of outflow percentages from origins and inflow percentages into destinations, summary measures of the extent of mobility have been devised, the best known of which is the "index of association" or "social distance mobility ratio."[13] The quantitative score of occupational status employed in our research makes it possible to utilize several more complex statistical procedures, such as regression techniques, which permit refined analysis of the data. These more elaborate methods of analysis are of special importance for the investigation of the simultaneous influence of several factors on occupational achievement and mobility. A major substantive difference between our inquiry and earlier mobility research is our concern with these factors that influence occupational mobility.

The predominant emphasis in mobility research has been on the analysis of the occupational mobility matrix as a self-contained entity. Although the results of this analysis describing the mobility pattern are occasionally related to other variables, such as education or fertility, the major preoccupation is typically the internal analysis of mobility tables, and relatively little attention is devoted to the systematic investigation of the relationships between other factors and occupational mobility. The tendency to conceive of mobility as a single variable and examine it largely without relating it to other variables has severely restricted the fruitfulness of mobility research. After all, the purpose of scientific inquiry is to establish, and then to explain, general relationships between variables, and not merely to delineate the population distribution of one variable, regardless of how important this variable may be. It is as if students of political behavior were merely to ascertain the shifts in party preferences between elections without investigating the factors associated with different party preferences and with shifts in them. Preoccupied with mobility as such, investigations have generally not supplied sufficient information on its correlates to make it possible to explain the observed mobility patterns.

The comparison of occupational mobility in different countries greatly enhances the substantive interest of the findings, because this comparison stimulates insights and speculations about other known variations between these countries that may have produced the differences in mobility patterns. Thus Carlsson relates his findings on mobility in Sweden to those of other investigators of mobility in Great

---

[13] Independently developed and differently labeled in Glass (ed.), *loc. cit.*, and Rogoff, *loc. cit.* Limitations of this measure are discussed in Chapter 3.

Britain and West Germany, and Miller presents a comprehensive secondary analysis of mobility in 18 different nations, although the data for some of these are unfortunately of questionable reliability.[14] The most extensive secondary analysis of social mobility in various industrial societies has been carried out by Lipset and Bendix, who investigate a variety of factors associated with mobility in different countries and derive from their analysis suggestive theoretical generalizations about social stratification in modern society.[15] The national studies of occupational mobility, despite their limited scope, have made the important contribution of laying the groundwork necessary for such comparative secondary analysis.

Whereas research on occupational mobility in a single society cannot make the comparisons needed to generalize about stratification systems, as previously noted, it can attempt to explain the observed patterns of mobility by ascertaining some of the other conditions associated with them. This is a basic objective of the present monograph. Although we, too, start the substantive discussion of our findings with an analysis of the intergenerational and intragenerational mobility tables themselves, we proceed to discern what other factors not contained in these tables affect the patterns reflected in them. After examining, in the next two chapters, the patterns of intergenerational and intragenerational mobility among occupational groups and historical trends in these patterns, the focus shifts to the study of the conditions that influence differential occupational success and some of its consequences.

A substantive problem of central concern to us, which mobility research in the past has largely neglected, is, therefore, how the observed patterns of occupational mobility are affected by various factors, such as a man's color, whether he has migrated, or the number of his siblings and his position among them. We found it advantageous, however, to reformulate this problem by decomposing the concept of occupational mobility into its constituent elements: social or career origins and occupational destinations. Rather than asking what influence a variable—community size, for instance—exerts on upward mobility, we ask what influence it exerts on occupational achievements *and* how it modifies the effect of social origins on these achievements. The main reason for this reformulation is that the likelihood

---

[14] Carlsson, *op. cit.*, pp. 116-120; and Miller, *loc. cit.* See also Thomas G. Fox and S. M. Miller, "Economic, Political and Social Determinants of Mobility," *Acta Sociologica,* 9(1965), 76-93.

[15] Seymour M. Lipset and Reinhard Bendix, *Social Mobility in Industrial Society,* Berkeley: Univer. of California Press, 1959.

of upward mobility depends, of course, greatly on the level from which a man starts; this makes the finding that a given factor is associated with mobility ambiguous, as will be more fully shown in Chapter 5. Such ambiguities are avoided by taking the level of social or career origins into account. To cite only one example at this point: the chances of upward mobility of Negroes, though lower than those of whites, appear misleadingly high unless the exceptionally low levels of origins are taken into consideration.

This reformulation of the problem enables us to dissect the process of occupational mobility by determining how various factors condition the influence of origins on occupational success. Thus we trace the interdependence between social origins, career beginnings, and education, and examine their direct and indirect influences on occupational achievements. This basic model is subsequently enlarged by investigating how a variety of other factors contribute to occupational achievement and mobility. The analysis of the characteristics of individuals and social conditions that affect occupational success serves to explicate the patterns of movement observable in the mobility matrix. A system of stratified occupations must include provisions for the allocation of persons to positions in order to maintain itself in the face of the birth and death of men, their maturation and retirement, the expanding need for some occupational services, and the declining demand for others. The process of occupational mobility refers to the social metabolism that governs this allocation of manpower and hence underlies the dynamics of the occupational structure. The specification of the factors that affect the occupational achievements of individuals seeks to account for this dynamic process. In sum, the conventional mobility matrix represents the structure of occupational allocations to be explained, and the analysis of the conditions that determine the process of mobility is designed to furnish the required explanation.

METHOD OF DATA COLLECTION

Following the lead of the subcommittee on stratification and mobility of the International Sociological Association, the data for our study were collected in a national sample survey. There is an important innovation in our procedure, however. Our survey of "Occupational Changes in a Generation" (OCG) was not organized as an *ad hoc* inquiry but was carried out as an adjunct to the monthly "Current Population Survey" (CPS) of the U. S. Bureau of the Census. The CPS, in continuous operation since 1942, has the primary function of producing monthly statistics on the labor force, unemployment, and related topics,[16] but it often collects data on a variety of other subjects, as illustrated in the information given in Appendix A, "Bibliography of Official Government Publications Relating to the Population Covered in OCG."[17]

The decision to secure our mobility data through the CPS had far-reaching consequences for the study design and analysis—largely benign consequences, but occasionally troublesome ones. The most attractive result of this decision was that we were able to obtain, at marginal cost, data on social mobility for a much larger sample than had ever been studied in such a national sample before. A second important advantage was that the investigators did not have to become involved in the creation and operation of a complex survey mechanism but could depend on the skills in sampling, questionnaire design, field operations, and data processing of a large staff of highly trained and experienced professionals.

The disadvantages and vexations attending this *modus operandi* stemmed largely from two circumstances: the lengthy lead-and-lag times required from initial planning to execution of field work, and from field work to data processing and statistical analysis, necessitated by having to work through a giant bureaucracy; and the severe restrictions on the amount of information that could be collected. For example, no attitudinal data could be obtained, because the field staff lacked the required experience; and no information on religion could be collected, because the present policy of the Bureau of the Census prohibits it.

Discussions with officials of the Bureau of the Census during the latter half of 1959 established that the Bureau recognized a general public interest in statistics on social mobility; that it would be feasible to include questions on this subject in the CPS; that such questions could be cross-tabulated with others normally obtained in the CPS; that this could be done at reasonable marginal costs; but that special financing would have to be obtained to support such work.

During the succeeding 12 months the investigators drafted proposals for financing and secured approval of two projects to be supported, respectively, by the National Science Foundation and the Public Health Service. The development of plans for the two projects re-

---

16 U. S. Bureau of Labor Statistics and U. S. Bureau of the Census, "Concepts and Methods Used in Household Statistics on Employment and Unemployment from the Current Population Survey," *BLS Report* No. 279 and *Current Population Reports*, Series P-23, No. 13, June 1964.

17 An instructive discussion of the value of the CPS as a resource for social research is presented in Daniel B. Levine and Charles B. Nam, "The Current Population Survey," *American Sociological Review*, 27(1962), 585-590.

quired considerable consultation with officials of the Bureau of the Census, inasmuch as it was necessary to anticipate in considerable detail what would be done and what it would cost. The essential features of the study were determined during this period. The grants for the study were officially approved early in 1961; the questionnaire was pretested in the summer of that year; and final decisions about all aspects of the study design had to be made soon thereafter, including specification of the actual statistical tables to be produced.

The data collection for the OCG survey took place in March 1962. The Bureau of the Census had already planned to obtain in this month not only the usual labor-force information, including occupation, industry, and class of worker of members of the experienced civilian labor force, as well as age, sex, and color, but also data on educational attainment, income, marital and household status, and number of children ever born. With this information available from the regular CPS interview, it was necessary only to determine what additional items would be required to serve the purpose of a study on social mobility.

As a matter of feasibility and economy, it was decided that the supplementary OCG information should be collected not in the course of the regular CPS interview but by means of a "leave-behind" questionnaire, which the eligible respondents were asked to fill out and mail to the regional headquarters of the Bureau of the Census. The pretest confirmed the supposition that this self-enumeration procedure would be workable. It was still necessary to impose strict limitations on the amount and detail of information to be requested in the OCG questionnaire. A two-page document, supposedly self-explanatory to the great majority of respondents, was developed to secure data on the following items: birthplace of respondent, his father, and his mother; number of siblings and birth order; educational attainment of respondent's oldest brother (if any); size of community of residence at age 16; type of school attended up to age 16; age at entering first job, and occupation, industry, and class of worker of that job; family living arrangements up to age 16; occupation of father (or other person who was the family head) when respondent was about 16 years old; educational attainment of father (or other family head); marital status; and, for married men living with their wives, the number of the wife's siblings and her father's occupation. The actual questionnaire is reproduced in Appendix B. The reader must remember, however, that it covers only the supplementary OCG items and not the whole array of information available from the regular CPS interview. There is no point in reproducing the CPS interview form itself; it is a complex document, fully intelligible only to trained interviewers, and designed for automated data processing.[18]

One of the hazards of self-enumeration is, of course, that respondents will not comply with the request to complete and return the document on schedule. Provision was made, therefore, for initial mail follow-up, and for a final follow-up by personal contact (telephone call or household visit) of a subsample of the remaining nonrespondents. Assuming a high completion rate for these final follow-up interviews, as was in fact obtained, it was possible to introduce differential sample inflation factors for the two groups in the sample: (a) those responding to the initial contact or to one of the mail follow-ups, and (b) those responding only on the final wave of personal follow-ups. The end result was a set of estimates essentially free of nonresponse bias. (This refers to potential bias resulting from failure to respond at all; a separate bias remains due to failing to answer particular questions when returning the questionnaire.)

We shall not attempt to supply details on the design and properties of the CPS sample, as a thorough technical discussion is available elsewhere,[19] and as each official report based on CPS carries notes on sampling procedures and estimates of sampling variability. In March 1962, as in each month since 1956, the CPS contacted some 35,000 occupied dwelling units or households. These contained approximately 25,000 men 20 to 64 years of age who were designated as eligible respondents for the OCG questionnaire. Complete questionnaires or follow-up interviews were obtained from almost exactly five-sixths of these men; that is, from about 20,700 respondents. Sample figures were inflated to independent estimates of the U. S. population by age, sex, and color, incorporating the differential weights for response status already mentioned. The 20,700 respondents represent the approximately 45 million men 20 to 64 years old in the civilian, noninstitutional population of the United States in March 1962 (including as "civilians" some 900,000 members of the Armed Forces living in families on military posts in the United States or off posts in civilian quarters). Unless otherwise specified, all tables refer to this sample.

The tabulations produced for the OCG study are in the form of

---

[18] Detailed specifications on regular CPS items can be found in the *Current Population Reports* and *Special Labor Force Reports,* such as those listed in Appendix A.

[19] U. S. Bureau of the Census, "The Current Population Survey: A Report on Methodology," Technical Paper No. 7, 1963.

estimates of population frequencies (in 1000's). Given the controls employed in the estimation process, we automatically enjoy near-perfect comparability of the OCG data with other CPS tabulations for the month of March 1962, although some minor discrepancies are unavoidable, given the difference in over-all completion rate for the regular interviews and the OCG supplement. (See Appendix C, "Notes on Coverage of OCG Tabulations and Comparability with Other Sources.") The advantage of comparability with several other sources makes the OCG statistics one element in a comprehensive set of social and demographic statistics describing the state and condition of American society at a particular point in time. We do not have to offer interpretations in a vacuum or resort to speculation as soon as we depart from the confines of the particular tables at hand; a cornucopia of reliable supporting information is at hand.[20]

What can we say of the quality of the OCG statistics? The first observation is that those portions of the data deriving from the regular CPS interview represent a product of survey procedures repeated literally scores of times in the past and refined and improved in the course of repetition. A large amount of information is available on their reliability and validity. We have detailed statistics, for example, on the correspondence between responses obtained in CPS interviews and those obtained independently in a full-scale census.[21] As survey data go, the CPS statistics must be presumed to be highly reliable and accurate by current standards.

We are in a less secure position with respect to the data secured in the OCG supplementary questionnaire. Questions resembling these had been asked in previous surveys, of course, but little work on the evaluation of the resulting statistics had been done. In the OCG study it was possible to design only a modest number of checks on data quality, although these go beyond what is usually available for the evaluation of survey data. The most significant evaluations are summarized here.

In the pretest carried out in the Chicago metropolitan area during the summer of 1961 an effort was made to ascertain addresses of respondents at the time they were 16 years old so that these identical respondents could be located in the records of one of the censuses of 1920, 1930, or 1940. Among 123 cases in which a census match was

20 See Appendix A, "Bibliography of Official Government Publications Relating to the Population Covered in OCG."

21 U. S. Bureau of the Census, "Accuracy of Data on Population Characteristics as Measured by CPS-Census Match," *Evaluation and Research Program of the U. S. Censuses of Population and Housing: 1960*, Series ER 60, No. 5, Washington: Government Printing Office, 1964.

achieved we found that there was 70 per cent agreement between the census report and the respondent's report of father's major occupation group. Although 30 per cent disagreement may appear high, this figure must be interpreted in the light of two facts. First, the date of the census and the date at which the respondent attained age 16 could differ by as much as five years; many fathers may actually have changed occupations between the two dates. Second, re-interview studies of the reliability of reports on occupation may find disagreements on the order of 17 to 22 per cent,[22] even though the information requested is current, not retrospective. Hence we are inclined to think that the reporting of father's occupation is perhaps not markedly inferior in reliability to the reporting of respondent's own occupation. (For further details, consult Appendix D, "Chicago Pretest Matching Study.")

Although the pretest afforded the only opportunity for a case-by-case comparison of OCG information with information from another source, some other checks were possible. Certain cohorts that were classified in 1910 and 1940 Census reports by father's occupation could be identified in the OCG data. The distributions of these cohorts by father's occupation in the two sources were compared. The comparisons suggest that the OCG distributions are reasonable, if allowance is made for the fact that the census classifications pertain to the time when the cohorts were under 5 years of age, whereas the OCG question asked for father's occupation at the time the respondent was age 16.

Another check of the same sort pertained to the distribution of men by father's educational attainment. Here a somewhat involved estimation procedure was used to impute distributions of respondents by father's year of birth. The latter then furnished a basis for estimating what the educational attainment distributions should have been had the fathers been typical of the cohorts from which they were drawn, as these cohorts were enumerated in the censuses of 1940, 1950, and 1960. Contrary to what might be expected, the comparison of imputed education distributions with those reported in OCG revealed no general tendency for the OCG respondents to exaggerate the attainment of their fathers, except that considerable numbers of OCG respondents appear to have classified their fathers as high-school graduates when they should have been reported as completing only one to three years of high school.

Both sets of results—reported in detail in Appendix E, "Census

22 *Ibid.*, Table 34; U. S. Bureau of the Census, "The Post-Enumeration Survey: 1950," Technical Paper, No. 4, 1960, Table 36.

Checks on Retrospective Data"—are, therefore, moderately reassuring. The conclusion, however, is not that the OCG data on socioeconomic background are free of error, but merely that they may be almost as reliable as the CPS data on current occupational status. Although this study took·some special pains to look into the incidence of data error, it must be conceded that very little was done to estimate the effect of such error on conclusions and inferences. In that respect, unfortunately, our investigation is all too typical of the current standards of social research.

Still another aspect of the problem of quality was subjected to special study. This is the matter of potential bias due to nonresponse on particular items in the questionnaire. The problem was examined with special reference to its impact on correlation coefficients. It is possible to set absolute limits on the possible extent of "NA bias" in a computed correlation, but these limits are so wide as to be rather uninformative. A particular correlation between father's occupational status and status of the respondent's first job, for example, was computed as .377 from cases reporting both variables. The extreme values that it could take if computed for all cases, on opposite extreme assumptions about the bivariate distributions of NA cases, are .190 and .464. However, on a reasonable rather than extreme allowance for variation between the reporting cases and the NA cases in respect to the correlation in question, it turns out that the correlation for all cases would probably not differ by more than ± .03 from the computed value. This is of the same order of magnitude as the standard errors of sampling for most of the correlations used in the analysis. Moreover, we are aware that the use of broad class intervals in our calculations and other approximations in computing can, by themselves, easily induce errors of the magnitude of .01. Again, we are somewhat reassured that normal precautions taken in the interpretation of small differences will suffice to avoid erroneous inferences from results affected by NA bias. (For details of this calculation, see Appendix F, "Effect of Nonresponse on Correlation Results.")

It should be mentioned that the problem of NA bias arises mainly for the supplementary OCG items, since the current practice in processing regular CPS items is to allocate NA's. The following summary account describes the procedure that is used:[23]

Assignment of years of school completed for those not reporting. When information on either the highest grade attended or completion of the grade

[23] U. S. Bureau of the Census, "Educational Change in a Generation: March 1962," *Current Population Reports*, Series P-20, No. 132, September 22, 1964, p. 5.

was not reported for respondents in the 1962 survey, entries for the items were assigned using an edit in the computer. Such assignments were not made where the education of brothers or fathers [OCG supplementary questions] was not reported. The general procedure was to assign an entry for a person that was consistent with entries for other persons with similar characteristics. The specific technique used in the March 1962 survey was as follows:

1. The computer stored reported data on highest grade attended by color and age, and on completion of the grade by age and highest grade attended, for persons 14 years old and over in the population.

2. Each stored value was retained in the computer only until a succeeding person having the same characteristics (e.g., same color and age, in the case of assignments for highest grade attended) and having the item reported was processed through the computer. Then, the reported data for the succeeding person were stored in place of the one previously stored.

3. When one or both of the education items for a person 14 years old and over were not reported, the entry assigned to this person was that stored for the last person who had the same characteristics.

One reason for dwelling on the matter of data quality is the suspicion that, in this study, biases in the data are more likely to lead to erroneous inferences than are random errors of sampling. Research workers have become sensitized to the problem of sampling error and are accustomed to presenting tests of statistical significance as a protection against the effects of such error. The sample size here, however, is so much larger than in most sociological studies based on surveys that it is largely a waste of time to compute significance tests. With some exaggeration, we can assert that almost any difference big enough to be at all interesting is statistically significant. Indeed, the data show all kinds of "significant differences" (not due to sampling error) that can be given no clear interpretation and that may be so slight as to be of no practical importance. There is always the chance, moreover, that a difference that is not a result of accidents of sampling may nonetheless be misleading in the sense that it could have arisen from response bias.

We have, therefore, largely refrained from using formal tests of significance and only occasionally make reference to standard errors. In any event, the only statistics for which we have reasonably good estimates of standard errors are percentages. Appendix G reproduces the table of standard errors computed by the sampling experts of the Bureau of the Census. If the reader studies this table he may discern that the standard errors are of about the magnitude that would be computed on the assumption of simple random sampling if the sample were about two-thirds as large as the OCG sample. This reflects the fact that the sample is not a simple random one but an areally clustered sample. We do not know, however, how other statistics, such as regression coefficients and F-ratios, are affected by the departure of the sample design from simple random sampling. Only very rough guesses about standard errors can be made, when we feel obliged to discuss sampling variation explicitly.

We can give few details about the complex job of collating records, bringing together information coded manually with that stored in a form suitable for automated data processing, compiling the final composite record, and programming the tabulation of the statistics we requested. All this work was done according to standard operating procedures of the regular staff of CPS. One special feature of the OCG survey was the requirement for detailed coding of occupations and industries, which is a prerequisite for the recoding into occupational status scores, to be described in Chapter 4. Such coding is not carried out in the usual CPS studies but is, of course, a feature of the decennial census. Hence elaborate coding instructions were already available.

By the time the data were actually collected the investigators had developed the first of two major sets of specifications for tabulations. It should be mentioned here that at no time have we had access to the original survey documents or to the computer tapes on which individual records are stored. This information is confidential and not available to private research workers. Consequently it was necessary for us to provide detailed outlines of the statistical tables we desired for analysis without inspecting the "raw" data, and to provide these, moreover, some 9 to 12 months ahead of the time when we might expect their delivery. This lead time was required for programming the computer runs that would produce the tables. Evidently this circumstance precluded our following the common strategy of looking at a few marginal totals before running some two-way tables and deciding on interesting three-way or higher-order tabulations after having studied the two-way tables. We had to state in advance just which tables were wanted, out of the virtually unlimited number that conceivably might have been produced, and to be prepared to make the best of what we got. Cost factors, of course, put strict limits on how many tables we could request. We had to imagine in advance most of the analysis we would want to make, before having any advance indications of what any of the tables would look like.

The general plan of the analysis had, therefore, to be laid out a year or more before the analysis actually began, although there turned out to be "serendipitous" elements in the tabulation specifications we drew up; some tabulations proved to be amenable to analytical procedures not initially contemplated. The reason some particular combination of variables that seems to be called for is not reported is usually that the need for it had not been anticipated. There are many combinations we might have desired but could not afford, and many others that we would later have liked to see but that we simply had not thought of when dummy tables were drawn up. We were conscious of the very real hazard that our initial plans would overlook relationships of great interest. However, some months of work were devoted to making rough estimates from various sources to anticipate as closely as possible how the tables might look. This time was well spent, for, on the whole, the tabulations have proved satisfactory. The specific design of the analysis, however, goes beyond our concern here, since it is part of the story of each of the substantive chapters in the volume.

ORGANIZATION OF THE BOOK

The analysis of the data collected in the survey constitutes the bulk of the material reported in the present book, although we draw occasionally on other sources as well. In concluding this introductory chapter we present a brief outline of the organization of the book and the topics of the various chapters.

The next two chapters deal with the structure of relations among occupational groupings and their changes through time. Here the conventional intergenerational and intragenerational mobility tables are analyzed, with little reference to any variables not already contained in them. A number of new procedures are used to explore the flow of manpower among occupational groups from different perspectives and to infer the underlying factors that govern these movements and that reflect the social distances between occupations. Having investigated the patterns of mobility in Chapter 2, we consider historical trends in them in Chapter 3. One of the contributions of this analysis is to demonstrate how difficult and hazardous it is to make inferences about changes in intergenerational mobility from a knowledge of the changes that have occurred in the occupational structure.

After this examination of the occupational structure itself we turn to the analysis of the processes of occupational achievement and mobility that find expression in this structure. The basic question is how the status individuals achieve in their careers is affected by the statuses ascribed to them earlier in life, such as their social origin, ethnic status, region of birth, community, and parental family. The relatively novel techniques employed for the purpose of this analysis are described in Chapter 4. Lest this methodological discussion appear intolerably abstract, we have incorporated into it some of the major findings of the study in the guise of illustrations, such as those on the relationship between education and occupational mobility.

The basic model of the process of occupational mobility is presented in Chapter 5. Occupational status in 1962, the survey date, is conceived as the outcome of a lifelong process in which ascribed positions at birth, intervening circumstances, and earlier attainments determine the level of ultimate achievement. A formalization in terms of a simple mathematical model permits an approximate assessment of the relative importance of the several measured determinants. In the following chapters this model is, in effect, modified and enriched by introducing estimates of the effects of several factors and contingencies not included in the initial formulation. The question recurrently asked is how an additional set of variables modifies the influences of social origins and earlier attainments on later achievements.

Thus Chapter 6 considers the inequalities of opportunities engendered by race, region of birth, and nativity, paying special attention to the question of whether the inferior chances of success of Negroes and other minorities are essentially due to their inferior background and education or persist when these factors are controlled. In the context of analyzing the relationship between migration and social mobility in Chapter 7 we investigate whether the migrant's community of origin or the community in which he lives and works has a greater influence on his occupational chances, and we derive some inferences about the impact the influx of rural migrants into large cities has on the occupational chances of the city natives. The significance of farm background for occupational achievements is examined in Chapter 8. The influences exerted on careers by number of siblings, sibling position, the relations among siblings, and the emphasis on education in the family are treated in Chapter 9. The analysis in Chapter 10 of the relationship between marriage and occupational life is particularly concerned with homogamy, the degree of similarity in background and education between husband and wife.

Attention shifts in the eleventh chapter to a variable usually considered to be a consequence rather than an antecedent of occupational status and mobility; that is, fertility or, more precisely, the number of children born to the respondent's wife. This topic serves to exemplify a procedure considered appropriate for abstracting the influence of mobility as such on a dependent variable from the influence of those statuses in terms of which mobility is defined. The substantive problem is whether the additive effect of social origin (either husband's or wife's) and present status can account for the fertility of the couple, or whether mobility itself exerts a further independent influence on their fertility. It would have been advantageous to ascertain also whether mobility exerts such an independent influence on a variety of other factors—for instance, political attitudes, prejudice, and anomie —but the limitations imposed by the method of data collection unfortunately make this impossible.

In the final chapter we not only summarize the main findings but also discuss some of their broader implications. At that point, we shall relate our findings to the comparative data on mobility in different industrial societies analyzed by Lipset and Bendix and suggest some reformulations in their theoretical generalizations that appear to be implied by our results. This concluding discussion gives us an opportunity to speculate about some general principles concerning the causes and consequences of occupational mobility in modern society.

CHAPTER 2

The Occupational Structure: I
Patterns of Movement

The study of social mobility may be approached from various perspectives. We can focus on changes in socioeconomic status, whatever the particular occupational base on which the status rests, or on movements between occupational groups (clerks, farmers), ignoring status differences within each group. Concern may be with the opportunities for success of individuals or with the occupational structure of the society. In subsequent chapters attention centers largely on socioeconomic status, and the investigation deals with the factors associated with individual opportunity and achievement. This first substantive chapter on our research findings, in contrast, presents an analysis of the American occupational structure at large, specifically, of the movements of manpower among occupational groups.

The occupational structure is conceived of as consisting of the relations among its constituent subgroups; and these occupational subgroups, not the individuals composing them, are the units of analysis. The labor force has been divided for the purpose of this analysis into 17 occupational categories, an extension of the 10 major occupational groups of the U. S. Bureau of the Census. The seven additional categories represent simple subdivisions of Census categories; self-employed "professional, technical, and kindred workers" are distinguished from salaried ones. Similarly, "managers, officials, and proprietors" are separated into the self-employed ("proprietors") and the salaried ("managers"). "Sales workers" are divided into retail and other salesmen. Finally, three groups of manual workers have been partitioned by industry: there are three categories of "craftsmen, foremen, and kindred workers"—in manufacturing, in construction, and in other industries—two categories of "operatives and kindred workers" —in manufacturing and in other industries—and the same two categories of "laborers, except farm and mine."

The structure of relations among these occupational groupings is defined in terms of the flow of manpower between them through time, either intergenerationally or intragenerationally. Each occupation is characterized by the inflow or recruitment of its manpower from various origins, on the one hand, and by the outflow or supply of sons to various destinations, on the other. For example, farmers are disproportionately recruited from their own ranks and from farm laborers, but they supply sons to a large variety of occupations in the next generation. This procedure of describing an occupation on the basis of its relations to the others in the social structure is analogous to the sociometric method, which also describes individuals in a group on the basis of their relations to the rest, and which also usually employs two criteria of relations: choices made and choices received. The analogy is intended to indicate that concern is with a structure of relations among units in a larger whole, but it must not be pressed too far. The units are large occupational groupings in our case, not individuals; and whereas self-choice is usually not considered in sociometric studies, self-recruitment and occupational inheritance occur, of course, and must be taken into account.

The flow of manpower among occupational groups reveals the dynamics of the occupational structure. To be sure, the 17 occupational categories used are not social groups in the conventional sense of the term. Most members of an occupational category are not in direct social contact and may not even share a common identification, because their occupational identification may be either broader ("professional") or narrower ("accountant") than the category delimited by the social scientist. Nevertheless, the occupational classes are meaningful social groupings and not entirely arbitrary categories. Their members share life chances and social experiences, and many of the direct social contacts of men at work and even at play are with others in a similar, if not necessarily the same, occupational category. The term "occupational grouping" might best convey the fact that although these are not corporate groups with distinct boundaries and pervasive social interaction among members, neither are they arbitrary categories, but they are meaningful social aggregates that affect the formation of many face-to-face groups.

The classification by father's occupation, however, raises additional problems. Whereas the occupational classification of sons represents actual groupings of individuals in 1962, the generation of fathers never existed at any one time. Many of these fathers still pursued their occupations in 1962, that is, are part of the labor force that has been sampled. The occupational distribution of fathers is not an actual distribution of men existing at any earlier period. Even if all fathers had been in the labor force at some one time, they provide a sample of that universe biased by differential fertility. Thus a farmer has more weight in the generation of fathers than a professional because the farmer's higher fertility gives him a greater probability of falling into the sample through his sons. However, although origin categories do not refer to distinctive groupings of fathers, they do refer to distinctive groupings of sons: those who have similar occupational backgrounds and home environments. What is under consideration, therefore, is the movement of manpower from groupings that have common social origins, defined by father's occupation, to occupational groupings in 1962.[1]

The occupational structure constitutes the framework of social mobility within which individuals must achieve occupational success or suffer failure.[2] Changes in the size of the various occupations reflect changes in the demand for different occupational services, which, in turn, often have their source in technological advances, as exemplified by the declining demand for farm workers consequent to improved farming methods and higher farm productivity. These structural changes require a redistribution of manpower. But the actual amount of occupational mobility observed far exceeds that necessary to effect the redistribution of manpower. Some of this additional mobility results from educational improvements that alter the quality of the manpower supplied, and some of it results from indirect repercussions of changes in demand. For example, a need for professionals is most likely to be met by those men who have acquired in their early environments the social skills and habits appropriate to professional pursuits, those aware of various professional careers and able to afford the prolonged education requisite to professional status, that is, by sons of other white-collar workers. If the need for these other white-collar workers does not decline at the same time as that for professionals is increasing, the outflow of sons will create a demand in the lower white-collar occupations, a secondary product of the demand for professionals. Moreover, a high demand for professionals may lead

[1] The same applies to first occupation in respect to intragenerational mobility. Classification by first occupation refers to groupings of men with common early career experiences, not to occupational groupings that actually existed at any one time, since different times are involved for men of different ages.

[2] This analysis is not concerned with the question of the socioeconomic mobility achieved by whole occupational groupings.

to the lowering of previously existing barriers to entry—for instance, by no longer restricting admission to professional schools to whites— with the result that more qualified men from lower strata can now move up into this level.

The flow of manpower in the occupational structure, rather than merely the net redistribution necessitated by shifts in demand, delineates the existential conditions governing the individual's chances of socioeconomic success. The analysis of this pattern of movement provides a baseline for the investigation, in subsequent chapters, of historical trends, the process of social mobility, and the factors associated with individual achievements.

THE FLOW OF MANPOWER

In order to determine whether movement from an occupational origin to an occupational destination entails upward or downward mobility, it is necessary to rank the occupations. Table 2.1 presents a rank order of the 17 occupational groupings and the data on which this ranking is based. The criteria are median income and median education. The percentage increase in income or education is indicated as one moves up the ranks.[3] Only five of these percentage differences are not in the same direction. In these cases the two are equally weighted, which means that the larger percentage difference determines the rank. The one exception is the placement of retail salesmen above craftsmen, which has been made to maintain the nonmanual-manual distinction.

Differences between manufacturing and other craftsmen, and between manufacturing and other laborers, are not available, and the mean difference across the same industry line for operatives is small. Hence, in considering upward and downward mobility, the industry partition of these three major occupational groups is treated as a horizontal one. To wit, movement between manufacturing and other industry within each of the three manual groups is considered to be horizontal and counted neither as upward nor as downward mobility.

This ranking differs in a few respects from the customary ranking of the ten major occupational groups. Nonretail salesmen fall between the two subgroups of "managers, officials, and proprietors" of the Census classification, so that only salaried managers remain above these other salesmen. Proprietors have descended to a point that may confound, or possibly delight, doctrinaire Marxists, though by virtue of their income levels they are still above clerks and retail salesmen

---

[3] The index of occupational socioeconomic status for individuals used elsewhere in the book is similarly based on income and education, but for specific occupations.

TABLE 2.1. RANKING OF SEVENTEEN OCC. CATEGORIES BY SOCIO-ECONOMIC STATUS, FOR MALES 14 AND OVER EMPLOYED IN 1962

Occ.	Income Median (dollars)	Income Percentage Difference	Years of Schooling Median	Years of Schooling Percentage Difference
Professionals				
Self-Empl.	$12,048		16.4	
		76.1		
Salaried	6,842			
		-5.5		28.1
Managers	7,238		12.8	
		20.5		-1.5
Salesmen, Other	6,008		13.0	
		8.3		7.4
Proprietors	5,548		12.1	
		7.2		-3.2
Clerical	5,173		12.5	
		69.9		1.6
Salesmen, Retail	3,044		12.3	
		-44.5		9.8
Craftsmen				
Mfg.				
Other	5,482[a]		11.2	
		4.1		9.8
Construction	5,265		10.2	
		13.6		2.0
Operatives				
Mfg.	4,636		10.0	
		10.2		-3.8
Other	4,206		10.4	
		30.1		1.0
Service	3,233		10.3	
		47.7		15.7
Laborers				
Mfg.				
Other	2,189		8.9	
		9.9		1.1
Farmers	1,992		8.8	
		308.2		6.0
Farm Laborers	488		8.3	

SOURCE: Current Population Reports, P-60, #41, Consumer Income: "Income of Family and Persons in the United States: 1962," October 21, 1963, and Special Labor Force Report, #30, "Educational Attainment of Workers, March, 1962," May, 1963. (Some figures include minor estimates entailed in combining detailed occupation groups. All data subject to sample error and to distortion due to inclusion of men outside age range 25-64.)

[a] Excludes foremen, who are concentrated in manufacturing and whose median income is $7073.

TABLE 2.2. MOBILITY FROM FATHER'S OCC. TO 1962 OCC., FOR MALES 25 TO 64 YEARS OLD: OUTFLOW PERCENTAGES

Father's Occupation	Respondent's Occupation in March, 1962																	Total[a]
	1	2	3	4	5	6	7	8	9	10	11	12	13	14	15	16	17	
Professionals																		
1 Self-Empl.	16.7	31.9	9.9	9.5	4.4	4.0	1.4	2.0	1.8	2.2	2.6	1.6	1.8	.4	2.2	2.0	.8	100.0
2 Salaried	3.3	31.9	12.9	5.9	4.8	7.6	1.7	3.8	4.4	1.0	6.9	5.2	3.4	1.0	.6	.8	.2	100.0
3 Managers	3.5	22.6	19.4	6.2	7.9	7.6	1.1	5.4	5.3	3.1	4.0	2.5	1.5	1.1	.8	.5	.1	100.0
4 Salesmen, Other	4.1	17.6	21.2	13.0	9.3	5.3	3.5	2.8	5.4	1.9	2.6	3.7	1.7	.0	.8	1.0	.3	100.0
5 Proprietors	3.7	13.7	18.4	5.8	16.0	6.2	3.3	3.5	5.2	3.9	5.1	3.6	2.8	.5	1.2	1.1	.4	100.0
6 Clerical	2.2	23.5	11.2	5.9	5.1	8.8	1.3	6.6	7.1	1.8	3.8	4.6	5.6	1.0	1.8	1.3	.0	100.0
7 Salesmen, Retail	.7	13.7	14.1	8.8	11.5	6.4	2.7	5.8	3.4	3.1	8.8	5.1	4.6	.1	3.1	2.2	.0	100.0
Craftsmen																		
8 Mfg.	1.0	14.9	8.5	2.4	6.2	6.1	1.7	15.3	6.4	4.4	10.9	6.2	4.6	1.7	2.4	.4	.1	100.0
9 Other	.9	11.1	9.2	3.9	6.5	7.6	1.5	7.8	12.2	4.4	8.2	9.2	4.6	1.2	2.8	.9	.3	100.0
10 Construction	.9	6.7	7.1	2.6	8.3	7.9	.8	10.4	8.2	13.9	7.5	6.2	5.2	1.1	4.3	.8	.6	100.0
Operatives																		
11 Mfg.	1.0	8.6	5.3	2.7	5.6	6.0	1.4	12.2	7.3	3.2	17.9	6.9	5.1	4.0	3.5	.8	.6	100.0
12 Other	.6	11.5	5.1	2.5	6.6	6.3	1.4	7.1	9.3	4.9	10.4	12.5	5.9	2.1	4.2	.9	1.1	100.0
13 Service	.8	8.8	7.4	3.5	6.0	9.0	1.9	8.0	6.4	5.4	11.7	8.1	10.5	2.7	3.3	1.0	.2	100.0
Laborers																		
14 Mfg.	.0	6.0	5.3	.7	3.3	4.4	.7	10.7	6.0	2.8	18.1	9.4	9.4	7.1	5.8	1.7	.9	100.0
15 Other	.4	4.9	3.5	2.5	3.5	8.7	1.7	7.7	8.2	5.7	12.7	10.6	8.1	3.4	9.9	.9	1.1	100.0
16 Farmers	.6	4.2	4.1	1.2	6.0	4.3	1.1	5.6	6.7	5.8	10.2	8.6	4.8	2.4	5.4	16.4	3.9	100.0
17 Farm Laborers	.2	1.9	2.9	.6	4.0	3.5	1.2	6.4	6.6	5.8	13.1	10.8	7.5	3.2	9.2	5.7	9.4	100.0
Total[b]	1.4	10.2	7.9	3.1	7.0	6.1	1.5	7.2	7.1	4.9	9.9	7.6	5.5	2.1	4.3	5.2	1.7	100.0

[a]Rows as shown do not total 100.0, since men not in experienced civilian labor force are not shown separately.
[b]Includes men not reporting father's occupation.

(who are nevertheless their educational superiors). Retail sales is the lowest white-collar occupation.

Table 2.2 presents the transition matrix of intergenerational mobility; that is, the movements between father's occupation and respondent's 1962 occupation. These movements can be considered to consist of two steps, from social origin to entry into the labor market, and from the latter to present occupation. The pattern of movement from father's to first occupation is shown in Table 2.3, and intragenerational mobility from first to present occupation is shown in Table 2.4.[4] The percentages in the tables, computed horizontally, reveal the outflow from occupational origins to occupational destinations. The total row in Table 2.2 indicates the per cent of men in the various occupational destinations. It is evident that the 17 occupational categories were not equal in size in 1962, ranging from $1\frac{1}{3}$ per cent of the total labor force for self-employed professionals to 10 per cent each for salaried professionals and operatives in manufacturing.

By and large the percentages are highest in the major diagonal and decrease with movement away from it, a reflection of a prevailing tendency toward self-recruitment and occupational inheritance. But the pattern is by no means entirely consistent. Fewer sons of retail salesmen become retail salesmen than become clerks, proprietors, other salesmen, managers, or salaried professionals. Sons of operatives outside manufacturing have a greater chance of becoming salaried professionals than the higher-status (hence closer to the diagonal) sons of craftsmen outside manufacturing, and nearly as good a chance as sons of proprietors. The intragenerational matrix (Table 2.4) shows that the likelihood of rising to the status of independent businessman is better for workers who begin their careers as either skilled craftsmen or semiskilled operatives than for men whose first jobs are as clerks, even though the latter are only one step below business owners in the socioeconomic status hierarchy. Perhaps manual workers are more likely than clerks to start working for self-employed fathers whose business they later inherit.

Although percentages within the same column can be compared, tables in this form do not permit meaningful direct comparisons across columns. Thus sons of self-employed professionals are nearly twice as likely to become salaried professionals as they are to become self-employed professionals (Table 2.2, row 1). But this is in part because of the fact that there are today seven times as many salaried as self-employed professionals, a fact indicated in the total row at the bottom

4 The raw data on which these tables are based are presented in Appendix J, Tables J2.1, J2.2, and J2.3.

TABLE 2.3 MOBILITY FROM FATHER'S OCCUPATION TO FIRST JOB, FOR MALES 25 TO 64 YEARS OLD: OUTFLOW PERCENTAGES

Father's Occupation	First Job																	Total[a]
	1	2	3	4	5	6	7	8	9	10	11	12	13	14	15	16	17	
Professionals																		
1 Self-Empl.	10.5	27.6	2.2	4.4	.8	17.9	4.4	2.6	3.2	.0	4.6	6.7	2.0	1.0	2.8	1.2	1.6	100.0
2 Salaried	1.2	29.5	3.7	2.1	.0	12.3	6.0	3.9	4.7	1.6	9.7	7.6	3.4	3.1	5.3	.5	2.0	100.0
3 Managers	1.9	18.2	2.8	3.5	.8	20.8	5.9	2.9	4.4	1.7	10.0	11.5	1.8	2.5	6.7	.5	1.1	100.0
4 Salesmen, Other	2.6	17.0	2.6	11.4	1.0	17.2	8.9	1.4	2.8	1.4	9.0	9.5	1.8	1.2	3.7	.0	2.3	100.0
5 Proprietors	1.9	14.0	3.9	5.1	4.4	12.5	11.0	3.7	3.8	2.5	10.1	9.4	3.4	2.4	5.9	.3	2.2	100.0
6 Clerical	.4	18.0	2.3	1.7	.2	21.9	4.3	2.8	5.7	1.0	13.2	9.4	3.1	4.8	5.7	.7	1.3	100.0
7 Salesmen, Retail	1.5	10.0	2.5	2.1	1.8	19.3	11.8	3.3	3.0	.1	15.5	8.0	2.1	3.9	8.0	.7	4.3	100.0
Craftsmen																		
8 Mfg.	.1	6.5	.8	.5	.1	14.4	5.2	9.6	3.6	2.6	25.3	8.9	4.4	8.5	4.8	.2	1.8	100.0
9 Other	.5	6.1	.4	.8	.3	13.9	6.0	3.9	10.1	1.6	15.0	13.6	3.6	3.9	10.9	.5	4.3	100.0
10 Construction	.1	5.7	.8	.6	.0	12.5	5.5	4.1	5.2	10.4	17.0	11.0	6.0	3.1	9.2	1.1	5.7	100.0
Operatives																		
11 Mfg.	.3	4.1	.4	1.0	.1	11.1	3.9	4.1	2.6	1.7	35.9	7.7	5.1	8.6	6.1	.2	3.0	100.0
12 Other	.3	5.5	2.2	.3	.1	10.9	4.6	3.4	4.1	1.6	13.2	28.6	3.5	4.6	8.7	.4	3.9	100.0
13 Service	.2	4.4	1.4	1.2	.3	13.8	4.2	2.8	6.0	2.2	18.2	12.9	10.1	6.7	8.4	.7	4.1	100.0
Laborers																		
14 Mfg.	.0	3.8	.1	.0	.0	5.3	4.8	1.1	4.1	1.1	23.2	9.1	4.1	22.2	7.5	.3	7.7	100.0
15 Other	1.1	3.2	.2	.5	.1	9.4	4.4	2.5	3.1	1.0	16.0	12.8	6.5	6.8	21.9	.7	6.3	100.0
16 Farmers	.2	3.3	.4	.4	.3	4.1	2.3	1.9	2.0	1.8	9.7	8.5	2.2	4.0	7.5	10.2	37.8	100.0
17 Farm Laborers	.2	.7	.2	.2	.3	2.4	1.1	.6	3.1	1.0	10.6	7.0	2.9	5.5	5.9	1.5	54.5	100.0

[a]Rows as shown do not total 100.0, since men not reporting first job are not shown separately.

TABLE 2.4 MOBILITY FROM FIRST JOB TO 1962 OCCUPATION, FOR MALES 25 TO 64 YEARS OLD: OUTFLOW PERCENTAGES

First Job	Respondent's Occupation in March, 1962																	
	1	2	3	4	5	6	7	8	9	10	11	12	13	14	15	16	17	Total[a]
Professionals																		
1 Self-Empl.	53.5	25.5	1.8	4.7	2.5	1.5	.0	1.5	.7	.0	.7	.0	.0	.0	2.5	.0	.7	100.0
2 Salaried	6.5	54.5	12.3	2.8	5.5	4.9	.4	1.6	2.0	.4	1.2	1.2	1.0	.1	.3	1.0	.1	100.0
3 Managers	1.2	20.4	35.7	4.3	9.1	6.6	2.3	2.3	4.1	2.9	2.1	1.4	1.2	.6	1.2	.6	.4	100.0
4 Salesmen, Other	.6	8.5	25.1	23.7	12.4	5.0	2.8	.6	3.3	1.3	5.4	3.9	2.8	.0	.0	.4	.0	100.0
5 Proprietors	.9	6.8	19.2	6.4	36.3	2.6	2.6	1.7	2.1	.4	4.3	4.3	3.0	.9	2.1	3.8	.0	100.0
6 Clerical	1.6	13.0	17.3	7.3	5.4	17.6	1.8	4.6	4.3	2.6	5.6	4.2	4.4	1.0	1.8	1.2	.2	100.0
7 Salesmen, Retail	2.1	10.0	15.6	7.4	11.6	11.6	5.1	4.5	4.8	2.9	6.1	7.4	3.1	1.1	1.9	1.0	.1	100.0
Craftsmen																		
8 Mfg.	.9	8.7	7.8	2.5	12.2	4.1	.7	22.5	7.5	4.3	9.1	3.5	3.7	.8	4.0	2.3	.0	100.0
9 Other	.3	9.0	6.6	1.9	10.3	4.1	3.4	10.9	21.3	4.7	7.1	5.5	3.6	1.4	1.7	1.2	.7	100.0
10 Construction	.3	5.6	3.4	1.6	11.1	3.1	.2	8.8	13.2	26.2	5.0	4.3	2.4	1.0	3.1	2.1	.8	100.0
Operatives																		
11 Mfg.	.4	6.1	5.3	2.0	7.0	6.2	1.7	13.4	6.7	4.6	18.8	7.6	4.7	3.2	3.5	2.0	.6	100.0
12 Other	.5	5.0	6.1	3.0	8.7	4.3	1.1	7.3	10.8	6.9	9.6	15.0	6.0	1.4	4.3	1.8	1.0	100.0
13 Service	.5	7.1	4.9	1.4	6.2	5.0	1.2	3.4	6.4	6.2	13.3	7.7	19.8	2.5	5.8	.4	.5	100.0
Laborers																		
14 Mfg.	.3	5.5	3.9	1.5	2.9	6.2	1.2	10.5	5.3	3.9	18.1	8.8	7.3	8.2	6.3	1.6	1.7	100.0
15 Other	.2	5.5	5.4	2.4	6.7	4.1	1.3	6.1	9.6	6.8	10.5	10.8	6.3	2.4	11.5	2.1	.9	100.0
16 Farmers	.2	2.3	2.6	1.8	3.8	3.0	1.2	4.2	5.9	5.4	8.3	5.0	4.6	1.4	3.6	30.0	5.0	100.0
17 Farm Laborers	.2	1.7	2.4	.8	4.7	2.7	1.1	5.3	6.3	5.5	10.4	9.3	5.8	2.8	6.7	19.3	7.0	100.0

[a]Rows as shown do not total 100.0, since men not in the experienced civilian labor force are not shown separately.

31

TABLE 2.5. MOBILITY FROM FATHER'S OCCUPATION TO OCCUPATION IN 1962, FOR MALES 25 TO 64 YEARS OLD: RATIOS OF OBSERVED FREQUENCIES TO FREQUENCIES EXPECTED ON THE ASSUMPTION OF INDEPENDENCE

Father's Occupation	Respondent's Occupation in March, 1962																
	1	2	3	4	5	6	7	8	9	10	11	12	13	14	15	16	17
Professionals																	
1 Self-Empl.	11.7	3.1	1.2	3.0	.6	.7	.9	.3	.3	.5	.3	.2	.3	.2	.5	.4	.5
2 Salaried	2.3	3.1	1.6	1.9	.7	1.2	1.1	.5	.6	.2	.7	.7	.6	.5	.1	.2	.1
3 Managers	2.5	2.2	2.5	2.0	1.1	1.2	.7	.8	.7	.6	.4	.3	.3	.5	.2	.1	.1
4 Salesmen, Other	2.9	1.7	2.7	4.1	1.3	.9	2.2	.4	.8	.4	.3	.5	.3	.0	.2	.2	.2
5 Proprietors	2.6	1.3	2.3	1.9	2.3	1.0[a]	2.1	.5	.7	.8	.5	.5	.5	.2	.3	.2	.2
6 Clerical	1.6	2.3	1.4	1.9	.7	1.4	.8	.9	1.0[a]	.4	.4	.6	1.0[a]	.5	.4	.2	.0
7 Salesmen, Retail	.5	1.3	1.8	2.8	1.6	1.0[a]	1.7	.8	.5	.6	.9	.7	.8	.1	.7	.4	.0
Craftsmen																	
8 Mfg.	.7	1.5	1.1	.8	.9	1.0	1.1	2.1	.9	.9	1.1	.8	.8	.8	.6	.1	.1
9 Other	.6	1.1	1.2	1.2	.9	1.2	1.0	1.1	1.7	.9	.8	1.2	.8	.6	.6	.2	.2
10 Construction	.6	.7	.9	.8	1.2	1.3	.5	1.4	1.1	2.8	.8	.8	.9	.5	1.0	.2	.4
Operatives																	
11 Mfg.	.7	.8	.7	.9	.8	1.0	.9	1.7	1.0[a]	.6	1.8	.9	.9	1.9	.8	.2	.4
12 Other	.4	1.1	.6	.8	.9	1.0[a]	.9	1.0	1.3	1.0	1.0[a]	1.7	1.1	1.0	1.0	.2	.7
13 Service	.5	.9	.9	1.1	.9	1.5	1.2	1.1	.9	1.1	1.2	1.1	1.9	1.3	.8	.2	.1
Labor																	
14 Mfg.	.0	.6	.7	.2	.5	.7	.5	1.5	.8	.6	1.8	1.2	1.7	3.3	1.4	.3	.5
15 Other	.3	.5	.4	.8	.5	1.4	1.1	1.1	1.1	1.2	1.3	1.4	1.5	1.6	2.3	.2	.7
16 Farmers	.4	.4	.5	.4	.9	.7	.7	.8	.9	1.2	1.0[a]	1.1	.9	1.1	1.3	3.2	2.3
17 Farm Laborers	.1	.2	.4	.2	.6	.6	.8	.9	.9	1.2	1.3	1.4	1.4	1.5	2.1	1.1	5.5

[a] Rounds to unity from above (other indices shown as 1.0 round to unity from below).

TABLE 2.6. MOBILITY FROM FATHER'S OCCUPATION TO FIRST JOB, FOR MALES 25 TO 64 YEARS OLD: RATIOS OF OBSERVED FREQUENCIES TO FREQUENCIES EXPECTED ON THE ASSUMPTION OF INDEPENDENCE.

Father's Occupation	Respondent's First Job																
	1	2	3	4	5	6	7	8	9	10	11	12	13	14	15	16	17
Professionals																	
1 Self-Empl.	15.2	3.8	1.8	3.3	1.4	1.7	.9	.8	.8	.0	.3	.6	.5	.2	.4	.4	.1
2 Salaried	1.8	4.1	3.0	1.6	.0	1.2	1.3	1.2	1.2	.7	.6	.7	.9	.6	.7	.2	.1
3 Managers	2.8	2.5	2.3	2.6	1.5	2.0	1.2	.9	1.2	.8	.7	1.0a	.5	.5	.8	.2	.1
4 Salesmen, Other	3.7	2.3	2.1	8.5	1.8	1.6	1.9	.4	.7	.7	.6	.9	.5	.2	.5	.0	.2
5 Proprietors	2.8	1.9	3.2	3.7	7.6	1.2	2.3	1.1	1.0	1.1	.7	.9	.9	.5	.7	.1	.2
6 Clerical	.6	2.5	1.9	1.2	.3	2.1	.9	.9	1.5	.4	.9	.9	.8	.9	.7	.2	.1
7 Salesmen, Retail	2.2	1.4	2.1	1.5	3.1	1.8	2.5	1.0a	.8	.1	1.0a	.7	.5	.8	1.0	.2	.3
Craftsmen																	
8 Mfg.	.1	.9	.7	.4	.2	1.4	1.1	3.0	1.0	1.2	1.7	.8	1.2	1.7	.6	.1	.1
9 Other	.7	.8	.3	.6	.5	1.3	1.3	1.2	2.7	.7	1.0a	1.2	1.0	.8	1.4	.2	.3
10 Construction	.2	.8	.7	.4	.0	1.2	1.2	1.3	1.4	4.8	1.1	1.0a	1.6	.6	1.1	.3	.4
Operatives																	
11 Mfg.	.4	.6	.3	.7	.1	1.0	.8	1.3	.7	.8	2.4	.7	1.3	1.7	.8	.1	.2
12 Other	.4	.8	1.8	.2	.1	1.0	1.0	1.1	1.1	.8	.9	2.6	.9	.9	1.1	.1	.3
13 Service	.3	.6	1.2	.9	.5	1.3	.9	.9	1.6	1.0a	1.2	1.2	2.7	1.3	1.0a	.2	.3
Laborers																	
14 Mfg.	.0	.5	.1	.0	.0	.5	1.0a	.4	1.1	.5	1.6	.8	1.1	4.4	.9	.1	.5
15 Other	1.6	.4	.1	.4	.2	.9	.9	.8	.8	.5	1.1	1.2	1.7	1.4	2.7	.2	.4
16 Farmers	.3	.5	.3	.3	.5	.4	.5	.6	.5	.8	.7	.8	.6	.8	.9	3.3	2.7
17 Farm Laborers	.3	.1	.2	.1	.5	.2	.2	.2	.8	.4	.7	.6	.8	1.1	.7	.5	3.8

a Rounds to unity from above (other indices shown as 1.0 round to unity from below).

33

TABLE 2.7. MOBILITY FROM FIRST JOB TO OCCUPATION IN 1962, FOR MALES 25 TO 64 YEARS OLD: RATIOS OF OBSERVED FREQUENCIES TO FREQUENCIES EXPECTED ON THE ASSUMPTION OF INDEPENDENCE

First Job	Respondent's Occupation in 1962																
	1	2	3	4	5	6	7	8	9	10	11	12	13	14	15	16	17
Professionals																	
1 Self-Empl.	37.3	2.5	.2	1.5	.4	.2	.0	.2	.1	.0	.1	.0	.0	.0	.0	.0	.4
2 Salaried	4.5	5.4	1.6	.9	.8	.8	.2	.2	.3	.1	.1	.2	.2	.0	.1	.2	.1
3 Managers	.9	2.0	4.5	1.4	1.3	1.1	1.5	.3	.6	.6	.2	.2	.2	.3	.3	.1	.2
4 Salesmen, Other	.4	.8	3.2	7.6	1.8	.8	1.8	.1	.5	.3	.5	.5	.5	.0	.0	.1	.0
5 Proprietors	.6	.7	2.4	2.0	5.2	.4	1.7	.2	.3	.1	.4	.6	.5	.4	.5	.7	.0
6 Clerical	1.1	1.3	2.2	2.3	.8	2.9	1.2	.6	.6	.5	.6	.6	.8	.5	.4	.2	.1
7 Salesmen, Retail	1.4	1.0	2.0	2.3	1.7	1.9	3.3	.6	.7	.6	.6	1.0	.6	.5	.4	.2	.0
Crafts																	
8 Mfg.	.6	.9	1.0	.8	1.7	.7	.5	3.1	1.0[a]	.9	.9	.5	.7	.4	.9	.4	.0
9 Other	.2	.9	.8	.6	1.5	.7	2.2	1.5	3.0	1.0	.7	.7	.7	.6	.4	.2	.4
10 Construction	.2	.5	.4	.5	1.6	.5	.2	1.2	1.8	5.3	.5	.6	.4	.5	.7	.4	.5
Operatives																	
11 Mfg.	.3	.6	.7	.6	1.0	1.0[a]	1.1	1.9	.9	.9	1.9	1.0	.9	1.5	.8	.4	.3
12 Other	.3	.5	.8	.9	1.3	.7	.7	1.0[a]	1.5	1.4	1.0	2.0	1.1	.7	1.0[a]	.4	.6
13 Service	.3	.7	.6	.4	.9	.8	.8	.5	.9	1.3	1.3	1.0[a]	3.6	1.2	1.4	.1	.3
Laborers																	
14 Mfg.	.2	.5	.5	.5	.4	1.0[a]	.8	1.5	.7	.8	1.8	1.2	1.3	3.8	1.5	.3	1.0
15 Other	.2	.5	.7	.8	1.0	.7	.8	.8	1.4	1.4	1.1	1.4	1.1	1.1	2.7	.4	.6
16 Farmers	.2	.2	.3	.6	.5	.5	.8	.6	.8	1.1	.8	.7	.9	.7	.8	7.0	3.0
17 Farm Laborers	.1	.2	.3	.2	.7	.4	.7	.7	.9	1.1	1.0	1.2	1.1	1.3	1.6	3.7	4.1

[a] Rounds to unity from above (other indices shown as 1.0 round to unity from below).

of the table. Whereas the ratio of self-employed to salaried professionals for the entire sample is 1:7, the ratio among sons of self-employed professionals is 1:2. These sons exceed the chance all sons have of becoming self-employed professionals even more than they exceed the chance all sons have of becoming salaried professionals. The sons of self-employed professionals who follow in their father's footsteps, though fewer in number than those who go into salaried professions, pre-empt a proportionately larger share of the positions in the free professions.

The influence of social origins on occupational destinations finds expression in the relative, not the absolute, proportion of men with the same origin who end up in a certain occupation, specifically, in the ratio of the per cent from a given origin in one occupation to the per cent of the total labor force in this occupation. The last row in Table 2.2, which presents the percentage distribution of the total labor force in the several occupations, serves as the standard against which all percentages in the body of the matrix are compared, the divisor in the desired ratio. By dividing each value in the matrix by the corresponding figure in the total row at the bottom of its column, we obtain an index of the influence of occupational origins on occupational destinations.[5] This ratio, which has been termed the "index of association" or "social distance mobility ratio,"[6] measures the extent to which mobility from one occupation to another surpasses or falls short of "chance"; that is, a value of 1.0 indicates that the observed mobility is equal to that expected on the assumption of statistical independence.

The model of "perfect" mobility, defined by statistical independence of origins and destinations, serves as a baseline for comparison, departures from it being reflected in the mobility ratios.[7] In the case of perfect mobility each destination group has the same distribution of origins as the total population, each origin group has the same distribution of destinations as the total population, and all indices are 1.0. The actual mobility ratios for intergenerational movements, corresponding to Table 2.2, are presented in Table 2.5; those for mobility

---

[5] The indices were not actually computed in this manner, which introduces unnecessary rounding errors, but by deriving the ratio of observed to expected frequency from the raw numbers in Tables J2.1, J2.2, and J2.3 in the Appendix.

[6] For previous use of this index, see David V. Glass (Ed.), *Social Mobility in Britain,* Glencoe: Free Press, 1956, pp. 177-217; and.Natalie Rogoff, *Recent Trends in Occupational Mobility,* Glencoe: Free Press, 1953.

[7] Some questionable assumptions underlying the model of perfect mobility and consequent limitations of the index of association for comparisons between periods or places are discussed in Chapter 3.

from father's to first occupation are presented in Table 2.6; and the intragenerational flow patterns from first to present occupation are shown in Table 2.7. In order to convey a visual impression of the over-all flow of manpower, values greater than 1.0 are underlined.

These three tables bring the main characteristics of the American occupational structure into high relief. First, occupational inheritance is in all cases greater than expected on the assumption of independence; note the consistently high values in the major diagonal. Second, social mobility is nevertheless pervasive, as revealed by the large number of underlined values off the diagonal. Third, upward mobility (to the left of the diagonal) is more prevalent than downward mobility (to the right), and short-distance movements occur more often than long-distance ones.

If occupational inheritance and fixed careers were dominating the stratification system, all excess manpower would be concentrated in the 17 cells in the major diagonal and the values in all other cells would fall short of theoretical expectation. In fact an excess flow of manpower is manifest in 101 cells of the father's-to-1962-occupation matrix, also 101 cells in the father's-to-first-job matrix, and 78 cells in the first-to-1962-job matrix. This indicates much movement among occupational strata. A rough indication of the prevailing direction of mobility is the number of such cells lying on either side of the major diagonal. For the intergenerational flow of manpower, as Table 2.5 shows, the underlined values to the lower left of the diagonal, which indicate disproportionate upward mobility, outnumber by more than three to one (64:20) those to the upper right, which indicate disproportionate downward mobility. Excessive upward movements outnumber excessive downward movements in the intragenerational flow five to two (44:17), as can be seen in Table 2.7. Table 2.6 shows, however, that the excessive flow of manpower from father's to first occupation is hardly more likely to go to higher than to lower occupations (46:38), undoubtedly because career beginnings often entail a temporary drop in status.[8]

Short-distance movements exceed long-distance ones. Most of the underlined values are concentrated in the area adjacent to the major diagonal, denoting short-distance mobility, and there are few in the areas surrounding the upper right and the lower left corners, which would be evidence of long-distance mobility. The values of the mobility ratios tend to be highest in the diagonal and decrease gradually with movement away from it. In general, the closer two occupations are to

---

[8] These patterns hold also if the cells indicative of horizontal movement are omitted.

one another in the status hierarchy, the greater is the flow of manpower between them.

There are, however, numerous exceptions to this basic tendency for the flow of manpower to occur predominantly between occupations similarly ranked, as revealed by the blank cells in areas that have predominantly underlined values and the underlined values in predominantly blank areas. The majority of these discrepancies in all three tables reflect industrial lines. Hence another distinctive pattern to which the tables call attention is that industrial lines constitute stronger barriers to mobility than do skill levels within an industry. Indeed, the expectation that industrial differences would affect the flow of manpower, partly because industries are concentrated in different geographical areas, was what prompted the decision to subdivide manual occupations by industry.

Finally, exceptional cases that are not covered by any of the above general patterns should be mentioned. Looking first at movements from father's to 1962 occupation (Table 2.5), we note that sons of craftsmen are more likely to move into higher than into lower white-collar occupations. This possibly reflects a reluctance on the part of men reared in the most affluent blue-collar homes to accept the lower income levels of the more menial nonmanual occupations. By and large, sons of manual workers outside manufacturing are more apt to be upwardly mobile than those in manufacturing. Lastly, service occupations contain relatively few sons of farmers.

The flow from father's to first occupation (Table 2.6), which often entails a temporary drop in status, reveals more discontinuities than that from father's to 1962 occupation. Sons of nonmanufacturing operatives and of service workers disproportionately often find first jobs as managers. The unexpectedly large movement of sons of nonmanufacturing laborers to first jobs as self-employed professionals may be due to sampling error resulting from the small number of cases involved—approximately six, possibly even fewer.[9] Even with a sample as large as this one, some cells have frequencies too low to assure reliable results. Sons of service workers start their careers in an unusually large variety of occupations, ranging from other laborers to salaried managers. Downward mobility to first job is most marked for those in the highest white-collar groups and for skilled craftsmen, and upward mobility to the first job is most common among both lower nonmanual and lower manual workers. This observation suggests that movements within the white-collar and within the blue-collar class

9 These might be men in such unusual "professions" as boxing.

are more prevalent than movements between these two classes, a notion that will be more systematically explored later in this chapter.

Intragenerational movements (Table 2.7) also reveal a few deviations from the main trends. First, men who start their careers as farmers, in sharp contrast to those starting as farm laborers, do not move in proportionate numbers to any nonfarm occupation, with the sole exception of skilled construction work. Second, proprietors are disproportionately recruited from skilled and semiskilled manual workers (except manufacturing operatives). Third, men who enter the labor force on higher white-collar levels and later move downward drop in excessive numbers down to retail sales, skipping the slightly higher status of clerk. Indeed, whereas men are recruited to clerical work from a wide variety of social origins, few move into clerical work after having started their careers (compare the columns for clerks in the three tables).

SUPPLY AND RECRUITMENT FROM ONE GENERATION TO THE NEXT

What is the outflow of manpower supplied by each occupational grouping to others? What is the inflow of manpower recruited from other occupational groups with which each occupation fills its ranks? These are the basic questions posed by a consideration of occupational supply and recruitment. In terms of the intergenerational volume of inflow and outflow these questions are answered by Tables 2.2 and 2.8. Table 2.2 presents the percentages of sons each social origin supplied to the various occupations in 1962. Thus every occupational origin above the level of construction craftsmen sends more than one-fifth of its sons to only two of the 17 occupations, salaried professionals and managers. A major reason is that these two occupational groups have been expanding rapidly while reproducing at a level somewhat lower than the rest of the population. Of the men sampled in 1962, 18 per cent are in these two occupational groupings, whereas only 6.5 per cent of their fathers were.

Table 2.8 shows what proportion of the men in each occupation was recruited from the various occupational origins. It indicates, for example, that every occupational group has recruited more than 10 per cent of its members from sons of farmers. Three evident reasons for this are the large size of the farm category in the past (in 1940 it was still the largest of the 17 occupational groups, accounting for 14.7 per cent of the working force); the rapid decline in the number of farmers in recent decades; and the exceptionally high fertility of farmers.

TABLE 2.8. MOBILITY FROM FATHER'S OCC. TO OCC. IN 1962, FOR MALES 25 TO 64 YEARS OLD: INFLOW PERCENTAGES

Father's Occupation	Respondent's Occupation in 1962																
	1	2	3	4	5	6	7	8	9	10	11	12	13	14	15	16	17
Professionals																	
1 Self-Empl.	14.5	3.9	1.5	3.8	.8	.8	1.1	.3	.3	.6	.3	.3	.4	.2	.6	.5	.6
2 Salaried	7.0	9.5	4.9	5.8	2.1	3.8	3.4	1.6	1.9	.6	2.1	2.1	1.9	1.4	.4	.5	.3
3 Managers	8.7	7.9	8.7	7.0	4.0	4.4	2.6	2.7	2.6	2.2	1.4	1.2	1.0	1.8	.7	.3	.3
4 Salesmen, Other	5.6	3.4	5.2	8.1	2.6	1.7	4.4	.8	1.5	.8	.5	1.0	.6	.0	.4	.4	.3
5 Proprietors	18.5	9.6	16.5	13.2	16.3	7.1	15.2	3.5	5.2	5.7	3.7	3.4	3.7	1.6	2.0	1.5	1.6
6 Clerical	4.9	7.3	4.4	5.9	2.3	4.5	2.6	2.9	3.1	1.2	1.2	1.9	3.2	1.5	1.3	.8	.0
7 Salesmen, Retail	.9	2.3	3.0	4.7	2.8	1.8	2.9	1.4	.8	1.1	1.5	1.1	1.4	.1	1.2	.7	.0
Craftsmen																	
8 Mfg.	3.8	8.3	6.1	4.3	5.1	5.7	6.3	12.0	5.1	5.1	6.2	4.7	4.8	4.5	3.2	.5	.4
9 Other	4.0	7.0	7.4	7.9	6.0	8.0	6.1	6.9	11.0	5.8	5.3	7.8	5.4	3.8	4.1	1.2	1.2
10 Construction	3.0	3.2	4.4	4.1	5.8	6.2	2.6	6.9	5.5	13.7	3.6	3.9	4.6	2.6	4.9	.8	1.8
Operatives																	
11 Mfg.	5.2	6.4	5.1	6.5	6.1	7.5	7.1	12.9	7.7	4.9	13.7	6.9	7.1	14.5	6.3	1.2	2.8
12 Other	2.8	7.5	4.2	5.4	6.2	6.7	6.0	6.5	8.6	6.6	6.9	10.9	7.1	6.5	6.4	1.2	4.4
13 Service	2.3	3.7	4.0	4.8	3.7	6.3	5.3	4.8	3.9	4.7	5.1	4.6	8.2	5.4	3.3	.8	.6
Laborers																	
14 Mfg.	.0	1.0	1.2	.4	.8	1.3	.8	2.6	1.5	1.0	3.2	2.2	3.0	5.9	2.4	.6	.9
15 Other	1.0	2.0	1.9	3.3	2.1	6.0	4.7	4.5	4.8	4.8	5.3	5.9	6.2	6.7	9.6	.7	2.8
16 Farmers	11.2	10.8	13.3	10.1	24.3	18.3	17.6	20.1	24.4	30.4	26.6	29.4	22.8	29.5	32.6	82.0	59.7
17 Farm Laborers	.3	.5	.9	.5	1.5	1.5	2.1	2.3	2.4	3.1	3.4	3.7	3.6	3.9	5.6	2.9	14.5
18 Total[a]	100.0	100.0	100.0	100.0	100.0	100.0	100.0	100.0	100.0	100.0	100.0	100.0	100.0	100.0	100.0	100.0	100.0

[a]Columns as shown do not total 100.0, since men not reporting father's occupation are not shown separately.

The less occupational inheritance there is in a given stratum, the greater is the outflow of sons supplied by this origin stratum to other occupational destinations. The five occupations with least inheritance, which supply more than 90 per cent of their sons to other destinations, are the two lowest white-collar, the two lowest blue-collar, and the lower of the two farm groups, as Table 2.2 shows. Sons of men in occupations near the bottom of one of the three broad occupational classes have exceptional opportunities for social mobility. The salaried professions, in contrast, exhibit the highest degree of inheritance, and this stratum of origin is, consequently, least likely to supply sons to other occupational destinations. The rapid growth of this prestigeful occupational group undoubtedly helped restrict the outflow of its sons.

The less self-recruitment there is in an occupational grouping, the more it tends to rely on the inflow of manpower recruited from other occupational origins. Variations in recruitment are greater than those in supply. Table 2.8 indicates that the two occupations with the largest inflow of outsiders, recruiting more than 95 per cent of their manpower from other origins, are clerks and retail salesmen, both of which also have a high rate of outflow. Farmers, on the other hand, reveal by far the highest rate of self-recruitment, recruiting less than 20 per cent of their manpower from different occupational origins, whereas no other occupation recruits less than 85 per cent from different origins.

There is a direct relationship between an occupation's rate of outflow or supply to others and its rate of inflow or recruitment from others. The rank correlation is .54.[10] This is the same as saying that occupational inheritance and self-recruitment are positively related, which is not inevitable despite the fact that both values depend on the number of men in a given occupational group whose fathers were in the same group. This number, the number of cases in the diagonal of the matrix in Table J2.1 in Appendix J, divided by the row total defines the index of occupational inheritance, or the per cent of the men in an occupational category whose fathers were in the same category. The same number divided by the column total defines the index of self-recruitment, the per cent of fathers whose sons continue in their occupational category. As the two marginals are positively related it follows that the two index values are too, although the latter would be fully determined by the former correlation only if it were 1.00 (actually the rank correlation between the marginals is .62 and

[10] Product movement correlation is an insignificant .19, undoubtedly in part due to the extreme deviant values for salaried professionals on supply and for farmers on recruitment.

the product moment correlation is .23).[11] Some occupations appear to be relatively self-contained and self-sufficient, whereas others supply disproportionate numbers of sons to different occupations and also recruit a disproportionate share of their own manpower from different occupations. What characteristics of occupations are associated with these contrasting tendencies?

The three occupational groups that manifest most occupational inheritance and self-recruitment are the only three that entail self-employment—independent professionals, proprietors, and farmers. It seems that proprietorship—of a farm, a business, or a professional practice—discourages sons from leaving the occupation of their fathers and makes it difficult for other men to move into an occupation. Even when proprietorship does not involve actual ownership of an establishment, as in the case of tenant farmers and of independent professionals who only own their equipment and the good will of their clientele, it may produce a stronger occupational investment and commitment than mere employment, and these are transmitted to sons. The fact that the very occupations that rest on proprietorship and that reveal little mobility in or out have either contracted in size or expanded less than the rest in recent decades may well be a factor that has contributed to the large amount of social mobility observable today. This decline in proprietorship may counteract other trends, such as decreasing immigration and lessening differential fertility, that would otherwise have depressed mobility rates.

The five occupations characterized by a high rate of inflow of manpower recruited from other origins in the last generation as well as by a high rate of outflow of manpower supplied to other destinations in the present generation are the two lowest white-collar and the three lowest blue-collar groups—clerical, retail sales, service, and the two kinds of nonfarm labor. These five occupational strata may be considered distributors of manpower, into which disproportionate numbers move from different origins, and from which disproportionate numbers of sons move to different destinations. The distributing occupations are channels for upward mobility, into which successful sons from lower origins tend to move and from which successful sons tend to move to higher destinations. Simultaneously, they provide a refuge for the downwardly mobile from higher origins (inasmuch as

[11] The measures of supply and recruitment are the sum of all nondiagonal frequencies, except the NA value, in the appropriate row or column of Table J2.1, divided by the row and column totals, respectively. Thus, except for the differential assignment of the NA cases, there is a perfect negative correlation between inheritance and supply as well as between self-recruitment and recruitment.

downward mobility into them exceeds theoretical expectations considerably more than does downward mobility into any lower occupations), thereby enabling unsuccessful sons of nonmanual fathers to maintain their white-collar status and unsuccessful sons of manual fathers to find jobs in the urban labor market, respectively. The skidder from a white-collar home, unfamiliar with the working class and possibly threatened by the prospect of becoming part of it, appears to be willing to pay the price of the lesser income offered by the lowest nonmanual occupations to preserve the cherished symbol of the white collar. The skidder from manual homes has probably also little inclination and certainly few qualifications or opportunities to work on a farm.

If occupations are divided into three broad classes, white-collar, blue-collar, and farm, it is evident that a position just above one of the two class boundaries is what tends to make an occupation a distributor in the intergenerational flow of manpower. Proprietorship, on the other hand, has the opposite effect, restricting the inflow and the outflow of manpower. Proprietorship and location in the occupational structure, therefore, are two important characteristics of an occupation that influence the proportionate volume of manpower it supplies to others and recruits from others. This is the case, however, only for the intergenerational flow from father's to 1962 occupation. Neither in the flow from father's to first occupation nor in that from first to 1962 occupation are the volumes of supply and recruitment directly related, which calls attention to the distinctive character of first jobs, a topic to be examined in the next section. But before doing so another aspect of intergenerational movements will be considered.

Whatever the volume of outflow or inflow, it may range from highly dispersed to highly concentrated. The outflow of manpower from a given origin may disperse to supply many different destinations or become concentrated to supply primarily a few. Correspondingly, the inflow of manpower into a given destination may be recruited from a wide base of different origins or largely from a narrow base of a few origins. Whereas the volume of supply and of recruitment depend directly on the number of men whose fathers had the same occupation, the degree of dispersion of supply and of recruitment do not. The first problem is to devise appropriate measures of dispersion of supply and dispersion of recruitment. The basic principle is to compare the distribution of outflow from or inflow into a given category with the distribution for the entire population.

To illustrate the construction of these measures, let us examine the outflow from social origin, defined by father's occupation, to occupational destination in 1962, presented in Table 2.2. Of all sons of self-employed professionals, 16.7 per cent entered this same occupation, 31.9 per cent became salaried professionals, 9.9 per cent took jobs as salaried managers, and 9.5 per cent went into nonretail selling. The corresponding percentages for all men (bottom row) are 1.4, 10.2, 7.9, and 3.1. These four occupations are the only ones in which men originating as self-employed professionals are overrepresented, that is, constitute a higher proportion than in the total population. A simple way to summarize this observation is that four of the 17 possible destinations contained disproportionate numbers of men with fathers who were self-employed professionals, which implies that the supply of manpower from this origin is relatively concentrated, excessive numbers going to only three destinations in addition to the self-employed professions themselves. Applying the same procedure to all categories of origins yields a crude measure of dispersion of supply, and applying this procedure with appropriate changes to the inflow percentages in Table 2.8 yields a crude measure of dispersion of recruitment. The *number* of underlined entries, whatever their value, in each row of Table 2.5 indicates dispersion of supply, using this rough procedure, and the number of underlined entries in each column indicates dispersion of recruitment.

A more refined index of the degree of concentration—or, inversely, dispersion—which takes the quantitative differences in percentages into account instead of merely dichotomizing them, and which ascribes neither special meaning nor equality to the 17 occupational categories, can be devised simply by summing the differences between the corresponding percentages given above (that is, all the differences of the same sign). Thus the degree of concentration in the destinations to which sons of self-employed professionals move is $(16.7 - 1.4) + (31.9 - 10.2) + (9.9 - 7.9) + (9.5 - 3.1)$, which equals 45.4. The range of values this measure can assume makes its meaning apparent. If father's occupation exerts no influence and the destination of sons from a given social origin is identical with that of the entire population, the index value is zero. If all men from a given origin were concentrated in a single destination, the index value would be close to 100.0; specifically, as much short of 100.0 as the per cent of the total population in this destination. Hence this index, the index of dissimilarity, measures how much more concentrated the destinations of men from a given origin are than those of all men in the sample, or what proportion of the sons of a given origin would have to change their 1962 occupation for their distribution to equal that of the total population. A high value indicates low dispersion whereas a high value on the crude measure indicates high dispersion. The corresponding index for inflow shows how concentrated (or dispersed) the origins of men in each occupational destination are.

Two further refinements have been introduced before actually computing the measures. The first is to exclude the men in the same occupational group as their fathers (those in the diagonal) from the analysis, since otherwise the index is again strongly influenced by occupational inheritance or self-recruitment, whereas concern is with the outflow from or the inflow into *different* occupations.[12] In addition, movements identified as lateral movements earlier in this chapter—mobility between manufacturing and other craftsmen, manufacturing and other operatives, and manufacturing and other laborers—have been excluded by the same blocking procedure, restricting the analysis to vertical mobility.

We have, then, a crude index of dispersion in the flow of manpower based on merely counting the observed values that exceed those expected on the assumption of statistical independence, and a refined measure that takes the precise degree of dispersion or concentration in vertical movements alone into account. These two measures do not behave in parallel fashion at all. The dispersion of supply and the dispersion of recruitment in the intergenerational flow of manpower are inversely related if the crude measures are used ($r = -.46$), whereas the two are directly related if the refined measures are used (.59). Moreover, the rate of growth of an occupational group between 1940 and 1960 reveals a pronounced positive correlation with the dispersion of its recruitment as indicated by the crude measure (.72), but not with dispersion in recruitment as indicated by the refined measure (.26).[13]

In a previous publication by one of the present authors,[14] which relied on the crude measures exclusively, the inverse relationship between dispersion in recruitment and dispersion in supply observed

---

[12] The procedure for computing expected values in such a model of quasi-independence in which the diagonal cells or some others are blocked has been developed by Leo Goodman, "On the Statistical Analysis of Mobility Tables," *American Journal of Sociology*, 70(1965), 564-585. If we compute an analogous measure of concentration that does not involve the block procedure, it can be shown to be a composite of occupational inheritance (or self-recruitment) and concentration of supply (or recruitment) for those undergoing mobility. Our procedure, therefore, was designed to yield a measure of concentration that is not mathematically dependent on the degree of inheritance or self-recruitment.

[13] To measure rate of growth, the distribution of the labor force in 1940 and that in 1960 were percentaged, and the difference between the two corresponding percentages, divided by the 1940 percentage, was taken as the index of rate of growth.

[14] Peter M. Blau, "The Flow of Occupational Supply and Recruitment," *American Sociological Review*, 30(1965), 475-490.

was interpreted as due to the forces that are set in motion by changes in demand for occupational services and that are reflected in changes in the relative size of various occupations. For an occupation to expand in response to an increased demand for its services, it must recruit more outsiders than previously, particularly if its fertility is not very high. Successful recruitment of outsiders requires improvement of working conditions, such as higher incomes or shorter hours than men with the requisite training can otherwise command. Superior economic conditions not only attract men from diverse other origins to an occupational group but also strengthen the attachment of its own sons to it, thus lessening the tendency of sons to move into widely different occupations. The opposite conditions in contracting or less expanding occupational groups weaken the attachments of sons and promote their dispersal to a variety of other occupations. These considerations would explain why the width of the base of recruitment of an occupation is related to its expansion, on the one hand, and to a lack of inclination on the part of its sons to disperse from it, on the other. The problem is, however, that the more refined measures do not yield this relationship.

The refined measures of concentration of supply and concentration of recruitment, the obverse of which indicates dispersion, are presented in Table 2.9. The data show that the outflow of sons of self-employed professionals is most concentrated in respect to occupational destinations in 1962, whereas the sons of operatives outside manufacturing have become most dispersed as adults (column 1). Farm laborers are recruited from the most concentrated social origins, whereas "other" craftsmen and proprietors are recruited from the most widely dispersed origins. Although the polar cases of dispersion in supply and dispersion in recruitment are not identical, the degree of dispersion in supply and in recruitment are directly related for the flow of manpower from father's to 1962 occupation, as previously noted. Indeed, positive correlations between these two factors are also obtained when movements between father's and first occupation (product moment, .77) and those between first and 1962 occupation (.51) are considered.

Why do two sets of measures that presumably refer to the same underlying variables yield opposite results? One possible reason is that the crude measure is not a reliable indication of dispersion. Another possibility, however, is that the two kinds of measure refer to entirely different aspects of dispersion. Thus dispersion of recruitment as defined by the crude measure indicates that an occupation attracts more than its proportionate share of men from *many* different occupational origins, whereas its operational definition by the

TABLE 2.9. INDEX OF DISSIMILARITY BETWEEN DESTINATION OR ORIGIN DISTRIBUTION OF VERTICALLY MOBILE MEN AND DISTRIBUTION EXPECTED ON THE MODEL OF QUASI-INDEPENDENCE, FOR SPECIFIED ORIGIN OR DESTINATION

Occ. of Origin or Destination	Concentration of Supply[a]			Concentration of Recruitment[b]		
	1 Father's Occ. to 1962 Occ.	2 Father's Occ. to First Job	3 First Job to 1962 Occ.	4 1962 Occ. from Father's Occ.	5 First Job from Father's Occ.	6 1962 Occ. from First Job
Professionals Self-Empl.	41.4	41.1	61.6	35.5	44.1	51.6
Salaried	22.9	20.4	45.5	23.7	27.9	23.1
Managers	30.1	27.0	39.2	23.1	42.1	31.0
Salesmen, Other	35.5	31.3	38.9	25.7	41.7	28.8
Proprietors	26.9	24.5	32.0	8.8	31.3	15.1
Clerical	24.0	21.0	27.5	9.5	20.4	16.1
Salesmen, Retail	20.7	20.3	25.5	14.8	18.1	17.0
Craftsmen Mfg.	9.9	23.9	14.7	13.5	16.4	20.7
Other	8.2	16.1	15.3	8.2	16.5	14.3
Construction	12.4	15.5	23.2	14.1	9.2	16.0
Operatives Mfg.	12.1	22.0	13.6	15.2	15.7	17.3
Other	7.5	17.3	13.8	15.9	8.2	16.7
Service	8.5	16.9	16.9	10.9	18.4	11.1
Laborers Mfg.	24.7	23.2	23.2	23.5	19.3	24.7
Other	18.8	17.9	14.2	22.8	8.9	20.6
Farmers	16.2	28.0	18.5	20.9	25.2	52.7
Farm Laborers	27.1	26.4	27.2	49.9	52.1	34.5

[a]Destination distribution for origin distribution listed in stub.
[b]Origin distribution for destination distribution listed in stub.

refined measure indicates that an occupation does *not* attract disproportionately large numbers from the various other origins. Although both measures reveal increasing dispersion as the origin distribution in a given occupation approaches that of the entire population, the two behave quite differently in response to some other conditions, including the changes in size to which the above interpretation refers. If employment conditions in a growing occupation have widened its appeal, we may surmise that men will be drawn into it in disproportionate numbers from more origins than before, but that the consequent greater competition for these desirable jobs makes it more difficult than it was previously for men from distant origins to move into the occupation. Such a change making an occupation more attractive to those from surrounding origins, and for this very reason less accessible to the rest, would find opposite expression in the two measures. It would be manifest as *more* dispersed recruitment in the crude measure, because an excess of men is recruited from a larger number of origins than before, while it would be manifest as more concentrated and hence *less* dispersed recruitment in the refined measure, since the origin distribution departs further than before from the random expectations based on the population. Parallel considerations apply to the two measures of dispersion of supply. The crude measure is indicative of the width of the recruitment base or the supply sector of an occupation, and these are affected by the superior economic rewards in expanding occupations according to the interpretation advanced. But the refined measure is indicative of the randomness of the origin distribution of the men recruited into an occupation or of the destination distribution of the men it supplies to other occupations, and other forces than those associated with expansion apparently govern how randomly dispersed the flow of manpower into and out of an occupation is.

The data in Table 2.9, in which occupations are ranked by their status, reveal a nonmonotonic pattern. The sons of skilled and semi-skilled workers tend to disperse widely in their careers. The sons of the higher white-collar strata as well as the sons of the lower unskilled workers and farm workers are more likely to become concentrated in relatively few occupational groups (column 1). Dispersion of recruitment reveals a similar pattern as that of supply, with the intermediate occupational groupings being recruited from less concentrated origins than either those near the top or those near the bottom, except that the lower nonmanual strata as well as the higher and middle manual ones are recruited from dispersed origins (column 4). Roughly the same nonmonotonic pattern is manifest in the data on dispersion of supply from father's to first occupation (column 2) and from first to present occupation (column 3), and also in the corresponding data on dispersion of recruitment (columns 5 and 6). The parallel patterns of these values account for the correlations between dispersion of supply and dispersion of recruitment.

Men in occupations in the middle of the status hierarchy come from more dispersed backgrounds than those in the highest or the lowest occupations, and men originating in these intermediate strata also move to more dispersed occupations in their careers than men originating at either extreme of the occupational hierarchy. This is the case whether origin is defined by father's occupation or by first job and whether destination is defined by first job or by 1962 occupation, that is, for intragenerational mobility as well as for intergenerational mobility of either kind (from father's to first job and from father's to 1962 occupation). The significance of status proximity for careers can help explain this pattern of findings.

The underlying principle of the interpretation suggested is that differences in economic conditions and styles of life between occupational groupings tend to reveal a gradient, being pronounced only for those far apart in the status hierarchy. The resources, training, education, and value orientations of men with a given occupational background do not differ generally very much from those with a somewhat higher or lower background, but differences between men, say, 10 or more steps apart are considerable in these respects. Moreover, there is much opportunity for social contact among men from different occupational groupings as long as these are not too widely apart in status, in which case there is little social contact. Without social contacts with representatives of an occupational group that stimulate interest in and provide knowledge about careers in it, men are unlikely to move into it. In brief, the assumption is that various conditions make movements to occupations within a given range of a man's origin more likely than movements to those outside this range. It follows from this assumption that intermediate occupational groups are recruited from more diverse origins and supply men to more diverse destinations than extreme groups at either end of the hierarchy. This is what the data show. The reason is that any given range of other occupations above and below a point of reference includes a larger number of different occupations if the point of reference is an intermediate occupation than if it is near the top or near the bottom, because in the latter case part of this range simply does not exist.

THE SIGNIFICANCE OF CAREER BEGINNINGS

The preceding discussion concentrated on intergenerational movements from father's to 1962 occupation with only occasional reference to first jobs; we now turn to an investigation of the significance of these career beginnings. This entails the study of intragenerational movements, but it includes more than that. Data on the first full-time regular job of men can be looked at from two perspectives, since the relationship between social origins and career beginnings can be examined, as can the movements from career beginnings to occupation in 1962.[15] This possibility introduces a time dimension into the analysis of occupational mobility. We can ask how the occupational origins of men starting their careers at various points in the occupational structure affect subsequent careers and deduce the significance of social origins for intragenerational movements.

Let us start by examining the role of career beginnings as intervening links between social origins and subsequent careers; specifically,

---

[15] The fact that different time periods are involved for men varying in age from 25 to 64 years should be kept in mind, since the differences are not the same for the various occupational groupings. Differences between age cohorts, which turn out to be usually minor, will be discussed in subsequent chapters.

is the influence of occupational origins on ultimate achievements mediated by entry into the labor market? It is possible that occupational origins influence the level on which men start their careers and that this starting level affects their subsequent occupational life, but that social origins have no additional direct effect on later careers. To test this hypothesis, indices of association have been computed between father's occupation and 1962 occupation within categories of first job. In effect, this procedure holds entry occupation constant, providing a basis for evaluating the remaining relationship between occupational origins and destination in 1962. If the hypothesis is correct and the entire influence of occupational origins is exerted through the first job, the index should be 1.0 in all cells. Table 2.10 presents the results of applying this procedure.

The data testify that social origins exert a direct effect on later careers in addition to that mediated by career beginnings. To be sure, comparison of the values in Table 2.10 and Table 2.5 reveals that those in Table 2.10 are generally, though not uniformly, closer to unity than those in Table 2.5. This demonstrates that career beginning is an intervening variable in the relationship between occupational origin and occupation in 1962. A good part of the influence of social origins on subsequent occupational life is due to the influence of origins on career beginnings, which in turn affect later careers. The deviations from an index value of 1.0 in Table 2.10, however, parallel those in Table 2.5, with values decreasing with movement away from the major diagonal. This indicates that even after a man has been launched on his career, his occupational origin continues to exert an influence on it.

We now turn to the investigation of the volume of supply in the intragenerational flow of manpower from first to 1962 occupation. The 17 occupations have been divided on the basis of whether the outflow of manpower each supplies to other occupations later in life exceeds or falls short of the average outflow for the total population (which is 80 per cent). Ten first occupations retain a disproportionate share of men and supply comparatively little manpower to other occupations in 1962 (as indicated by a high percentage in the diagonal of Table 2.4). Once men start to work in these occupational groupings, they tend to remain in them. The other seven groupings are disproportionate suppliers which men leave at above average rates in the course of their careers. These occupational groupings are clerical, retail sales, both groups of operatives, both groups of manual laborers, and farm laborers. What distinguishes these occupational groupings from others?

TABLE 2.10. MOBILITY FROM FATHER'S OCC. TO OCC. IN 1962, FOR MALES 25 TO 64 YEARS OLD: RATIOS OF OBSERVED FREQUENCIES TO FREQUENCIES EXPECTED ON THE ASSUMPTION OF INDEPENDENCE WITHIN OCC. GROUPS OF FIRST JOB

Father's Occupation	Respondent's Occupation in 1962																
	1	2	3	4	5	6	7	8	9	10	11	12	13	14	15	16	17
Professionals																	
1 Self-Empl.	2.1	1.4	.9	2.0	.7	.6	1.1	.4	.4	.9	.5	.4	.5	.4	1.0	1.1	1.3
2 Salaried	1.0	1.4	1.2	1.5	.7	1.1	1.2	.6	.8	.3	1.0	1.0	.8	.7	.2	.4	.3
3 Managers	1.2	1.3	1.7	1.4	1.1	1.0	.7	.9	.8	.8	.5	.4	.3	.8	.3	.3	.2
4 Salesmen, Other	1.3	1.0	1.7	2.1	1.2	.7	1.9	.6	.8	.6	.4	.6	.4	.0	.3	.6	.4
5 Proprietors	1.4	.9	1.6	1.2	1.8	.9	1.8	.6	.8	1.0	.7	.6	.6	.3	.4	.6	.6
6 Clerical	1.1	1.4	1.0	1.5	.7	1.1	.8	1.0	1.1	.5	.5	.8	1.2	.6	.6	.7	.0
7 Salesmen, Retail	.3	1.0	1.3	2.0	1.5	.8	1.4	.9	.6	.8	1.0	.8	1.0	.1	.9	.9	.0
Craftsmen																	
8 Mfg.	.8	1.4	1.0	.7	.8	.9	1.1	1.6	.9	.9	1.0	.9	.9	.7	.7	.2	.2
9 Other	.7	1.1	1.1	1.1	.9	1.1	.8	1.0	1.5	.9	.8	1.2	.8	.6	.7	.4	.3
10 Construction	.8	.7	.9	.8	1.1	1.2	.5	1.3	1.0	2.0	.8	.8	1.0	.6	1.1	.3	.6
Operatives																	
11 Mfg.	1.0	1.0	.7	.9	.8	.9	.9	1.3	1.0	.7	1.4	.9	.9	1.5	.9	.3	.7
12 Other	.5	1.2	.6	.8	.9	1.0	.9	.9	1.2	.9	1.0	1.4	1.0	1.1	1.0	.4	1.1
13 Service	.7	.9	.9	1.1	.8	1.3	1.2	1.0	.8	1.1	1.1	1.0	1.6	1.2	.8	.4	.2
Laborers																	
14 Mfg.	.0	.7	.8	.3	.5	.7	.4	1.2	.8	.6	1.4	1.1	1.5	2.0	1.2	.5	.6
15 Other	.3	.6	.5	.8	.5	1.4	1.1	1.0	1.1	1.1	1.2	1.2	1.3	1.4	1.8	.3	1.0
16 Farmers	.8	.7	.8	.6	1.1	1.0	.8	.8	1.0	1.1	1.0	1.0	.9	1.0	1.0	1.4	1.1
17 Farm Laborers	.4	.4	.7	.4	.7	.9	1.0	.9	.9	1.1	1.2	1.2	1.2	1.1	1.6	.5	2.2

The clue is provided by the net mobility into and out of first occupations. If the number of men in an occupational grouping in 1962 is subtracted from the number who started their working life in this grouping (see the totals of Table J2.3 in the Appendix), an index of net mobility during these men's working lives is obtained, which may reveal either a net outflow or a net inflow. Similarly, if the number of men who started to work in an occupation is subtracted from the number whose fathers were in this occupation (Table J2.2 in the Appendix), an index of net mobility from father's to first occupation is obtained, which also may show either net outflow or net inflow. With one exception—the rapidly expanding salaried professions, which manifest an inflow in both cases—there is a perfect negative relationship between these two indices. Occupations that more men leave than enter after having started their careers (outflow) exhibit an inflow of manpower from social origins, and those occupations that more men enter than leave after they have begun to work (inflow) reveal an outflow of manpower from social origins. In other words, some occupations have more men starting in them than either the number of men pursuing this line of work later in life or the number with fathers who pursued this line of work, and other occupations constitute career beginnings for fewer men than are found in them at later career stages in either generation.

Seven occupations may be considered distinctive entry occupations or career beginnings, since the number of men who started to work in them exceeds both the number whose fathers and the number who themselves worked in them in later career stages. These are the same seven entry occupations whose disproportionate supply of manpower to other occupational groups later in life was noted above: clerks, retail salesmen, both groups of operatives, and all three groups of laborers. It is noteworthy that these distinctive career beginnings consist of the lowest white-collar occupations, the lowest blue-collar ones (except for service), and the lowest farm occupation. More men start their careers in the lowest strata of each of the three occupational classes than remain in them or later move into them. The data pertaining to fathers suggest that in the last generation, too, comparatively few men stayed in these lines of work as adults. These entry occupations dominate the intragenerational flow of manpower, supplying disproportionate numbers to other occupations in later career stages. The importance of distinctive entry occupations for the intragenerational flow of manpower is an important factor differentiating the intragenerational from the intergenerational flow.

Having identified the entry occupations that supply a large *volume* of manpower to other occupations later, the next question posed is from which first jobs men are most likely to *disperse* to many different career lines later in life. Specifically, we want to inquire whether the origin composition of an occupational grouping influences the inclination of its members to disperse to other occupations later. The hypothesis may be suggested that the more thoroughly the men entering an occupation are integrated into it, the less likely they are to disperse to other occupational groups in the course of their careers.

Homogeneity of social background is expected to promote social integration. The hypothesis implies, therefore, that the homogeneity in social origins of the men in an entry occupation is inversely related to their tendency to leave it for a large variety of other occupations. The operational definition of homogeneity in background is that any two randomly chosen men in an entry occupation have the same social origin (father's occupation), whatever this origin is.[16] The measures of homogeneity corresponding to this definition are presented in the first column of Table 2.11. The dependent variable is measured by the previously discussed crude index of dispersion of supply in movements from first to 1962 occupation.[17] The hypothesis predicts a negative association between the homogeneity of entry occupations and the dispersion of supply of manpower from them. But in fact the product moment correlation is close to zero (—.07), negating the hypothesis. Homogeneity of social origins of the men starting their careers in the same occupational grouping apparently does not discourage them from moving into many different lines of work later in life.

As the original hypothesis is discredited by the data, it must be modified: for integration into an occupation to prevent subsequent dispersal into a variety of different occupations, homogeneity in background is not sufficient, but men must have common social roots in this particular occupational group that precede their own actual entry into it and firmly tie them to it. The percentage of all men in an entry occupation whose fathers were in the same occupation furnishes an index of common social roots. These values, derived from Table J2.2 in the Appendix, are presented in column 2 of Table 2.11.

[16] The procedure used to arrive at the index of homogeneity of occupational origins is to sum the probabilities that two men in a given entry occupation are from the same particular occupational background, a sum of 17 probabilities, each produced by squaring the probability that a single man in a given grouping had a father in any specific grouping. Operationally, this is a summation of the squares of the vertically computed percentages, by columns, in Table J2.2.

[17] The crude measure of dispersion of supply in movements from first to 1962 occupation is used, because the refined measure with its blocked diagonal is not affected by the proportion remaining in an occupation, which is important here. The correlation is also close to zero (.08) when the refined measure is used.

TABLE 2.11. FIRST OCCUPATIONS: MEASURES OF HOMOGENEITY SELF-RECRUITMENT, NET MOBILITY, AND GROSS MOBILITY, FOR MALES 25 TO 64 YEARS OLD

Occ.	1 Homogeneity of Origins	2 Occupational Self-Recruitment	3 Net Mobility Father's Occ. to 1962 Occ.[a]	4 Per Cent in First Job Mobile to First Job[b]	5 Per Cent in First Job Mobile from First Job to 1962 Occ.[b]	6 Difference Between Columns 4 & 5
Professionals						
Self-Empl.	11.3	18.9	57.6	81.1	46.5	34.6
Salaried	8.1	12.3	49.3	87.7	45.5	42.2
Managers and Officials	10.6	8.2	43.5	91.8	64.3	27.5
Salesmen, Others	12.7	16.5	31.8	83.5	76.3	7.2
Proprietors	32.1	53.8	37.2	46.2	63.7	-17.5
Clerical	7.0	6.5	36.7	93.5	82.4	11.1
Salesmen, Retail	8.2	4.2	32.8	95.8	94.9	.9
Craftsmen						
Mfg.	9.5	16.9	24.0	83.1	77.5	5.6
Other	8.6	17.1	26.4	82.9	78.7	4.2
Construction	13.2	23.4	25.6	76.6	73.8	2.8
Operatives						
Mfg.	9.8	18.3	20.5	81.7	81.2	.5
Other	10.3	17.2	24.7	82.8	85.0	-2.2
Service	8.5	11.4	25.3	88.6	80.2	8.4
Laborers						
Mfg.	10.0	7.7	23.0	92.3	91.8	.5
Other	11.0	11.4	27.0	88.6	88.5	.1
Farmers	71.6	84.5	50.5	15.5	70.0	-54.5
Farm Laborers	48.6	10.0	55.4	90.0	93.0	-3.0

[a] In percentages.
[b] Or NA.

The new hypothesis is that the greater solidarity in those occupational groupings in which a large proportion of the men who enter have common social roots lessens the likelihood that men will disperse from these occupations to a large variety of others in the course of their careers. The inverse relationship predicted between the values in column 2 of Table 2.11 and the number of underlined values in each row of Table 2.7 is confirmed, though not strongly, by the data, which reveal a product moment correlation of —.50. The larger the proportion of men starting their careers in an occupation whose background gives them common social roots in it, the less likely men are to leave it later for many different occupations. To be sure, this correlation over occupational groups does not demonstrate that *individuals* who enter the same occupation as their father's are more likely than others to remain in this occupation. But the correlation observed is of great interest even if it is not a result of such an underlying individual correlation, because in that case it implies that social solidarity, or a similar social mechanism, is the intervening variable that connects the proportion of men with social roots in an entry occupation with the disinclination of other men to disperse from this occupation.

According to the interpretation advanced, cross-generational occupational solidarity restricts the tendency of men who have started their careers in a certain line of work to leave it later for others. Indeed, different manifestations of the underlying variables from those previously used support this interpretation. The proportion of sons from a given origin who enter their father's line of work is another indication of cross-generational solidarity. (This measure of occupational inheritance—the values in the diagonal of Table 2.3—is not significantly related to the measure of self-recruitment employed in the preceding analysis, the product moment correlation being —.24.) The proportion of men entering an occupation who have remained in it until 1962 (the values in the diagonal of Table 2.4) is a measure of the disinclination to leave that is different from the crude dispersion measure previously used. These two factors are highly related; the product moment correlation between the values in the two diagonals is .89. The greater the proportion of sons originating in an occupational group who themselves start careers in it, the greater is the tendency of men once they have entered this occupational group to remain in it. This is also a correlation over occupational groups. Note that the two measures of the dependent variable—the proportion of men who remain in an entry occupation and the degree of dispersion among those who leave it—are based on the behavior of entirely different individuals. The fact that two different correlations yield parallel results strengthens confidence in the conclusion that social mechanisms, not merely personal feelings of attachment, are responsible for the relationship observed. Cross-generational occupational solidarity seems to increase the reluctance of men from all origins to move out of the occupational group they have entered.

Finally, the role played by career beginnings in the intergenerational movements from social origins to 1962 occupations will be examined. The specific question asked for each category of first occupation is how dissimilar its distribution of father's occupations and its distribution of 1962 occupations is. The index of dissimilarity employed to answer this question is based on the same procedure as the refined measures of dispersion. For men with a given first job, the distribution of father's occupations and the distribution of 1962 occupations are reduced to percentages, and the differences between corresponding percentages are calculated. The sum of all positive (or all negative) differences yields the index of dissimilarity, which is presented in column 3 of Table 2.11, and which shows how different the occupational destinations of men starting their careers on a certain level were from their social origins.[18] In effect, this index of dissimilarity reveals the net intergenerational mobility experienced by men who started their careers in a certain occupational group.

Men who start their working lives in manual jobs experience relatively little intergenerational mobility. At least, the net mobility reflected in the dissimilarity between their fathers' and their 1962 occupations is small, and there is little difference in this respect between the various manual occupations, with the index ranging only from 20.5 to 27.0. Although this low volume of *net* intergenerational mobility of men who entered the labor force on blue-collar levels does not necessarily mean that few of them moved to levels different from their fathers' or that few of them experienced mobility during their lifetimes, it does show that the occupations in which these men ended up as adults were, in the aggregate, little different from their fathers'. Although these men experience in fact a considerable amount of mobility into and out of first jobs (columns 4 and 5 in Table 2.11), the movements into first jobs in one direction are largely compensated by movements out of first jobs in the opposite direction, with the result that the destination distribution differs little from the origin distribution.

Men who began their careers either in white-collar jobs or on farms experience much more net intergenerational mobility between social origins and 1962 destinations than those who started by working in manual jobs. The distribution of occupations in which these white-collar and farm entrants end up are very different from those of their fathers, in contrast to the similarity between the two distributions for men whose first job is in one of the blue-collar categories. The interesting phenomenon is that the *gross* amount of mobility experienced by white-collar and by farm starters, both from origin to first job and between first job and 1962 occupation, is no greater than that experienced by blue-collar starters (see columns 4 and 5 of Table 2.11); but the two segmental movements of the former groups do not largely compensate each other, whereas those of the latter do, so that only the white-collar and farm starters experience much *net* mobility and arrive at destinations that differ considerably from their origins. The net rates of an occupational group are indicative of the mobility experience of the entire collectivity, while the gross rates are indicative

18 It is also possible to calculate the dissimilarity between first and 1962 occupation for each social origin, and the dissimilarity between father's and first occupation for each 1962 occupational grouping. These values, which have less substantive meaning, and which do not reveal consistent patterns, are not presented.

of the mobility experience of its individual members. The *collectivities* of men who start work on various manual levels experience little mobility, notwithstanding much movement on the part of their individual members, in contrast to the collectivities of men starting in white-collar jobs or on farms, which experience much net mobility. Moreover, the higher the status of a white-collar occupation into which men enter, the greater is the net mobility experienced by them as a collectivity, increasing, with a single exception, from 33 per cent for retail sales to 58 per cent for self-employed professions.

Despite the fact that men who start their careers on blue-collar levels experience no less mobility than other men, their movements effect less change in the aggregate from one generation to the next, so that the distribution of occupational positions at which they arrive differs little from that of their fathers. The implication, then, is that the two segmental gross movements of men who enter the labor force in blue-collar occupations merely serve to take these man back to the occupations of their origins, whereas first jobs in white-collar and farming occupations carry men away from their origins. The occupational world of these blue-collar starters seems to be epitomized by the remark the Queen made to Alice: "Now, *here,* you see, it takes all the running *you* can do, to keep in the same place. If you want to get somewhere else, you must run at least twice as fast as that!" The large amount of upward mobility of men holding blue-collar first jobs observable in the data must not be misinterpreted. It does not basically alter the occupational situation of blue-collar starters as a class from one generation to the next, since there is much compensating downward mobility. The case of white-collar and farm entrants is fundamentally different, inasmuch as the mobility of individuals in these occupational groups effects a net change of the aggregate positions in each group, and from other data we know that this change is largely an improvement. In the aggregate, the men who enter careers in the highest white-collar strata or in the farm strata are most likely to experience intergenerational mobility, with those entering the lower white-collar strata being intermediate, and with the entrants on blue-collar levels being at the opposite extreme.

In the preceding section we found that the inflow into and the outflow from blue-collar groups is more dispersed than that for either white-collar or farm groups. This finding seems at first to contradict the present one that blue-collar starters experience *less* net mobility than either white-collar or farm starters, but actually the two findings are by no means incompatible. The very fact that blue-collar starters, who experience no less mobility than other men, exhibit more dispersed movements helps to explain why these movements produce less net change in the occupational distributions. The more diverse the movements, the more likely they are to neutralize one another.

First occupations that manifest much net intergenerational mobility may do so primarily as the result of much movement from social origin to first job, or of much movement from first job to 1962 occupation, or of both kinds of movement. The percentage of men in each starting occupation who had moved there from different social origins is presented in column 4 of Table 2.11, and the percentage in each starting occupation who moved to different occupations in 1962 (the complement of the value in the diagonal of Table 2.4) is presented in column 5. The difference between these two percentages in column 6 reveals whether a given group experienced more mobility before it had entered these careers or subsequently in intragenerational movements to 1962 occupation. Most differences for blue-collar starters are small, corresponding to their low rates of net mobility (although small differences do not necessarily reflect low net rates, as they may be a result of many noncompensating movements of both kinds). Of major interest are the differences for white-collar and farm starters, which enable us to explore what the source of the high net mobility of these groups is.

Whereas men who start their careers on high white-collar levels and those starting on farms have similar high rates of net intergenerational mobility, the kinds of movement producing this result are quite different. Men entering high white-collar occupations have already experienced much movement from social origins, which must entail mostly upward mobility, and experience less movement subsequently in their own careers. Men entering farm occupations, in contrast, have as yet experienced little movement from social origins but experience much movement in their own careers, which must be primarily upward mobility off the farm. (Although the value for farm laborers in column 4 is high and the negative difference in column 6 is small, this is primarily due to the fact that 68.5 per cent of them had farm fathers; if movements between farm and farm labor are excluded, the negative difference in column 6 becomes pronounced.) Men starting careers as proprietors are the only white-collar group who experience more mobility after having started their own careers than before. Men entering on the lowest white-collar levels have already experienced very high rates of mobility from social origins and also experience very high rates of mobility subsequently in their own careers. These movements are partly, though not entirely, compensating, yielding a moderate amount of net mobility. In sum, the high rates of net intergenerational mobility of men starting careers in high white-collar strata are due to much upward mobility from social origins; those of men starting on farms are due to much subsequent movement in their own lifetimes, as are those of men starting as proprietors; the lower rates of men starting on low white-collar levels are associated with much movement of both kinds, which is partly compensating; and the still-lower rates of blue-collar starters are due to a still-greater degree of compensation in their movements.

MOBILITY AND CLASS BOUNDARIES

The direction of movement among occupational groupings is, of course, crucial to an understanding of the occupational structure. It is not enough to know that the men in a certain occupational group experience much mobility, but we also want to know whether this involves primarily upward mobility or downward mobility or both. The foregoing discussion that showed that much gross mobility can be associated with little net mobility, owing to compensating movements, directs attention to the importance of taking the direction of movements into account. As a convenient starting point for the study of the direction of movements among occupational groupings, Tables 2.5, 2.6, and 2.7 will be re-examined here, centering attention more explicitly and systematically than before on the ranking of occupational groupings and the direction of mobility among them.

A distinctive pattern is revealed by the data on intergenerational movements among occupations in Table 2.5. Assume that two coordinates are drawn in the major diagonal. There are 16 such pairs of coordinates that can be drawn. Whereas 14 of these reveal some underlined values, indicating excessive downward mobility, in the upper-right field, two of them have no such values indicative of downward mobility in excess of expectation across the boundary. They are the division between retail sales and crafts in manufacturing and that between labor outside manufacturing and farm. Although these two reveal some underlined values in the lower-left field—that is, some cases of disproportionate upward mobility across the boundary—there are no coordinates at all for which this would not be the case.

In short, two distinctive boundaries limiting downward mobility are in evidence, one between blue-collar and white-collar occupations, the other between blue-collar and farm groups. The application of the same procedure to Table 2.6, flow of manpower from occupational origins to first occupations, does not yield similarly clear results, which reflects the tendency of white-collar sons to start their careers on levels below their origins and move up later. However, the two boundaries are again in evidence for intragenerational mobility (Table 2.7), although in this case three additional dividing lines would also satisfy the boundary criterion of no disproportionate downward movements.

The American occupational structure appears to be partitioned by two semipermeable class boundaries that limit downward mobility between generations as well as within lifetime careers, though they permit upward mobility. To be sure, many *individuals* experience downward mobility across these boundaries. Ours is not a caste system in which birth secures permanent status. Thus more than one-quarter of the sons of white-collar workers are in manual or farm occupations, yet this is disproportionately few, for more than three-fifths of the entire labor force are in these occupations. The concern of the present analysis, moreover, is not the success or failure of individuals but the flow of manpower among occupational groups, specifically, the excess of this flow over what would be expected under conditions of independence. There is virtually no such excess flow between any two occupations downward across either boundary, whether we examine movements from one generation to the next or those within lifetime careers. As far as the exchange of manpower among occupations is concerned, therefore, it seems warranted to speak of the two boundaries as one-way screens that permit a proportionate flow only in the upward and not in the downward direction.

The manifest pattern is that two class boundaries restrict downward mobility between occupational groupings, but do not restrict upward mobility, at least not between adjacent classes. Upward mobility between all farm groupings and all white-collar groupings is disproportionately low (see Tables 2.5 and 2.7). The underlying forces producing this pattern, however, are more complicated than simply barriers to downward mobility.

To understand these forces, historical developments in the period to which the data refer must be taken into consideration. The data pertain to men 25 to 64 years old in March 1962. Occupational origins are defined by father's occupation at the time the respondent was 16 years old. Father's occupation, therefore, covers the period between 1913 and 1952, and the period covered by first job is probably slightly longer, particularly because it ends later. These years cover the final phase of the transition from an agricultural to an industrial economy in this country. In 1910, 11,300,000 persons were gainfully employed in agriculture in the United States, which is the peak of agricultural employment in absolute numbers over the entire period for which we have reliable estimates (1820 to the present). Since 1910 there has been a steady decline in agricultural employment, which has become greatly accelerated since World War II. As the demand for farm workers declined the natural increase of the farm population further and further outstripped replacement needs. Hence movements away from farms greatly exceeded movements to farms.

Demographic and economic conditions resulting from high fertility and rising labor productivity on farms during the preceding half century have produced what is, in effect, a barrier to mobility into farm occupations. There is simply a shortage of farm work, and men originating elsewhere are at a competitive disadvantage for obtaining these farm positions in short supply. More than one in four members of the labor force in 1962 originated on a farm, but only one in 12 was engaged in farm work himself. Men reared off the farm are not so well qualified for farm work as those reared on the farm and, consequently, are disadvantaged in the competition for positions on farms. Most of them, however, probably never experience this handicap, because they have little interest in engaging in such competition. The ideology of an expanding industrial society does not furnish strong incentives for urban workers to move to farms.[19] Furthermore, the expansion of the industrial economy made industrial jobs much more abundant than farm jobs.

These social conditions have created a boundary between the industrial and the agricultural sectors of the labor force, which is manifest in the finding that both intergenerational and intragenerational movements from any nonfarm occupation to either of the two farm groups fall short of what would be expected under conditions of statistical independence. Such a consistent pattern of disproportionately low movements between occupational groups is all that is meant by a class boundary here.

A schematic table may facilitate the analysis of the dynamics of occupational mobility among the three classes. In the table below, men are divided by present occupation and by social origins into three

| | | Son's Occ. | |
Father's Occ.	*W*	*B*	*F*	*T*
White-collar	1	2	3	*a*
Blue-collar	4	5	6	*b*
Farm	7	8	9	*c*
Total	*d*	*e*	*f*	*N*

[19] Although most of the automobile workers interviewed by Eli Chinoy wished to get out of the factory, for instance, only one-tenth of them expressed interest in farming, and even for most of these the idea to become a farmer seemed to be merely an unrealistic fantasy; *Automobile Workers and the American Dream*, Garden City: Doubleday, 1955, pp. 82-93.

categories—nonmanual, manual, and farm occupations—yielding a ninefold cross-classification. The marginals of this table are assumed to be fixed, respectively, by the existing occupational distribution and by fertility—specifically, the origins of sons.

The table has four degrees of freedom. It has just been indicated that the values in cells 3 and 6 should be very low, as they are observed to be in the data. The values in these cells can be fixed at an arbitrary low figure or might be assumed to be zero and tolerance of departures from zero might be specified, such as a tolerance of .5.[20] In either case, given these two values, that of cell 9 is determinate by subtraction. Two of the four degrees of freedom have thus been accounted for.

The pressures of a declining demand for farm workers and high fertility in these occupations compel many sons of farmers to leave the farm. Having to leave the place for which their skills best equip them —the farm—where do they go? Some manual work requires few skills; other manual work, such as construction, requires skills also used on the farm. The skills required for white-collar work, in contrast, tend to be far removed from those acquired on a farm.[21] Men reared in an urban environment, even those originating in the working class, have had more opportunities than farm youths for contact with white-collar occupations. Moreover, urban school systems offer training explicitly designed for nonmanual occupations, training less likely to be available in rural schools. Hence farmers and their sons are at a disadvantage in the competition for white-collar jobs. This implies that migrants from the farm will not move into cell 7 but into cell 8.

This prediction, however, is not strongly confirmed by the data.[22] To be sure, the indices of association for movements from farm origins to white-collar destinations are lower than those to blue-collar destination, and the ratio of white-collar to blue-collar destinations is less for men with farm origins (.42) than for men with blue-collar origins (.60). But the international data assembled by Lipset and Bendix show that, in all six countries investigated, the ratio of white-collar to blue-collar destinations is *greater* for men with farm than for those with blue-

[20] With this model, applying the .5 criteria, there is one negative case among 30 in the intergenerational table and two exceptions in the intragenerational table, which is a very good fit.

[21] Although lower white-collar occupations require few specialized skills—fewer than many industrial and farm jobs—the generalized skills in dealing with people they require are peculiarly urban, thus disadvantaging men with farm backgrounds.

[22] Applying the criterion that all indices of association in cell 7 should be no more than .5, of the 14 cases, there are six exceptions in Table 2.5, intergenerational mobility, and four exceptions in Table 2.7, intragenerational mobility. This is not a good fit.

collar origins,[23] which contradicts the assumption that men reared on a farm are at a competitive disadvantage compared to those reared in working-class homes in respect to white-collar careers. In other countries, in short, nonfarm men with farm origins are more likely than nonfarm men with blue-collar origins to go into white-collar occupations, whereas the reverse is true in the United States, possibly as a product of both the unusually rapid contraction of employment opportunities on farms in the United States and the disproportionate number of highly disadvantaged Negroes among Americans moving off farms.[24] In any case, the original assumption concerning migrants off the farm should be modified to state that their likelihood to become white-collar workers is fairly low but *not* as close to zero as is the likelihood of mobility from urban origins to farm occupations. Besides, the argument may be applicable only to the United States.

To summarize briefly, the oversupply of men reared on farms, their superior experience with and orientation towards farming, and their competitive disadvantage for white-collar work, even if it is not much greater than that of men from blue-collar homes, together explain much of the pattern of mobility observed. A boundary restricting mobility from the two other classes into farm occupations accounts for two of the four degrees of freedom in the table. An upward push on farmers' sons, coupled with a bridle on their movements into non-manual occupations, accounts for a third degree of freedom. One degree of freedom and four cells in the table—cells 1, 2, 4, and 5— remain unexplained. What accounts for the pattern of preponderant movements between white-collar and blue-collar occupations? Four alternative explanations are possible, depending on which of the four frequencies are theoretically derived, rendering the other three determinate. The interpretation here will focus on the relative values in cells 1 and 2.

White-collar occupations in general enjoy high prestige, inasmuch as many of these occupations require the rarest skills, command the highest salaries, and exercise most authority. However, the prestige claimed by many white-collar occupations produces a halo effect that reflects onto those nonmanual jobs that require little skill and command less income than many blue-collar occupations. Particularly

[23] Seymour M. Lipset and Reinhard Bendix, *Social Mobility in Industrial Society,* Berkeley: Univer. of California Press, 1960, pp. 19-21.

[24] As far as the earlier data presented by Lipset and Bendix show, the United States does not differ from the other countries in this respect, but, according to the more reliable OCG data, the United States does differ. For some systematic comparison of the OCG findings and those of the earlier United States surveys, see the following chapter.

men reared and socialized in the white-collar class tend to place much significance on nonmanual work and often prefer it to better-paid jobs involving manual labor. White-collar occupations as a whole also have been expanding much more rapidly than blue-collar occupations, increasing their proportion of the total employed labor force 23.5 per cent between 1940 and 1960, whereas blue-collar occupations increased only 8.6 per cent. At the same time, white-collar fertility has remained below that of blue-collar workers. In addition, many blue-collar positions are occupied by men who had moved off the farm. Men originating in white-collar strata have little interest in moving into manual occupations, and there is less need for them in the manual than in the nonmanual class.

These conditions discourage downward mobility from white-collar to blue-collar strata, but of particular importance in this respect is the large spread in status among white-collar occupations and the overlap between them and blue-collar occupations. Some white-collar occupations require much less skill and command considerably less income than many blue-collar occupations. This makes it possible for men with inferior abilities who want to remain in the white-collar class to do so. Men raised in white-collar homes are often strongly identified with the symbols of white-collar status. The unsuccessful ones among them are, therefore, willing to pay a price for being permitted to maintain white-collar status. The existence of relatively unskilled white-collar occupations, such as retail sales and clerical jobs, makes it possible for the unsuccessful sons of white-collar workers to remain in the white-collar class by paying the price of accepting a lower income than they might have been able to obtain in a manual occupation. The unskilled white-collar occupations tend to absorb most of the downwardly mobile from the higher nonmanual strata, which makes these occupations a boundary that creates relative protection against the danger of downward mobility from the white-collar to the blue-collar class.

The argument advanced is that the boundary between nonmanual and manual occupations would make the value in cell 2 particularly low.[25] Given this assumption that disproportionately few men move from nonmanual to manual occupations, and the previous assumption that most men originating in farming who cannot stay there move to manual occupations, it follows that the remaining manual occupations must be filled by sons of manual workers. That is, knowl-

---

[25] Applying the same criterion previously used, there are 20 exceptions in 56 cases in the intergenerational matrix (Table 2.5) and 13 exceptions in the intragenerational matrix (Table 2.7). The fit is fairly good.

edge of cells 2 and 8 makes cell 5 determinate. All remaining men with manual origins must move up to nonmanual occupations, cell 4. These considerations also determine the frequency in cell 1. All men originating in the white-collar class, except the low proportion permitted by the model to move down, remain in white-collar occupations.

In short, the theoretical interpretation predicts low values in cells 3, 6, 7, and 2. The rest of the pattern of movement can be inferred from these theoretical premises. A theory that would provide a basis for predicting the actual values in these four cells would furnish a complete explanation for the entire pattern of movement among the cells. Such a quantitative model does not presently exist.

These class boundaries do not reveal, however, whether the movements out of and into the various occupational groupings are predominantly upward or downward, which is the question raised at the beginning of this section. To answer this question, we consider only movements between a given occupational group and any higher one, that is, the outflow of men from given origins into any higher destinations, and the inflow of men into given destinations from any higher origins. The observed number of men in each of these categories is divided by the number expected on the assumption of independence when the cells for nonmobile men and lateral movements are blocked. The index obtained, which refers to the excess over expectations in the outflow to higher or the inflow from higher strata, is presented in Table 2.12. The outflow involves upward and the inflow downward mobility, because movements between given occupations and all those above it are considered in either case. The values for outflow into lower and inflow from lower strata are inverse functions of those shown and hence do not furnish any additional information, because the exclusion of the diagonal makes the dichotomous standardized values pertaining to movements in opposite direction complementary.

The first pattern noticeable in Table 2.12 is that the values for both the outflow into and the inflow from higher strata, in all three types of movements, decrease as we go down the status rank order of occupations. The higher the status of an occupational group, the more the flow of manpower between it and higher strata in both directions exceeds the volume expected on the assumption of independence. This finding reflects the preponderance of short-distance over long-distance movements. The higher the rank of an occupation, the shorter is the average distance between it and all higher strata, and the pattern in the table simply indicates that movements entailing such shorter distances occur with disproportionate frequency. To be sure, there are some noteworthy exceptions to the pattern. Thus men

TABLE 2.12. SUPPLY TO AND RECRUITMENT FROM HIGHER RANKING OCCUPATIONAL CATEGORIES, FOR MALES 25 TO 64 YEARS OLD: RATIO OF OBSERVED FREQUENCY TO FREQUENCY EXPECTED ON THE MODEL OF QUASI-INDEPENDENCE

	Supply to Above			Recruitment from Above		
	1	2	3	4	5	6
Occ.	Father's Occ. to 1962 Occ.	Father's Occ. to First Job	First Job to 1962 Occ.	Father's Occ. to 1962 Occ.	Father's Occ. to First Job	First Job to 1962 Occ.
Professionals Self-Empl.	...	...	...	...	...	...
Salaried	3.01	2.42	10.62	3.40	4.08	7.22
Managers	2.44	2.39	3.35	1.77	3.01	2.64
Salesmen, Other	2.27	2.59	2.38	2.31	2.60	1.80
Proprietors	1.87	2.32	2.17	1.12	2.16	1.48
Clerical	1.59	2.22	1.73	1.09	1.42	1.47
Salesmen, Retail	1.44	1.70	1.66	1.49	1.59	1.19
Craftsmen Mfg.	1.11	1.03	1.20	.64	1.08	.55
Other	1.10	1.08	1.22	.75	1.16	.60
Construction	1.07	1.05	1.20	.73	.98	.59
Operatives Mfg.	.98	1.05	1.04	.73	1.06	.64
Other	.99	1.15	1.03	.73	1.01	.65
Service	1.02	1.13	1.02	.86	1.10	.87
Laborers Mfg.	1.00	1.08	1.03	.83	1.04	.88
Other	1.01	1.11	1.03	.69	.98	.81
Farmers	.97	.67	.92	.83	.91	.37
Farm Laborers	1.00	1.00	1.00	1.00	1.00	1.00

originating in the lower manual strata experience somewhat more upward mobility than those originating in the strata above them (columns 1 and 2). The inflow of men from higher origins into sales occupations in 1962 is exceptionally high, indicative of much downward mobility (column 4). Of special interest is the complete reversal of the pattern in the inflow from higher strata into the various blue-collar occupations, whether inflow from social origins (column 4) or from career beginnings (column 6) is considered. Within the blue-collar class, and only there, the standardized rate of downward mobility into an occupation is inversely related to its rank. This means that another force must counteract the preponderance of short-distance movements, which has the opposite effect and produces a direct relationship.

That other force is apparently the restrictive influence of the boundary between the white-collar and the blue-collar class on downward mobility. This class boundary produces a sharp break in the rates of downward mobility into the various occupations, with those into white-collar occupations exceeding and those into blue-collar occupations falling short of the expected values (columns 4 and 6). As there is proportionately little downward mobility across the class boundary, the inflow from above into the higher blue-collar strata is depressed, effecting a reversal within the blue-collar class of the otherwise observable positive relationship between such inflow and rank.

The standardized rates of outflow to higher occupations and inflow from them are highly correlated. The product moment correlation is .93 for movements from father's to 1962 occupation (columns 1 and 4), .85 for those from father's to first occupation (columns 2 and 5), and .99 for intragenerational movements from first to 1962 occupation (columns 3 and 6). These positive relationships are merely another reflection of the predominance of short-distance movements, which produces excessive values for all kinds of movements between more highly ranked occupations and the relatively few others above them.

A surprising feature of the outflow values is that the large majority of them reveals an excess of upward mobility. Most of these values are greater than 1.0, the only exceptions being those for farm origins and, in the case of outflow from father's to 1962 occupation, also those for the two groups of operatives (column 1). The outflow of manpower from various origins is predominantly in the upward direction. What is the source of all this upward mobility? It may well be the change in the relative size of different occupational groups, which technological developments have produced in recent decades.

Technological advances have reduced the need for manpower to till the soil and perform menial labor, increasing the human resources available to furnish professional services and manage complex organizations. The two occupational groupings that expanded most between 1940 and 1960 are salaried professionals and managers, and the three that contracted most in proportionate size are farm laborers, farmers, and laborers in manufacturing. The fact that the contracting occupations are near the bottom of the hierarchy and have high fertility, whereas the expanding ones are near the top and have low fertility, creates an upward push in the flow of manpower. But we have seen that short-distance movements prevail over long-distance ones. Few of the displaced farm workers or laborers fill the growing number of professional and managerial positions. What seems to happen is rather that the pressure of displaced manpower at the bottom and the vacuum created by new opportunities at the top start a chain reaction of short-distance movements throughout the occupational structure.[26] This push of supply at the bottom and pull of demand at the top create opportunities for upward mobility from most origins, as the vacancies left by sons moving up can be filled by sons from lower strata. But

[26] See on this point also the discussion of migration from rural areas to large cities in Chapter 7.

men who start their working lives in blue-collar jobs are least likely to benefit from these opportunities, as previously indicated.

DIMENSIONS OF SOCIAL DISTANCE

The systematic study of the direction of social mobility poses serious problems. Simple measures do not convey significant information. It is hardly a revelation to ascertain that the proportion upwardly mobile is greater for sons of farm laborers than for sons of salaried professionals, since the former have so many more places they can move up to. More complex measures, like the one used in the last few pages, cannot easily be conceptualized and may therefore result in misleading conclusions. Besides, the impact of ceiling effects limits their usefulness. These problems are the major reason why the analysis in this chapter has largely relied on measures that are independent of direction, making inferences about direction by relating these measures to the rank order of occupations. Another approach of this kind is designed to indicate the social distances between occupational groups and the dimensions underlying it.

Let us examine again the intergenerational movements from father's to 1962 occupation in Table 2.2. For any pair of origins the percentage distributions of destinations differ to a greater or lesser degree. If the two distributions in any two rows of Table 2.2 were identical it would indicate a minimum of dissimilarity or social distance with respect to destinations between the two origin groups. At the opposite extreme, if there were no overlap between the two distributions the two origins would have a maximum distance from one another with respect to their destinations. The empirical cases fall between these two extremes of 0 and 100 per cent distance in regard to destinations. The index of dissimilarity previously encountered (the sum of the positive percentage differences) can represent this distance between origins with respect to destinations, or the distance between destinations with respect to origins. For example, the index of dissimilarity between rows 8 and 9 in Table 2.2 is 15.3, whereas that between rows 4 and 15 is no less than 55.5. There is little social distance, in terms of 1962 occupations, between sons of craftsmen in manufacturing and in "other" industries, but there is much social distance between sons of salesmen outside the retail field and laborers outside manufacturing. The index of dissimilarity between any two social origins in regard to 1962 occupations and between any two 1962 occupations in regard to social origins is presented in Table 2.13.

It should be noted that the calculation of the social distance between occupational groups by the procedure outlined does not in any

TABLE 2.13. INDEX OF DISSIMILARITY FOR MALES 25 TO 64 YEARS OLD. ABOVE DIAGONAL: BETWEEN FATHER'S OCC. GROUPS WITH RESPECT TO 1962 OCC.; BELOW DIAGONAL: BETWEEN 1962 OCC. GROUPS WITH RESPECT TO FATHER'S OCC.

Occupation	1	2	3	4	5	6	7	8	9	10	11	12	13	14	15	16	17
Professionals																	
1 Self-Empl.	...	22.8	30.3	31.8	38.7	28.8	37.4	44.9	45.7	54.5	53.6	51.0	51.3	60.4	61.3	60.5	66.0
2 Salaried	24.7	...	17.6	26.9	25.3	14.2	24.9	29.8	29.7	38.8	39.3	36.8	35.0	49.4	45.9	49.6	55.9
3 Managers	18.8	17.2	...	15.3	16.6	14.9	23.4	30.6	30.0	37.3	40.8	37.2	36.2	51.9	48.5	49.7	58.2
4 Salesmen, Other	22.3	15.1	13.6	....	16.0	26.5	23.0	36.5	37.2	44.5	46.5	43.0	43.0	56.5	55.5	54.5	63.0
5 Proprietors	32.8	27.0	17.7	25.3	...	26.0	16.5	29.7	28.9	36.1	38.8	34.6	34.8	50.0	47.1	47.0	55.4
6 Clerical	38.7	23.2	21.9	24.3	18.2	...	22.9	24.0	22.5	30.6	31.8	28.6	26.6	42.5	37.3	43.2	48.6
7 Salesmen, Retail	31.2	24.3	15.8	21.1	12.9	14.9	...	22.0	21.1	28.9	30.0	26.0	26.0	40.1	38.5	37.5	45.9
Craftsmen																	
8 Mfg.	50.5	33.3	34.1	37.3	24.4	17.2	22.6	...	15.3	20.5	15.3	17.0	16.5	28.5	27.8	31.0	37.6
9 Other	47.0	32.5	31.7	34.3	17.4	14.4	21.9	16.7	...	17.8	20.2	11.6	14.2	30.4	23.1	28.9	35.9
10 Construction	51.4	40.0	37.7	41.0	21.7	22.7	27.4	22.7	17.1	...	20.3	19.6	18.5	29.4	23.9	29.1	36.6
Operatives																	
11 Mfg.	52.8	38.3	38.6	41.3	24.3	21.9	24.7	14.5	16.4	18.0	...	16.8	15.6	14.6	21.0	28.3	30.8
12 Other	52.4	38.1	37.5	38.6	23.7	20.5	26.2	20.7	12.4	15.4	12.2	...	14.4	24.5	16.4	22.5	26.6
13 Service	50.5	36.4	36.0	38.3	21.4	16.4	23.8	17.9	12.2	18.9	11.3	12.0	...	21.2	15.3	25.9	28.4
Laborers																	
14 Mfg.	57.0	47.3	47.5	48.6	32.1	29.6	32.5	22.6	23.8	21.6	10.4	16.0	17.8	...	19.0	28.5	24.4
15 Other	57.1	46.7	46.3	48.1	29.5	29.7	35.1	28.1	23.3	19.5	19.2	15.8	18.5	18.3	...	24.4	16.2
16 Farmers	76.2	76.0	72.6	77.1	60.0	66.3	66.2	63.8	58.4	52.0	55.6	52.8	58.1	53.3	46.7	...	20.4
17 Farm Laborers	72.9	69.4	66.4	70.0	53.4	58.9	58.8	56.5	51.1	44.2	47.4	44.4	49.6	44.0	35.6	22.2	...

way depend on external information about the relative status of the various occupational groups, since the index of dissimilarity is not affected by the rank order in which the categories are presented. The index does depend, however, on the classification scheme, and a different set of categories would yield different index values. Thus, if the 17 occupational categories were collapsed into a smaller number, the values would become smaller, whereas further subdivision would increase these values.

The measure of social distance, inasmuch as it is independent of the rank order of occupations based on average income and education, provides an independent check for validating this rank order. The general pattern is that the magnitude of the values increases with movement away from the diagonal in either direction. The further apart two occupational groups are in income and educational status, the more distance there is generally between them in terms of either origin composition or occupational prospects of sons. Numerous exceptions to this basic pattern can be noted, however. To mention only a few conspicuous ones: the 1962 occupations of the sons of laborers outside manufacturing are not as dissimilar as might be expected from those of the sons of the various white-collar strata and of craftsmen (column 15); the origin composition of craftsmen in manufacturing reveals an unexpectedly great distance from that of all white-collar groups (row 8), whereas the origins of service workers exhibit unexpectedly little distance from that of the white-collar groups (row 13). The occurrence of such exceptions invites systematic analysis to ascertain the factors other than status that influence social distance between occupational groupings.

The "Guttman-Lingoes Smallest Space Analysis I" provides a technique suited for this purpose, although it is still in the experimental stage and not all its properties are fully known.[27] The triangular matrix of distance measures (one half of Table 2.13 at a time) is used as input in a computer program employing this technique, the output of which defines underlying dimensions of distance. In our case two dimensions appeared to be sufficient. The results of the analysis of distances between social origins with respect to 1962 occupations are presented in Figure 2.1. The scale on the two coordinates is arbitrary, provided that their relative values are preserved. The distance on a straight line between any two occupations can be ascertained. These

---

[27] Louis Guttman, "A General Nonmetric Technique for Finding the Smallest Euclidean Space for a Configuration of Points," *Psychometrika* (1966, in press); J. C. Lingoes, "An IBM 7090 Program for Guttman-Lingoes Smallest Space Analysis —I," *Behavioral Science,* **10**(1965), 183-184.

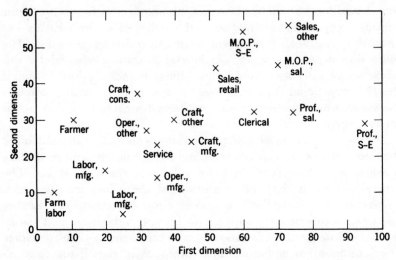

Figure 2.1. Two-dimensional Guttman-Lingoes solution for distances between fathers' occupations with respect to 1962 occupations (outflow).

distances supplied by the model can then be compared with the observed distances, and the relationship between the two indicates the goodness of fit of the model. The measure used to determine the fit of the derived model is called the coefficient of alienation, which approaches zero as the solution improves. Laumann and Guttman accepted as adequate a three-dimensional solution with a coefficient of alienation of .13, after finding that the coefficient for the best two-dimensional space was .26.[28] For our model in Figure 2.1, the coefficient of alienation is .07, an appreciable improvement over the one-dimensional solution with a coefficient of .15. It is highly questionable whether additional dimensions would be meaningful. Rotation is permissible, as the orientation of the axes as well as the scale of distances is arbitrary.

A physical analogy may help the reader not familiar with this type of procedure, which resembles factor analysis. Let us represent the 17 occupations by 17 objects and the differences between them by wires of varying length. Every occupation is tied by a wire of a specified length to each one of the 16 others, so that 136 wires connect the 17 objects. The task the computer program performs is analogous to placing the 17 objects into positions that make all the wires taut. If

28 Edward O. Laumann and Louis Guttman, "The Relative Associational Contiguity of Occupations in an Urban Setting," *American Sociological Review*, **31** (1966), 169-178.

this can be done by stretching the objects along a straight line, a one-dimensional solution is found. If there is too much slack in the wires, spreading them out on a table might make them all taut, which would correspond to a two-dimensional solution. Excessive slack in two dimensions might require distributing the objects in a three-dimensional space to straighten out all the wires, and although the physical analogy breaks down at this point, introducing further dimensions may be necessary to make all wires taut. The coefficient of alienation would indicate the amount of looseness of the wires remaining with a given solution. In our case, two-dimensional solutions seemed to be adequate.

The first dimension in Figure 2.1 evidently represents the socio-economic status of occupations. When occupational origins are classified in terms of the potential mobility of sons into various occupational destinations, the ordering of the similarity among them corresponds closely to their status rank order when status is defined by average income and education. There are only four inversions to a perfectly monotonic relationship between position on the horizontal dimension and socioeconomic status. "Other" salesmen and service workers have unexpectedly high positions on the first dimensions, reflecting high mobility potentials, and proprietors (MOP, S-E) and craftsmen in construction have unexpectedly low ones. We might suspect that these inversions are due to distortions introduced when the status ranking based on information from the present population is applied to the generation of fathers. Perhaps proprietors and construction craftsmen did not occupy so high a status a generation ago as they do today. Since the fathers do not include any very young men, it may well be that fathers classified as other salesmen or as service workers contain disproportionately few men in such low-status jobs as newsboy or bootblack, thus raising the average status of these groups of fathers. If this interpretation in terms of generational differences is correct, the same deviations should not be observable when men are classified by their own occupational status rather than that of their fathers. We shall return to this question. What should be re-emphasized here is that the first dimension reproduces rather accurately the status rank order of occupations, which itself is not entirely unambiguous, as has been noted.[29]

The two class boundaries are clearly manifest in the distances between social origins with respect to their destinations presented in Figure 2.1. It should be noted that interpretation of the diagram is

[29] See also, Robert W. Hodge, "The Status Consistency of Occupational Groups," *American Sociological Review*, 27(1962), 336-343.

not restricted to the two orthogonal dimensions but may include any configurations of positions in the two-dimensional space. A line drawn obliquely to the horizontal axis separates white-collar from blue-collar occupations, with appreciable distance between the two. Another line, at an acute angle from the first one and having the opposite orientation to the horizontal axis, separates blue-collar from farm occupations. There is considerable distance between the destinations of men originating in different occupational classes, revealing variations in mobility potential between origin classes. The class boundaries are not unrelated to the status hierarchy, but neither are they merely direct expressions of it. Rather, they constitute dimensions of social distance that are oblique to the status dimension, a fact that corresponds exactly to the accepted notion that social class is generally associated with socioeconomic status but has additional distinguishing features. Thus the style of life of a class depends on income and education without being exclusively determined by them. The acute angle between the two dividing lines implies that somewhat though not entirely different factors are responsible for the social distance at the two boundaries, which is plausible given the geographical separation of farm workers and the influence of socioeconomic factors in both cases.

The figure reveals self-employed professionals to be an occupational group isolated by considerable social distance from any other. The lowest index of dissimilarity for this origin group with respect to destinations is 22.8 (row 1, Table 2.13), whereas every other occupational origin except farmers has a minimum distance to at least one other occupational origin that is no larger than 20. The separation of self-employed professions from the rest is along the horizontal dimension indicative of socioeconomic status, which corresponds to the great difference in average income between this and any other occupational group (see Table 2.1). The self-employed professionals as a whole constitute a distinct economic elite in our society, whereas the business elite, which is undoubtedly more affluent as well as more powerful, comprises only a small segment of managers and is, therefore, not observable in our data.

The meaning of the second dimension is not easily discernible, but Figure 2.1 provides a few clues for speculating about it. The three origin groups of workers in manufacturing are set apart from the manual groups outside manufacturing along a line roughly parallel to the second dimension, though at a slight angle to it. The other three groups set apart in the same direction from the rest are the two professional categories and clerks. At the opposite extreme along this line are farmers, construction craftsmen, and proprietors, followed by the two groups of salesmen.

A possible interpretation of the distinction between these two extremes is in terms of the principles that govern the organization of work and the acquisition of skills necessary to perform it. On the one hand, work may be organized on the basis of rational principles explicitly formulated; the performance of individuals is expected to conform to these universalistic standards. Such conformance is brought about either by placing individuals into circumscribed roles in complex structures that are organized in accordance with rational principles or by training them to acquire abstract rational standards of performance. The former is the case for workers in large manufacturing concerns and for clerks in bureaucracies, and the latter for professionals. On the other hand, general principles for dealing with the diverse, idiosyncratic problems encountered at work may not have been formulated, and individuals must acquire the so-called intuitive knowledge required for dealing with these problems through apprenticeship and trial and error.[30] This description, we claim, applies fairly well to running a farm or a business in a competitive economy, selling, and the construction industry. The conclusion these speculations suggest is that whether the work of men is organized in terms of universalistic rational principles or rests on particularistic skills acquired through apprenticeship influences the orientations toward work that they transmit to their sons, and hence the social distance between the sons' occupational destinations.

Applying the same procedure to the inflow into own occupation, instead of the outflow from father's occupation, yields the two-dimensional solution for distances between 1962 occupational groups with respect to their social origins presented in Figure 2.2. Although the two figures are based on the same data, the asymmetry between outflow and inflow produces differences between them. (The values on which Figure 2.2 is based are shown in the lower left half of Table 2.13.) The coefficient of alienation for this solution is .08, only a slight improvement over the coefficient of .10 for the one-dimensional solution. The unimportance of the second dimension is indicated by the relatively low degree of dispersion of the various occupations on this dimension.

The first dimension approximates again fairly closely the socio-economic rank order of occupational groups. Indeed, when the same procedure is applied to the outflow and the inflow of movements

---

[30] See on this distinction Eugene Litwak, "Models of Bureaucracy Which Permit Conflict," *American Journal of Sociology*, **67**(1961), 177-184.

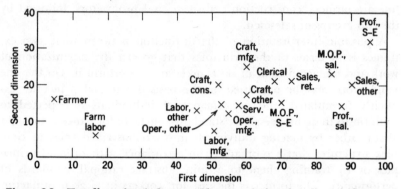

Figure 2.2. Two-dimensional Guttman-Lingoes solution for distance between 1962 occupations with respect to fathers' occupations (inflow).

from father's to first and those from first to 1962 occupation, the first dimension in all four cases, as well as in the original two, represents the status hierarchy.[31] Evidently socioeconomic status is a fundamental dimension of the social distance between occupational groups. The groups whose position on the first dimension in Figure 2.2 deviates from their status rank are largely the ones that also occupy deviant positions in Figure 2.1. The position of "other" salesmen and service workers is once more too high, and that of proprietors and craftsmen in construction is once more too low. The finding that the pattern of deviations in this analysis of 1962 occupations parallels that of the analysis of father's occupations discredits the interpretation of these deviations in terms of generational differences. A possible alternative interpretation is that nonretail salesmen and service workers have more social contact with and more resemblance to higher strata than their income and education would lead us to expect, whereas construction craftsmen with their strong unions, and proprietors, many of whom are former manual workers, have higher incomes than most men in their social circles, and these departures of social associations from economic levels are reflected on the distance dimension. Whether or not this interpretation of the few exceptions is correct, it is clear that the degree of dissimilarity in social origins between occupations corresponds quite closely to the status differences between them, just as the dissimilarity in destinations between origin groups does.

The class boundaries are manifest in Figure 2.2, but in a form that

[31] These four solutions—outflow and inflow from father's to first and from first to 1962 occupation—are not presented, since they reveal little beyond the fact that the location of occupations along the first dimension, though not along the second, is similar in all cases.

differs from that in Figure 2.1. First, they are much less oblique to the first dimension, thus representing essentially differences in hierarchical status. Second, the distance separating white-collar from blue-collar occupations has narrowed, whereas that separating blue-collar from farm occupations has widened. The dissimilarity in social composition between white-collar and blue-collar strata today is hardly greater than that between strata differing in status within each class, but the origin composition of farm workers is very dissimilar to that of any other occupational group. As before, self-employed professionals occupy an isolated position at the high end of the scale, being considerably dissimilar in composition from the next-highest occupational groups. In sum, most of the differences in background composition between 1962 occupations are along the status continuum, with the self-employed professionals and the two farm groups located at opposite extremes and separated by appreciable distances from the 14 intermediate groups.

The second dimension in Figure 2.2 not only discriminates little between occupations but also fails to reproduce the pattern of relative positions observed on the second dimension in Figure 2.1. A scatter plot of the 17 values on the two first dimensions reveals a strong positive relationship, whereas one of the values on the second dimensions reveals scarcely any relationship. Moreover, no common properties of the occupations similarly located along the second dimension in Figure 2.2 are readily discernible. These characteristics of the second dimension make it doubtful that it reveals significant forces affecting occupational mobility.[32] Whether this tentative conclusion that the second dimension in Figure 2.2 has little substantive significance invalidates the interpretation of the second dimension in Figure 2.1 advanced earlier is an open question. On the one hand, confidence in the interpretation is weakened by the fact that the results it implies are not replicated by the inflow values. On the other hand, the considerable differences in outflow values along the second dimension call for some explanation, even if it has to remain speculative, and it is not impossible, given the asymmetry between outflow and inflow, that similar work experiences of fathers induce sons to move into similar occupations without being reflected in the total origin compositions of the various occupations.

32 It is of interest in this connection that Laumann and Guttman (*op. cit.*, p. 177) were similarly unable to offer convincing interpretations of the second and third dimensions for the solution for Laumann's data on associational contiguity of occupations, while the first dimension clearly approximated prestige rather closely. Their only tentative interpretation of another dimension conforms to ours of the second dimension in Figure 2.1.

CONCLUSIONS

The focus of this chapter has been on the relations among occupational groups in the American occupational structure as defined by the flow of manpower among these groups. The analysis has centered on various aspects of two major relational characteristics of occupational groupings, the outflow of manpower from one supplying others, and the inflow of manpower into one recruited from others. This emphasis on occupational groups as units of analysis and the structure of relations among them is distinct from the concern of much of the rest of the book with the socioeconomic status of individuals and the factors influencing occupational achievement. The occupational structure viewed in over-all perspective here provides the framework for the processes of mobility to be examined in greater detail later.

The analysis of intergenerational movements reveals that the volume of supply and of recruitment are directly related. At one extreme are self-contained occupations, which neither supply to other career lines in the next generation nor recruit from others in the last a proportionate share of men. These are the three occupations resting on self-employment: independent professionals, proprietors, and farmers. At the other extreme are five occupations that serve as distributors of manpower, which supply disproportionate numbers of men to other occupations in the next generation and recruit disproportionate numbers from the last. These are the five occupations located just above the two class boundaries: the two lowest white-collar and the three lowest manual groups.

To study the degree of dispersion in the flow of manpower, a crude and a refined measure were used, since the refined measure turned out not simply to be an improvement on the crude one but to reflect a different aspect of dispersion. The crude measure is indicative of the width of the recruitment base of an occupation, *from how many* different origins it recruits a disproportionately large share of manpower, or the width of the supply sector of an origin, *to how many* different destinations it supplies a disproportionately large share of manpower. The refined measure, on the other hand, refers to the degree of variation in the origins from which the men in an occupation are recruited or the degree of variation in the destinations to which sons are supplied from an origin. Using the crude measure, the dispersion of recruitment and supply are inversely related for intergenerational mobility. Occupations that recruit from a wide base in the last generation supply only to a narrow sector in the next, and those recruiting from narrower bases supply more broadly. This has been interpreted as an indirect result of changes in demand for occupational services that are reflected in the expansion or contraction of occupational groupings. For increasing demand to effect an occupation's expansion requires recruitment of outsiders, which in turn depends on economic conditions that attract men from diverse origins. Indeed, effective demand is positively associated with the recruitment of members from a wide variety of origins. Superior employment conditions, however, are not only attractive to outsiders but also to the occupational group's own sons, reducing their tendency to leave it for a variety of other occupations. The superior economic conditions in expanding occupations broaden their appeal, thus encouraging disproportionate numbers from other origins to move into these occupations and disproportionately few of their own sons to disperse to various others.

In contrast to this inverse relationship between the width of the recruitment base and of the supply sector of an occupation, the degree of variation in recruitment and in supply, as indicated by the refined measure, are directly related. This positive relationship is a result of the fact that both dispersion in recruitment and dispersion in supply reveal a nonmonotonic relationship with the status rank order of occupations. The highest white-collar strata and the lowest strata of unskilled workers and farm workers are less varied in social origin than the intermediate occupational groups, and men from the highest and lowest origins also move into less varied destinations than those originating in the intermediate ranks of occupations. This result is partly an indirect manifestation of the prevalence of short-distance movements. If most men tend to move relatively short distances, those in the highest and lowest positions of the status hierarchy are less likely to come from or move into as many different occupations than those in intermediate positions, because part of the range from which or into which the former would be likely to move just does not exist. But the greater dispersion of the intermediate, blue-collar levels also has another implication.

There is a large amount of upward mobility in the American occupational structure. Upward movements far exceed downward movements, whether raw numbers, percentages, or departures from standardized expectations are considered. An important source of this extensive upward mobility is the fact that some of the occupational groups near the top of the hierarchy have expanded most rapidly, whereas some of those near the bottom have contracted most in relative size during recent decades. Because few sons of men at the bottom move all the way to the top, the oversupply of men at the bottom and the demand for manpower at the top have repercussions throughout the occupational structures, with the upward movements of sons from one stratum opening up opportunities for upward movements to the sons of the strata below. Sons from all occupational origins participate in this predominant upward movement. Men who enter the labor force on blue-collar levels, however, benefit least from the prevailing intergenerational upward mobility, whereas the highest white-collar strata as well as farm workers benefit most from it. Although blue-collar entrants are as likely to experience *some* mobility as other men, the finding that there is more dispersion in their movements implies that many of these moves are likely to be in opposite directions. As a result, the movements of men starting careers on blue-collar levels effect little change in their ultimate occupational distributions compared to those of their fathers, whereas the movements of men starting on higher white-collar and farm levels achieve considerable improvements in their positions over those of their fathers. The men who most benefit from the expansion of the highest white-collar strata are those who move into them from other social origins, and the men who most benefit from the contraction of the farm strata are those who start to work there and then move out. Men who start their working lives in manual jobs suffer most relative deprivation in the expanding economy, notwithstanding their rising wage rates.

Cross-generational occupational solidarity encourages the men who have entered careers in a certain line of work to remain in it. If disproportionate numbers of the men who start to work in an occupational group have roots in it that solidify social integration, there is little tendency to leave it later, during the course of a career, for diverse other occupations. Two findings support this hypothesis. The degree of occupational inheritance of entry occupations is highly associated with the degree of career stability from first entry to 1962. Besides, the greater the proportion of men entering the labor force in their fathers' occupational group, the lower is the degree of dispersion from this entry occupation to others subsequently (using the crude measure).

The patterns of mobility reveal the existence of two class boundaries, which divide the American occupational structure into three classes—white-collar, blue-collar, and farm. Each boundary limits both intergenerational and intragenerational downward mobility between any two occupations on either side of it to levels below theoretical expectation but permits upward mobility in excess of chance. No other possible division among occupations sets such clear-cut limits on downward movements between occupational groupings. Different procedures confirm the conclusion that the two class boundaries restrict downward mobility. The lowest occupations in each class serve as distinctive entry occupations, from which disproportionate numbers move but into which relatively few men move later in life. In brief, the conventional division of the structure into middle class, working class, and agricultural class is reflected in the flow of manpower between occupations.

The underlying dynamics producing these class boundaries may well have its source in the decline of farm workers in the last half-century, which, together with the high fertility of farmers, has resulted in an oversupply of farmers' sons. These men are better qualified for and more interested in the relatively few available farm jobs than are sons of either blue-collar or white-collar workers. Therefore, there is little mobility either from nonmanual or from manual origins to farm occupations, and most farm jobs are occupied by sons of farmers.[33] The excess farmers' sons must move off the land. Because they are less qualified for white-collar jobs than men reared in cities, most of them cannot compete effectively for white-collar positions, and thus move into manual work. These conditions account for three of the four degrees of freedom in the 3×3 mobility table and explain the data in 5 of the 9 cells, leaving 4 cells and one degree of freedom to be explained.

Sons of white-collar workers seem to be disinclined by their upbringing to move into manual work and prefer to remain in the white-collar class, even at the cost of a lower income than they might obtain elsewhere. Men of blue-collar background are presumably not so willing to sacrifice economic advantages for white-collar status, or possibly are less able to do so. The existence of nonmanual jobs requiring little skill and commanding meager salaries, like sales clerk or file clerk, provides failures from higher white-collar origins with opportunities to remain in their parental class, with its status symbols that are so meaningful to them. Hence there are relatively few movements from white-collar origins to blue-collar destinations. This assumption, which the data fairly well support, uses up the last degree of freedom in the mobility table, and the rest can be mathematically deduced. Most sons of white-collar origins remain in white-collar occupational groupings, since few move downward. Sons of blue-collar workers fill the blue-collar positions not filled by sons of farmers, allowing—indeed, requiring—the remaining number raised in blue-

---

[33] Less than 3 per cent of men with other origins worked on farms in 1962.

collar homes to move up into the expanding white-collar class. These dynamic forces find expression in an occupational structure divided by two class boundaries.

When the social distances between occupational origins with respect to their destinations, or between occupational destinations with respect to their origins, are calculated, the major underlying dimension is socioeconomic status. The location of occupations along this dimension closely approximates their rank order based on average income and education, with self-employed professionals and the two farm groups, respectively, occupying somewhat isolated positions at opposite extremes. Since the calculation of distance does not depend on the rank order, the finding confirms the validity of this ordering. The exceptions suggest that salesmen outside the retail field and service workers are closer to higher strata and that proprietors and construction craftsmen are closer to lower strata than their economic-educational level indicates. The class boundaries are in evidence on the distance charts, being somewhat oblique to the status dimension, which accords with the accepted assumption that social class is not synonymous with broad differences in socioeconomic status though clearly related to them. Although the second dimension does not reveal a consistent pattern for all data, that for the outflow data has stimulated us to speculate that whether the work of men is organized in terms of rational universalistic principles or not may influence the orientation they transmit to their sons and consequent similarities in the sons' occupational destinations.

CHAPTER 3

The Occupational Structure: II
Historical Trends

It is a commonplace observation that the redistribution of the working force over categories of industry or occupation, occurring in the course of economic development, instigates both intergenerational and intragenerational mobility. Yet it turns out to be very difficult indeed to say just how this happens. The source of the difficulty is that the "generation" concept as applied in mobility studies is not commensurate with the "cohort" concept, which is central to the analysis of change in occupational structure.

The case for the cohort approach has been well stated by Jaffe and Carleton:[1]

Each age cohort has its own historical pattern of occupational change which will influence its 1960 occupational distribution. The occupational composition of men aged 55 to 59 years in 1960, for example, will be different from that of men aged 45 to 49 in 1960, not only because of the differences in age, but also because the two cohorts have had different occupational histories. These differences in occupational history can be traced back to the period in which they first entered the working force. Men aged 55 to 59 years in 1960 for the most part entered the working force in the period around World War I. The cohort ten years younger in 1960 entered the working force during the boom of the later 1920s and the early part of the depression of the 1930s. Having entered at different periods, they were confronted by varying types of job opportunities and thus entered various occupations. Once having entered

[1] A. J. Jaffe and R. O. Carleton, *Occupational Mobility in the United States: 1930-1960*, New York: King's Crown Press, 1954, p. 3. See also, Norman B. Ryder, "The Cohort as a Concept in the Study of Social Change," *American Sociological Review*, 30(1965), 843-861.

the working force, their subsequent careers were variously affected by prosperity and depression, by peace and war. Each of these influences affected their occupational distribution and added to the history which helped mold their subsequent occupational experiences.

The importance of this viewpoint in studying the transformation of occupation structures over time is suggested by the observation that entries into the working force during a given period typically are concentrated in a few young cohorts, while exits (resulting from death and retirement, in particular) are concentrated among older cohorts. As each cohort ages, it replaces (in a sense) the immediately preceding cohort, while itself undergoing mobility in terms of occupation or industry of employment. A comparison of aggregate changes in occupation distribution with intercohort differences in proportions in various occupations and with intracohort net mobility suggests that it is the succession of cohorts that is the primary source of aggregate redistribution, although mobility within a cohort's career is not a negligible source.[2]

COHORTS VERSUS GENERATIONS

In conventional intergenerational analysis of the kind permitted by the OCG tables, we may take advantage of the fact that the sons can be regarded as belonging to one or several well-defined birth cohorts. But the "fathers," in this event, definitely do not comprise a set of actual cohorts participating in economic activity contemporaneously. This point is obvious once it is stated, yet it proves difficult to appreciate its force in the absence of concrete illustration. Hence Table 3.1 was prepared to exemplify the way in which cohorts cross-cut generations. The table simultaneously classifies men 25 to 64 years old in 1960 (analogous to the OCG population of such men in 1962) by years in which these men were born and years in which their fathers were born. The figures are only rough estimates. For the older cohorts we could only assume that births were distributed by age of father in each year in the same way as for certain of the younger cohorts. Several other approximate procedures are required in deriving the estimates, as is explained in Appendix E, "Census Checks on Retrospective Data." If the highly approximate character of these estimates is borne in mind, they will serve quite adequately for the immediate purpose.

The crucial observation illustrated in Table 3.1 is that father's age at son's birth has a large variance. We know that the median is around

[2] Otis Dudley Duncan, "Occupation Trends and Patterns of Net Mobility in the United States," *Demography*, 3(1966), 1-18.

TABLE 3.1. ESTIMATED DISTRIBUTION OF SELECTED MALE COHORTS IN THE 1960 LABOR FORCE BY YEAR OF FATHER'S BIRTH (IN PERCENTAGES)

Father's Year of Birth	Cohort Identification: Year of Birth (Age in 1960)				
	1925–34 (25–34)	1915–24 (35–44)	1905–14 (45–54)	1895–1904 (55–64)	1895–1934 (total 25–64)
Total	100.0	100.0	100.0	100.0	100.0
1915–19	0.1	...	...	...	0.0[a]
1910–14	4.6	...	...	...	1.3
1905–09	16.0	0.1	...	...	4.6
1900–04	23.4	4.0	...	...	7.8
1895–99	21.8	15.1	0.1	...	10.7
1890–94	16.5	24.1	4.2	...	12.9
1885–89	9.9	23.0	15.3	0.1	13.6
1880–84	4.8	16.6	24.2	4.4	13.1
1875–79	1.9	9.8	22.9	16.0	11.9
1870–74	0.7	4.6	16.5	24.4	9.8
1865–69	0.2	1.8	9.7	22.6	6.8
1860–64	...	0.7	4.6	16.2	4.1
1855–59	...	0.2	1.8	9.4	2.1
1850–54	...	...	0.6	4.4	0.9
1845–49	...	...	0.2	1.7	0.3
1840–44	...	...	...	0.6	0.1
1835–39	...	...	...	0.1	0.0[a]

[a]Less than 0.05 per cent.

30 years—the length of a generation. Thus for the birth cohorts of 1925 to 1934 we should expect a concentration of father's birth years in the period 1895 to 1904. The first column of Table 3.1 reveals such a concentration, but it accounts for less than half (45.2 per cent) of the cases. Fathers born in this decade were, of course, 55 to 64 years old in 1960. Hence comparisons between the 1925 to 1934 and 1895 to 1904 birth cohorts involve, in part, a comparison of sons with fathers. But the translation from intercohort to intergenerational comparisons is extremely inexact. Not only does the 1895 to 1904 cohort fail to include over half the fathers of the 1925 to 1934 cohort; it includes many men besides such fathers—both fathers of sons born at some other time and men who had no sons at all.

The other factor that complicates any effort at generation-cohort translation is that some fathers have more than one son, whereas a substantial number of the contemporaries of any given group of fathers have no sons at all. It is easier to illustrate this point with respect to the proportions of potential mothers who have no sons, but the principle is, of course, the same for potential fathers. Consider, for example, 1950 census reports on women 55 to 59 years old (born in 1890 to 1894) by number of children ever born. We assume that all the never-married women and all the ever-married women reporting no children ever born had no son. One-half of those reporting one child, a quarter of those reporting two children, one-eighth of those reporting three children, and, in general $(\frac{1}{2})^k$ of those reporting k children are assumed to have borne no son. On this very rough basis, we reach the estimate that 38.5 per cent, or about thr e-eighths, of this cohort of women never had a son. A similar figure no doubt applies to a cohort of potential fathers born at about the same time. Evidently, there is a very substantial number of men who themselves move into and out of the working force but who are not represented at all in intergenerational data like the OCG mobility tables.

The unfortunate fact is that the demographic theory of population replacement is not yet sufficiently developed to permit a rigorous formulation of the generation-cohort translation problem. Pending such a development, the most we can do is to avoid drawing unwarranted analogies between aggregate and cohort data of the kind available in comparisons between successive censuses and intergenerational data of the kind obtained in the OCG survey.

In Figure 3.1 the OCG data have been juxtaposed with the more familiar data revealing aggregate trends in the occupational structure of the male working force. The aggregate data pertain to all male "gainful workers" in the censuses of 1900 to 1930 and all male members of the experienced civilian labor force in the censuses of 1940, 1950, and 1960. In representing the OCG data on a time-series chart it is necessary to choose arbitrary dates for plotting father's occupation and first job, since these questions were not time-specific. Along with the 1962 occupations of OCG cohorts, the figure includes 1952 data on the same cohorts, as estimated from CPS (Current Population Survey) figures for that year and 1950 census data. The derivation of these estimates is described more fully elsewhere.[3] In addition to the problem of temporal specificity, the interpretation of the data in Figure 3.1 must take account of problems of comparability between

---

[3] *Ibid.*

OCG-CPS data and census figures. The CPS, for example, overstates the number of managers, officials, and proprietors relative to census data for the same year. The retrospective OCG data, moreover, are subject to errors of recall. (See Appendix D, "Chicago Pretest Matching Study.") In view of such problems, we shall here focus on just the more salient contrasts between the two sets of data as they reveal the tempo of aggregate, intercohort, intergenerational, and intracohort (intragenerational) changes.

A convenient introduction to the discussion is provided by the series on percentage of farmers and farm managers, since these series produce some pronounced contrasts. A decided decrease in the proportion pursuing this occupation is revealed in the aggregate trend. The same general trend is revealed in intercohort comparisons based on either father's occupation or first job. But these two series give quite different impressions as to the rapidity of the decline, and neither agrees in this respect with the aggregate data. For each of the four OCG cohorts the sharp drop in percentage of farmers, from father's occupation to first job, agrees as to direction of change with the aggregate trend. But the rise from first job to 1952 or 1962 is in the opposite direction. This is only the first of several examples in which intracohort (or "intragenerational") changes do not move in the same direction as the aggregate, the intercohort, or the intergenerational changes.

How far the intergenerational basis of measuring change can deviate from the aggregate basis is indicated by the following comparison. Almost two-fifths (38.2 per cent) of the 1897 to 1906 OCG cohort reported their fathers were farmers, whereas only one-tenth (9.7 per cent) of these men were farmers themselves in 1952. Over the thirty-year period, 1920-1950, the aggregate trend underwent a decline from 18.4 to 10.0 per cent of all economically active men engaged in farming. The intergenerational net change of 28.5 percentage points (38.2 — 9.7) was, therefore, far larger than the intercensal change, over a period about one "generation" in length, of only 8.4 (18.4 — 10.0) percentage points. Indeed, Figure 3.1 reveals that all the intergenerational changes for OCG cohorts occurred much more rapidly than could be inferred from the aggregate data.

Our first inclination is to suppose that the OCG data greatly overstate the proportions of men whose fathers were farmers. But this point can be subjected to a rough check on the accuracy of the OCG reports on father's occupation (Appendix E, "Census Checks on Retrospective Data"). This check shows that the OCG data, if anything, understate the proportions whose fathers were farmers. Any reasonable allowance for errors and factors of noncomparability leaves intact

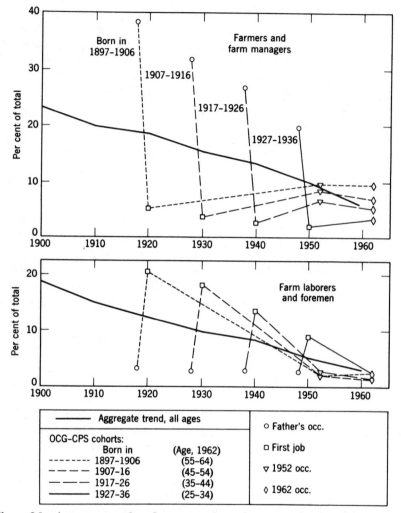

Figure 3.1. Aggregate trend and patterns of net intergenerational and intra-generational mobility: percent of men in each major occupation group. (Source: Duncan, "Occupation Trends and Patterns of Net Mobility in the United States," *op. cit.*)

the conclusion that the intergenerational decline in farming considerably exceeded the decline as measured by the aggregate time series.

The data on farm laborers afford an instructive contrast. Here there is a sharp intergenerational increase, from father's occupation to first job, counter to the aggregate trend. Subsequent net intracohort

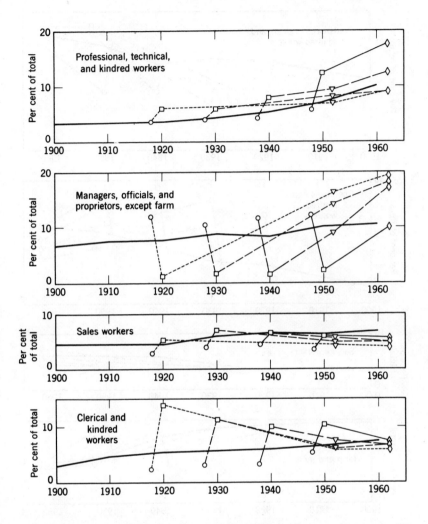

("intragenerational") movement out of the occupation conforms with the aggregate trend but occurs at a more rapid pace.

In the case of the professional-technical group of occupations all movements are consistent as to direction. For the two older OCG cohorts the net intergenerational movement into these occupations by 1962 was less rapid than the increase in the aggregate trend over a comparable time period. For the two younger cohorts, however, intergenerational change was more rapid than aggregate change. For all four cohorts, the influx into professional first jobs was rather more rapid than could be inferred from the aggregate data.

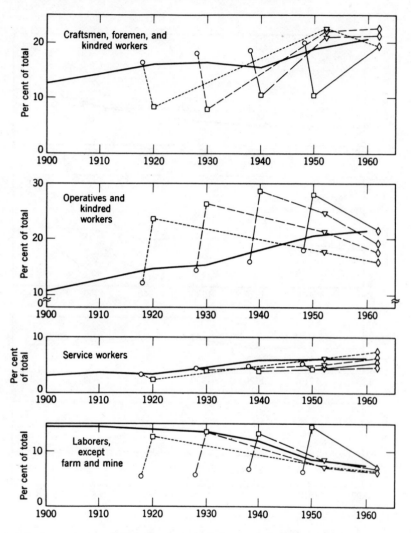

The data on nonfarm managers, officials, and proprietors resemble those for farm proprietors in terms of general career pattern: a sharp drop from father's occupation to first job, followed by a marked rise to the proportion engaged in this sort of work at ages 25 and over. This pattern for the nonfarm managerial group, however, interacts with a generally rising aggregate proportion in the occupation, whereas the aggregate trend moved in the opposite direction for farming.

The two lower white-collar groups—sales workers and clerical and kindred workers—share a similar pattern, although the movements are more pronounced for clerical workers. The intergenerational movement into these occupations, which conforms with the aggregate trend, is accomplished entirely via first jobs. Intracohort ("intragenerational") net movement subsequent to the first job is out of these occupations and, consequently, opposite to the direction of the aggregate trend.

The first two manual groups—craftsmen, foremen, and kindred workers; operatives and kindred workers—exhibit opposite career patterns superimposed on similarly rising aggregate trends. The intergenerational net movement into craft occupations occurs subsequently to a pronounced drop from father's occupation to first job. For operatives, on the contrary, the intergenerational increase occurs at the beginning of the work career; subsequent net mobility involves losses to this occupation group, counter to the rising trend of the aggregate data.

Service employment, like craft pursuits, recruits men in the course of their careers subsequently to the intergenerational decline in attachment to this kind of work from father's occupation to first job. In this regard, the pattern is similar to that noted for craft workers, although the amplitude of the changes is smaller.

The last occupation group, laborers, tends to recapitulate the pattern of farm laborers. It has been a declining occupation in the aggregate. The sharp rise from father's occupation to first job—counter to the aggregate trend—is followed by an intracohort decrease thereafter. For three of the OCG cohorts intergenerational mobility to 1962 apparently left slightly larger proportions in this occupation than had originated there (in terms of father's occupation). We may suspect some underreporting of laborer as a father's occupation, and our checks on the OCG data do not rule out this possibility. It is certainly curious that intercohort comparisons for either father's occupation or first job fail to reveal the declining importance of this occupation as indicated in the aggregate trend. Whether or not the explanation lies in problems of response error and comparability, this example shows that caution is required in reasoning from facts ascertained in intercensal comparisons to patterns that may be expected in mobility statistics.

In all the foregoing discussion the treatment of mobility, whether intergenerational or intragenerational, has been in net terms. If, as it appears, it is impossible to deduce with any accuracy the patterns of net mobility from a knowledge of aggregate trends alone, it is *a fortiori* impossible to infer patterns of gross mobility and changes therein merely from a knowledge of the over-all direction of change in occupation structure. Mobility trends require study in their own right. Unfortunately such study is beset by certain pitfalls not successfully avoided in previous research. We must at this point make room for a methodological digression.

MOBILITY TRENDS

It is only recently that the problem of measuring mobility trends has been investigated in a very methodical way. Sorokin's brief treatment[4] of the problem served only to open up the subject for investigation. The lively discussion of it during and immediately after World War II, begun by Sibley's provocative paper[5] and summarized in Chinoy's review,[6] succeeded mainly in demonstrating both the lack of relevant information and a need for greater clarity in posing the question itself.

If we confine attention to the more systematic attempts to measure directly or to infer mobility trends, we still are confronted with a variety of criteria for establishing changes in mobility patterns. Lenski's work relies mainly on an inspection of *transition matrices*, after making various estimates for the cohorts to be compared.[7] Somewhat earlier, Rogoff had presented an argument for using *social distance mobility ratios* in assessing trends.[8] Such ratios are used in an attempt to infer mobility trends from cross-sectional comparisons of age groups.[9] Both of these techniques are employed in the assessment of trends by Jackson and Crockett (along with sundry other summary indices of association and of amount of mobility).[10] Finally, a technique yet to be employed on any considerable scale has lately been proposed, which involves a model of *proportional adjustments* of the rows and columns of a mobility table.[11]

[4] Pitirim A. Sorokin, *Social Mobility*, New York: Harper, 1927, pp. 419-424.

[5] Elbridge Sibley, "Some Demographic Clues to Stratification," *American Sociological Review*, 7(1942), 322-330.

[6] Ely Chinoy, "Social Mobility Trends in the United States," *American Sociological Review*, 20(1955), 180-186.

[7] Gerhard E. Lenski, "Trends in Inter-Generational Occupational Mobility in the United States," *American Sociological Review*, 23(1958), 514-523.

[8] Natalie Rogoff, *Recent Trends in Occupational Mobility*, Glencoe: Free Press, 1953.

[9] Peter M. Blau, "Inferring Mobility Trends from a Single Study," *Population Studies*, 16(1962), 79-85.

[10] Elton F. Jackson and Harry J. Crockett, Jr., "Occupational Mobility in the United States," *American Sociological Review*, 29(1964), 5-15.

[11] Otis Dudley Duncan, "Methodological Issues in the Analysis of Social Mobility," in N. J. Smelser and S. M. Lipset (Eds.), *Social Structure and Mobility in Economic Development*, Chicago: Aldine, 1966.

Let us make explicit the rationale of each of the foregoing approaches, It is actually easier, though seemingly less natural, to state the problem in terms of criteria for recognizing no change in mobility patterns than in terms of criteria for measuring amount or degree of change.

Suppose, for concreteness and simplicity, that we have two intergenerational mobility tables, one for an "initial" time, t_0, and the other for a subsequent time, t_1. Let the matrix of cell frequencies in the first table be (m_{ij}) and in the second table (n_{ij}). If the total of all cells in the first is M and in the second N, we can perhaps agree that the comparison of the two tables registers "no change" in the volume, rate, or pattern of mobility if $(M/N)n_{ij} = m_{ij}$ for all i, j. That is, we presumably wish to abstract from the sheer increase (decrease) in size of the two cohorts whose mobility is to be compared (or from the difference in size of the two samples taken to represent the respective cohorts), so that we are studying relative, not absolute amounts of mobility.

The next question to face is whether there is any other sense in which we would be willing to agree that the comparison reveals "no change." Let us consider the three possibilities already mentioned.

(*i*) The two tables have the same transition matrix. That is, $n_{ij}/n_i. = m_{ij}/m_i.$ for all i, j. (We follow the convention that $\sum_j n_{ij} = n_i.$, etc.) This is the point of view of models in which mobility is viewed as a probability process and the transition matrix is taken to define a Markov chain.[12]

(*ii*) The two tables have the same matrix of social distance mobility ratios. That is, $Nn_{ij}/n_i.n_{.j} = Mm_{ij}/m_i.m_{.j}$ for all i, j. This criterion is implicit in Rogoff's study of "trends in mobility rates"; she writes:

In each time period, the differences in the occupational structure of the sons' and the fathers' generation influence the pattern of mobility. In order to remove these differences, and to make the two time periods comparable with respect to occupational structure, we will measure social distance mobility, or that mobility which is due to personal and group characteristics, rather than to variation in the occupational structure.[13]

(*iii*) The matrix (n_{ij}) is produced by a simultaneous proportional adjustment of the rows and columns of (m_{ij}). That is,

---

12 J. G. Kemeny and J. L. Snell, *Finite Markov Chains*, Princeton: Van Nostrand, 1960, section 7.6 (written with J. Berger); Judah Matras, "Comparison of Intergenerational Mobility Patterns," *Population Studies*, 14(1960), 163-196.

13 Rogoff, *op. cit.*, p. 43.

$$n_{ij} = \frac{N}{M} (1 + \lambda_i + \mu_j) \, m_{ij} \qquad \text{for all } i, j,$$

where λ_i is an adjustment factor that applies to all cells in row i while μ_j similarly applies to all cells in column j. The adjustment factors are secured by the procedure involved in "adjusting sample frequencies to expected marginal totals" developed by Deming in another context.[14]

Other criteria of "no change" could be entertained. We might, for example, require the inflow matrix rather than the transition or out-flow matrix to be the same at t_1 as at t_0. The three criteria listed will, however, suffice to illustrate the kinds of decision that must be made when conclusions are to be drawn from trend comparisons.

The identity of the transition matrices, criterion (i), is appealing in view of the elegant mathematics available for Markov-chain models. Such models are, indeed, instructive. Yet their applicability in the empirical analysis of intergenerational mobility is slight. For the chain model to work, the destination distribution for the first time period must be the origin distribution for the second period. But this involves a contradiction of the basic demography of labor force recruitment and replacement. If "sons" are a well-defined cohort, then neither their fathers nor their offspring can comprise a cohort in the same sense—a point that is developed earlier in this chapter and elsewhere.[15] We cannot, therefore, accept the availability of Markov-chain models as a justification for criterion (i). An alternative is simply to regard the transition matrix "as a descriptive device," in the apt phrasing of Carlsson.[16] It is also possible, however, to employ the transition matrix in making projections, assuming the matrix observed for one cohort applies to the (known or assumed) origin distribution of another. Where the destination distribution or the entire mobility table for the second cohort is known, the hypothesis on which the projection is made can be checked, and discrepancies may be attributed to "change" in mobility patterns.[17] Note that two mobility tables may have the same transition matrix—and thus register "no change" in their comparison—without having either set of marginals identical or proportional. However, it is not possible for both sets of marginals to be changed in an arbitrary way while the transi-

[14] W. Edwards Deming, *Statistical Adjustment of Data*, New York: Wiley, 1943, Chapter 7.

[15] Duncan, "Methodological Issues . . . ," *loc. cit.*

[16] Gösta Carlsson, *Social Mobility and Class Structure*, Lund, Sweden: CWK Gleerup, 1958, p. 73.

[17] Otis Dudley Duncan, "The Trend of Occupational Mobility in the United States," *American Sociological Review*, **30**(1965), 491-498.

tion matrix remains unchanged. There is, in fact, only one destination distribution compatible with the assumption of a given transition matrix and a given origin distribution. Hence, if our notion of the causal process at work entails the assumption that the destination distribution is a function of exogenous determinants (such as the demand for workers in various occupations or the educational qualifications of the men in a cohort), then the transition matrix must be altered to accommodate to the given origin distribution and the exogenously determined destination distribution. We can show, for example, that the intergenerational transition matrix for men 25 to 34 years old in 1952 cannot have been the same as the one for men of the same age in 1962 (even though the former is unknown), since the known origin and destination distributions of the two cohorts do not permit identity of their transition matrices.

Criterion (*ii*) leads us to recognize "change" as the occurrence of differences between two matrices of mobility ratios. The verbal argument on behalf of this criterion, quoted above from Rogoff, sounds plausible. It is perhaps doubtful, however, whether an investigator will wish to endorse this criterion when he realizes its crucial property.

This property may be stated as follows: *a matrix of mobility ratios implies a unique set of marginals for the corresponding mobility table.* The converse, of course, is not true—for a given set of marginals there is an exceedingly large (though finite) number of distinct possible matrices of mobility ratios.

The proof of the foregoing property follows at once from the definition of the mobility ratio, R_{ij}:

$$R_{ij} = \frac{M m_{ij}}{m_{i.} m_{.j}}.$$

Let us suppose M and R_{ij} known, the remaining quantities unknown. We may write

$$R_{ij} m_{i.} = M m_{ij} / m_{.j}, \quad \text{and hence}$$
$$\sum_i R_{ij} m_{i.} = (M/m_{.j}) \sum_i m_{ij} = M.$$

If we are working with a $c \times c$ mobility table, then the foregoing provides us with c equations, as j varies from 1 to c, in c unknowns (one for each $m_{i.}$). These may be solved simultaneously for the $m_{i.}$, yielding the origin distribution. Analogously, the expression

$$\sum_j R_{ij} m_{.j} = M$$

provides c equations ($i = 1, \ldots, c$) which may be solved for the c

unknown values of $m_{\cdot j}$. Once we know the two marginal distributions, of course, the cell values are readily obtained:

$$m_{ij} = R_{ij} \frac{m_{i\cdot}m_{\cdot j}}{M}.$$

If the mobility ratios rigorously imply the marginals, it is difficult to see in what sense the "effect" of the marginals has been "controlled" in computing the ratios. To put it another way, if it is impossible to observe "no change" on the assumptions being made in the analysis, the actual changes observed must have only an ambiguous meaning. Hence we must note an important implication of the property just demonstrated: one cannot have two mobility tables with identical matrices of mobility ratios if the respective marginal distributions of the two tables differ in an arbitrary fashion. The supposition that the mobility ratios "remove the differences," making "the two time periods comparable with respect to occupational structure" leads to a contradiction.

We may illustrate the point with some data used later in this chapter to investigate trends (Table 3.2). The mobility ratios from the SRC 1957 table were multiplied by the frequencies expected on the assumption of independence obtained from the marginals of the OCG 1962 table. This yields a set of imputed frequencies that would be the actual frequencies in the latter table if the two tables had identical mobility ratios. But these imputed frequencies do not sum to the actual marginals, as they must to avoid inconsistency. Indeed, they do not even sum to the correct grand total. The table of imputed frequencies, for example, implies that 2339 out of 38,006 OCG men 25 to 64 years old were farm workers (or 6.2 per cent), whereas the actual figures are 2897 out of 37,677 (or 7.7 per cent).

One might suppose that this disconcerting outcome could be avoided by following Carlsson's suggestion and computing the mobility ratio or, as he calls it, the c-value for the aggregate of all diagonal cells.[18] In this case he uses the notation c_d. But it is equally logical to compute such a ratio for the aggregate of off-diagonal cells; call it c_o. As an experiment, both ratios were computed for the SRC 1957 table, and the values were 1.562639 for c_d and .723296 for c_o. To use c-values for studying mobility trends, one would entertain (as a "null hypothesis") the assumption that the 1962 OCG table had the same values of c_d and c_o as the 1957 SRC table. Since the c-values are obtained as ratios of observed frequencies to frequencies expected on the

18 Carlsson, op. cit., p. 75.

TABLE 3.2. ILLUSTRATIVE DATA ON INTERGENERATIONAL MOBILITY

Item, Source,[a] and Father's Occ.	Respondent's Occ.			
	White-Collar	Manual	Farm	Total
SRC: 1957, Mobility ratios				
White-collar	1.869657	.576898	.257146	...
Manual	.858149	1.279875	.154418	...
Farm	.620579	.974267	2.288394	...
OCG: 1962, Observed frequencies (thousands)				
White-collar	6,313	2,644	132	9,089
Manual	6,321	10,883	294	17,498
Farm	2,495	6,124	2,471	11,090
Total	15,129	19,651	2,897	37,677
OCG: 1962, Independence frequencies (thousands)				
White-collar	3,649.64	4,740.50	698.86	...
Manual	7,026.23	9,126.34	1,345.43	...
Farm	4,453.13	5,784.15	852.71	...
SRC Mobility ratios multiplied by OCG independence frequencies				
White-collar	6,823.57	2,734.79	179.71	9,738.07
Manual	6,029.56	11,680.57	207.76	17,917.89
Farm	2,763.52	5,635.31	1,951.35	10,350.18
Total	15,616.65	20,050.67	2,338.82	38,006.14

[a] See Table 3.5.

hypothesis of independence, the latter must be obtained for the OCG data in Table 3.2:

expected stable	13,628.7
expected mobile	24,048.3
total	37,677.0

We may now multiply the OCG "expected stable" by SRC c_d and the OCG "expected mobile" by SRC c_o to see what frequencies of mobility and stability would be in the OCG data if there had been no change in mobility ratios; here are the results:

implied stable	21,296.74
implied mobile	17,394.04
total	38,690.78

But the actual total, given above, is 37,677. Hence the hypothesis of "no change" in both c-values gives rise to a logical contradiction. It would be *impossible* for the OCG table to have the same c-values as the SRC table, that is, to have the same mobility ratios both off and on the diagonal. Of course, one could posit that only one of the two c-values showed no change; but then the other would, of necessity, be different from that observed in the SRC table.

We must concede that an index that cannot logically attain values corresponding to no change is a poor one for purposes of measuring change. To put it another way, to suppose that a set of c-values represent a pattern of "rigidity" in the occupational structure that can remain invariant while "opportunity" changes owing to shifts in demand is to suppose a self-contradictory hypothesis. This property of the mobility ratio seems a somewhat more serious defect than the properties about which controversies have revolved since the ratio first was proposed.[19]

Criterion (iii) is suggested as perhaps the simplest approach to a model in which there is no change in mobility frequencies other than that induced by alteration of marginal distributions. We may, if we like, use this criterion to create a projection model. We shall then have to think of the destination distribution of the second table as being exogenously determined. If this distribution has already been observed, it may simply be taken as given. If the projection refers to a future date, the prospective destination distribution might be independently projected on the basis of anticipated manpower demand or worker qualifications. It would then be taken as one of the constraints on the projected mobility table. Whether such an approach would have value for purposes of forecasting is a moot question, and one not dealt with here. The idea of a projection is broached only for the insight it may convey as to the nature of the problem of analyzing past trends. In the example taking the approach of criterion (iii), Rogoff's 1910 table was adjusted to the marginals of the 1940 table.[20] This produced a reasonable facsimile of the actual 1940 table but one with some discrepancies that could not easily be attributed to "chance." A net summation of these discrepancies indicated that 7 per cent of the men in the 1940 table were in different cells than they would have been in had there been "no change" on criterion (iii).

Let us observe at this point that there *could* have been "no change" on criterion (iii), given the observed changes in the marginal distribu-

19 See Edward Gross, "On Controlling Marginals in Social Mobility Measurement," *American Sociological Review*, 29(1964), 886-887; Saburo Yasuda, "Reply to Gross," *idem*, 887-888; and literature there cited.

20 Duncan, "Methodological Issues . . . ," *loc. cit.*

tions. But in this case there would have been changes on both the previous criteria, that is, in the transition matrix and in the matrix of mobility ratios.

Evidently the choice of criteria on which to recognize and measure change cannot be reduced to a problem in arithmetic. It requires that conceptual considerations be brought into play. The social distance mobility ratio, although it has some attraction as an indication of departure from the hypothesis of "perfect mobility," is evidently unsuited to the problem of comparisons between time periods and, for that matter, for comparisons between places. The model of proportional adjustments is appropriate on a particular hypothesis as to the exogenous determination of marginal distributions. It is, however, best suited to comparisons involving only two time periods. As we shall later look at data for four different dates, a full analysis would involve no less than six paired comparisons. Moreover, the statistics for the earliest date are the least satisfactory and thus afford an unpromising basis for calculations depending on this model.

A direct comparison of transition matrices (outflow tables), therefore, may well be the best strategy for measuring trends in mobility, though perhaps not for investigating hypotheses about their causes. In the following analysis we shall depend on this approach, supplementing it with some summary measures of mobility or of the degree of association between origin and destination status, following the example of Jackson and Crockett.

DIRECT COMPARISONS BETWEEN YEARS

At the national level we have no time series on intergenerational mobility so designed as to secure strict comparability between time periods. The one example of a study with adequate standardization of statistical procedures applied to data from different periods pertains to a single metropolitan county and provides data for years around 1910 and 1940.[21] On the basis of the 1910 to 1940 comparisons, Rogoff concluded that

. . . no great change has taken place in recent times in the extent to which men may move from the occupational origins represented by their fathers' positions. The channels to social mobility afforded by the contemporary occupational structure are about as easily traversed now as they were at the beginning of the century.[22]

[21] Rogoff, *op. cit.*

[22] Natalie Rogoff, "Recent Trends in Urban Occupational Mobility," in P. K. Hatt and A. J. Reiss, Jr. (Eds.), *Reader in Urban Sociology,* Glencoe: Free Press, 1951, p. 417.

On the other hand, Rogoff's detailed analysis reveals some changes in specific *patterns* of mobility—as contrasted to over-all ease of movement. Some further analysis of Rogoff's data—employing regression techniques and the model of proportional adjustments by rows and columns—supports both conclusions and suggests that changes in mobility pattern were in large measure induced by changes in occupation structure or shifts in opportunities for mobility.[23]

In the absence of other research specially designed for temporal comparisons, Jackson and Crockett ventured an estimate of trends in analyzing tables derived from national surveys conducted in 1945, 1947, 1952, and 1957.[24] With the severe qualifications required because of factors of noncomparability and sampling error, the authors concluded that "the rate of occupational mobility in the United States has increased somewhat since the end of World War II. At the least, we found scant evidence that the system of occupational inheritance is growing more rigid."[25]

We are still in the position of Jackson and Crockett. Apart from the OCG data in which first job is the destination status (discussed subsequently), the only direct evidence of nationwide changes in amount or pattern of intergenerational mobility must come from the comparison of studies conducted independently with no regard to the building up of a comparable time series. In fact, we can do little more than add one more item—the OCG results—to the set that Jackson and Crockett compiled.

Before proceeding to this task, we are well advised to reflect on the hazards of comparison. If, as seems probable, any changes in mobility have been relatively small, their detection requires highly precise comparisons. It is all too likely that real changes are of a smaller order of magnitude than the errors in the data being used. One investigator has already recorded his perplexity in the face of apparent inconsistencies among four sets of U. S. survey data, noting that he was not able to verify the previously published calculations on one of these sets after having the data retabulated.[26] In turn, having access to the 1956 data that Miller accepts as "least objectionable," we are unable to "verify" his frequencies. The first hazard of comparison, then, is that successive secondary analyses of what is ostensibly the same information may turn up inconsistent results. There are several reasons for this: (1) Different tabulations may refer to slightly different defini-

23 Duncan, "Methodological Issues . . . ," *loc. cit.*

24 Jackson and Crockett, *loc. cit.*

25 *Ibid.*, p. 15.

26 S. M. Miller, "Comparative Social Mobility," *Current Sociology,* 9(1960), 27.

tions of the universe, for example, household heads or chief earners in one case but all male respondents in another. (2) Minor differences may occur in the way in which occupational subcategories are combined into larger groups and in the handling of NA cases. (3) Mechanical errors are inevitable when punched cards are repeatedly reproduced and tallied.

Needless to say, such factors producing discrepancies within one set of data may likewise operate to compromise comparisons between sets. In the latter case, moreover, there are additional problems in the variation between surveys in population coverage, concept, and coding procedures. Each survey is subject to sampling error as well. Before proceeding to substantive trend comparisons, therefore, we wish to supply some evidence on the magnitude of errors resulting from noncomparability.

In Table 3.3 we take advantage of the fact that four OCG age groups provide an approximate cohort match with the 1957 SRC (Survey Research Center) data analyzed by Jackson and Crockett. The period of five years between the two studies could well have witnessed actual changes in the occupations of respondents. There should, however, have been no change in their distribution by father's occupation. The SRC question was, "What kind of work did your father do for a living while you were growing up?" This closely resembles the OCG question on father's occupation, ". . . when you were about 16 years old?" We cannot be sure, however, that the two surveys were equally comparable in their handling of cases when the respondent did not live with his father.

Looking first at the total group aged 25 to 64 in 1962 or 21 to 59 in 1957 (disregarding the omission of 20-year-old men in the latter), we should expect identical distributions by father's occupation from the two sources—assuming comparability of survey procedures and negligible selectivity in losses to respondent cohorts over the five-year period, 1957-1962. Instead, there is a relative deficiency of 4 per cent of SRC men with manual origins, compensated by a 4 per cent excess with farm origins. We might be inclined to attribute the difference to sampling error alone, except for the fact (shown in the last line of Table 3.3) that another SRC survey conducted only one year earlier shows just the same discrepancies.

We may comment briefly on the comparisons for the four 10-year cohorts in Table 3.3. Here we find further discrepancies, not all in the same direction as those noted for the total OCG and SRC 1957 samples. No doubt these represent sampling variation for the most part. But such variation is relevant, for when we compare the OCG and SRC

TABLE 3.3. PERCENTAGE DISTRIBUTION OF OCG COHORTS BY BROAD
CATEGORIES OF FATHER'S OCCUPATION, AS REPORTED IN OCG SURVEY,
1962, AND IN SURVEY RESEARCH CENTER (SRC) SURVEYS, 1957 AND 1956

| Source, Date, and Respondent's Age | Total | Father's Occ. | | | (SRC Sample Size) |
		White-Collar	Manual	Farm	
OCG: 1962[a]					
Total, 25–64	100	24	45	31	...
25–34	100	27	51	22	...
35–44	100	24	46	30	...
45–54	100	22	43	35	...
55–64	100	21	38	41	...
SRC: 1957[b]					
Total, 21–59	100	24	41	35	(802)
21–29	100	28	47	25	(166)
30–39	100	18	46	36	(241)
40–49	100	29	35	36	(223)
50–59	100	21	37	42	(172)
SRC: 1957[c]					
Total, 21–64	100	23	40	37	(911)
SRC: 1956[d]					
Total, 21–64	100	24	40	36	(749)

[a]U.S. Bureau of the Census, "Lifetime Occupational Mobility of Adult Males:
March 1962," Current Population Reports, Series P-23, No. 11 (May 12, 1964).

[b]Elton F. Jackson and Harry J. Crockett, Jr., "Occupational Mobility in the
United States: A Point Estimate and Trend Comparison," American Sociological
Review, 29 (February, 1964), Table 2.

[c]Source same as [b]. Estimate for respondents 60-64 taken as one-half of respondents 60 and over.

[d]University of Michigan Survey Research Center, Project #417, Personal Data
Card VI, tabulated by staff of the University of Michigan Population Studies
Center.

mobility tables we shall have to break down the marginal distribution
of father's occupation just as it is here broken down by age.

A final test of comparability, in Table 3.4, concerns the distribution
of respondents by their own occupations. Here we have as the standard
of comparison the annual series of labor force data obtained in the

TABLE 3.4. OCCUPATION DISTRIBUTION OF RESPONDENTS IN THREE MOBILITY SURVEYS, COMPARED WITH CURRENT POPULATION SURVEY ESTIMATES, 1947 TO 1957 (IN PERCENTAGES)

Date and Source[a]	Total	Respondent's Occ.		
		White-Collar	Manual	Farm
1957				
SRC	100	35	53	12
CPS, Experienced labor force, annual average	100	34	55	11
1952				
SRC	100	34	51	15
CPS, Experienced labor force, annual average	100	31	56	13
1947				
NORC	100	41	43	16
CPS, Employed men, April	100	30	53	17
CPS, Employed men 20-59, April	100	30	56	14

[a] SRC and NORC from Jackson and Crockett, loc. cit. CPS from Bureau of the Census, Current Population Reports, Series P-20, No. 9, Table 10; P-20, No. 18, Table 19; P-50, No. 45, Table D; and Bureau of Labor Statistics, Special Labor Force Reports, No. 14, Table B-6.

Current Population Survey (CPS) of the Bureau of the Census since the late 1940's. The CPS data are themselves subject to error, of course; but they are based on much larger samples than the SRC and NORC figures. The CPS series, moreover, is reasonably comparable between years. We find some discrepancies, large enough to be disquieting, between SRC and CPS in 1952 and 1957. Whatever their source, we could expect similar differences between SRC and our OCG data in 1962, if there had been a 1962 SRC mobility table.

The really serious and egregious discrepancy, however, concerns the 1947 NORC (National Opinion Research Center) data. As compared with either all employed men or those 20 to 59 years old in CPS, the NORC table greatly overrepresents white-collar respondents and underestimates manual respondents. The differences are so great that we are inclined simply to dismiss the NORC results as untrustworthy. It is sobering to reflect on the fact that a number of social scientists have used the NORC figures without taking the precaution of checking the plausibility of the marginal totals.

TABLE 3.5. OUTFLOW PERCENTAGES FOR FOUR U.S. INTERGENERATIONAL
MOBILITY TABLES, BROAD OCCUPATION GROUPS, 1947 TO 1962

| Source, Date, and Father's Occ. | Total | Respondent's Occ. | | | (Sample Size) | Per Cent by Origin |
		White-Collar	Manual	Farm		
OCG: 1962[a]						100
White-collar	100	69	29	2	...	24
Manual	100	37	62	2	...	47
Farm	100	23	55	22	...	29
SRC: 1957[b]					1,023	100
White-collar	100	67	30	3	236	23
Manual	100	30	68	2	393	38
Farm	100	22	52	26	394	39
SRC: 1952[c]					747	100
White-collar	100	65	34	1	153	20
Manual	100	31	67	2	280	38
Farm	100	22	44	34	314	42
NORC: 1947[d]					1,153	100
White-collar	100	71	25	4	319	28
Manual	100	35	61	4	430	37
Farm	100	23	39	38	404	35
NORC: 1947, Adjusted[e]					1,153	100
White-collar	100	59	37	4	280	24
Manual	100	24	73	3	465	40
Farm	100	16	50	34	408	36

[a] Respondents 20 to 64 years old; omits father's occupation not reported.

[b] As reported by Jackson and Crockett, op. cit., Table 4 (percentages rounded).

[c] Idem. Note that this version of SRC-1952 differs slightly from that reported by Miller, op. cit., p. 27, and both differ from figures purportedly from the same primary source, as given by S. M. Lipset and R. Bendix, Social Mobility in Industrial Society (Berkeley: Univer. of California Press, 1959), Fig. 2.1, p. 21.

[d] National Opinion Research Center data, as reported by Jackson and Crockett, loc. cit., and by Lipset and Bendix, loc. cit.

[e] See text for method of adjustment.

Instead of discarding the NORC data, however, we have entertained the idea of a simple adjustment. The percentage distribution of the April 1947 CPS for men 20 to 59 years old was assumed to be correct. The columns of the NORC table were inflated or deflated so as to sum to the correct totals. This, of course, results in new estimates from the NORC data of the outflow percentages and of the proportions by father's occupation. In Table 3.5 both the original and the adjusted

NORC outflow tables are shown for comparison with the other three sets. The adjusted NORC figures are not to be taken too seriously as estimates. The adjustment corrects only for NORC sampling bias or coding bias in respect to respondents; it does not correct for coding bias (if any) with respect to father's occupation. The adjusted figures are, nonetheless, more nearly free of several anomalies that render the original data highly suspect.

Concentrating mainly on the 10 years, 1952 to 1962, we can quickly summarize such trends as are suggested by a literal reading of the data: (1) a decreasing proportion of men with farm origins remained on farms, whereas an increasing proportion achieved manual status; (2) an increasing proportion from manual origins moved up into white-collar positions; (3) yet there was no compensatory increase in downward mobility from white-collar origins; on the contrary, increasing proportions of those originating at this level remained there. Apparently the occupational structure changed continuously over this brief period in such a way as to provide greater opportunity for upward mobility for everybody.

One does not, of course, extrapolate such a trend without qualification. If off-farm movement has indirectly induced (or at least facilitated) manual-to-white-collar movement, then the declining proportion with farm origins must ultimately limit one major source of mobility. The argument here is the one Sibley used in his 1942 forecast (which was somewhat premature, even though cautious) of a "slackening of the upward tide of vertical circulation" consequent to the cessation of large-scale immigration of manual workers.[27] Still, the argument may cease to be correct at about the time it becomes relevant. If we are to believe that "automation" will abolish many manual jobs, it is perhaps just as well not to have an oversupply of farmers' sons ready to enter such jobs.

Besides inspecting outflow tables, there are various other ways to summarize trend comparisons. Table 3.6 presents several summary measures on the mobility tables being compared, following the pattern of Jackson and Crockett. The first row suggests there was no change, from 1952 to 1962, in the proportion having moved from the broad occupation group of origin; but all three of the later tables show a slightly higher percentage of movement than the 1947 NORC table. The second line reports the net mobility, or minimum proportion of movement required to effect the intergenerational change in marginal distributions. In view of our earlier evidence on errors in the marginal

27 Sibley, *loc. cit.* See the discussion of this point in Chapters 7 and 12.

TABLE 3.6. SUMMARY MEASURES OF MOBILITY FOR FOUR U.S. INTER-GENERATIONAL MOBILITY TABLES, BROAD OCCUPATION GROUPS, 1947 TO 1962

Measure of Mobility [a]	Source and Date [b]				
	OCG 1962	SRC 1957	SRC 1952	NORC: 1947	
				Observed	Adjusted
Per cent mobile					
Observed	47.8	48.5	47.4	44.4	44.2
Minimum (structural movement)	21.8	27.0	26.9	19.1	21.0
Observed minus minimum (circulation)	26.0	21.5	20.5	25.3	23.2
Expected, hypothesis of independence (full-equality model)	63.8	67.0	67.6	67.0	65.1
Contingency coefficient					
(Cramer's V)	.336	.348	.372	.390	.375

[a] Terms in parentheses are those used by Jackson and Crockett, loc. cit.

[b] See notes to Table 3.5; figures for SRC-1957, SRC-1952, and NORC-1947 (observed) computed by Jackson and Crockett, loc. cit.

distributions, we have to be cautious in interpreting the somewhat puzzling figures in this row.

In any event, the interest in calculating net mobility is primarily in using it to interpret the gross volume of mobility. If we subtract the second from the first row we obtain a residual that Jackson and Crockett term "circulation." This figure is higher in the OCG data than in any of the earlier tables. At the same time, observed (gross) mobility in the OCG table approximates most closely the amount of mobility to be expected if respondent's occupation were independent of father's occupation—the so-called model of "perfect" or "full-equality" mobility (fourth line of Table 3.6). For example, the difference between "expected" and observed mobility in 1952 was 67.6 — 47.4 = 23.2 per cent; in 1962 it was 63.8 — 47.8 = 16.0 per cent. (Perhaps we should note that this calculation is not subject to the problem of interpretation encountered with the aggregate c-values suggested by Carlsson, as discussed in the preceding section of this chapter.)

Finally, as an over-all measure of association between origin and destination, Jackson and Crockett suggest a certain contingency coefficient, Cramér's V. This index declines regularly from .375 in 1947 to .336 in 1962 (last row of Table 3.6). In sum, the data suggest that mobility has slightly increased in the last 10 or 15 years. At least there is no indication of increasing rigidity in the class structure.

INDIRECT INFERENCES

Waiving all problems of comparability and systematic error, we are still limited in making direct trend comparisons to an exceedingly crude occupational classification. The SRC and NORC samples are simply too small to afford reliable comparisons on a finer breakdown. We can circumvent this problem in some measure and, at the same time, provide partial corroboration of the changes in outflow patterns by taking an indirect route to the estimate of trends. The somewhat tedious methodological details have been presented elsewhere,[28] so that only a sketch of the technique need be given here.

In the OCG data we have transition matrices (outflow tables) for four main cohorts: men 25 to 34, 35 to 44, 45 to 54, and 55 to 64 years of age in 1962. Now, if we apply the transition matrix for men 25 to 34 to the origin distribution (father's occupation) of the men 35 to 44 years old, we can compute where the latter cohort would have been in 1952 (10 years earlier) if they had experienced the same pattern of mobility up to age 25 to 34 as did the younger cohort. We can then independently estimate from census and CPS data what was the actual occupation distribution of men 25 to 34 years old in 1952. The difference between the inferred distribution and the actual distribution in 1952 shows in *net* terms how the mobility patterns of the two groups differed.

In the first column of Table 3.7, for example, we see that if men born in 1917 to 1926 had been subject to the same outflow percentages up to age 25 to 34 as men born in 1927 to 1936, though starting from a different distribution of origins, 6.6 per cent more of them would have been salaried professional and technical workers in 1952 than there actually were in such jobs at the time. Similarly, the 1962 mobility matrix was somewhat more favorable for movement into salaried managerial positions. These two occupations, in fact, account for most of the excess movement into white-collar jobs. In compensation, the 1962 matrices involved lower proportions taking up farming (allowing for the difference in proportions originating there) and the skilled and semiskilled manual occupations.

Clearly, the 1962 outflow tables were more favorable than the 1952 tables for upward movement in general. The margin of superiority was greatest in terms of mobility at the younger ages, least at age 45

---

[28] Duncan, "The Trend of Occupational Mobility . . . ," *loc. cit.*

TABLE 3.7. DIFFERENCES IN PERCENTAGE POINTS BETWEEN OCCUPATIONAL DISTRIBUTIONS FOR MEN OF SPECIFIED AGES PRODUCED BY 1962 INTER-GENERATIONAL MOBILITY MATRICES AND BY UNKNOWN MATRICES FOR 1952

Major Occ. Group	1962 Minus 1952, by Age		
	25 to 34	35 to 44	45 to 54
Professional, technical, and kindred workers			
Self-employed	0.1	0.3	-0.1
Salaried	6.6	3.5	1.5
Managers, officials, and proprietors, except farm			
Salaried	1.7	2.4	0.7
Self-employed	-1.2	0.0	1.0
Sales workers	-0.2	0.1	0.3
Clerical and kindred workers	-0.5	0.4	0.6
Craftsmen, foremen, and kindred workers	-1.9	-0.8	0.1
Operatives and kindred workers	-2.6	-2.0	0.0
Service workers	0.9	-0.3	-0.3
Laborers, except farm and mine	-0.5	-0.5	-1.0
Farmers and farm managers	-2.6	-2.6	-2.3
Farm laborers and foremen	0.2	-0.5	-0.5
(Index of dissimilarity)	(9.5)	(6.7)	(4.2)

SOURCE: Duncan, "The Trend of Occupational Mobility in the United States," op. cit.

to 54, as is summarized by the indexes of dissimilarity (sum of positive percentage differences) at the bottom of the table.

In confirming the previous general observation as to the recent increase in over-all chances of upward mobility, we have also made it somewhat more specific: it is the higher salaried positions (rather than all white-collar jobs) that have expanded to accommodate the upward flow, and it is the younger men in particular who have been able to take advantage of this expansion.

The implication of this finding is that the amount of upward intergenerational mobility has increased in the last decade. Although the comparisons are not given here, we may mention in conclusion that much the same generalization is reached in regard to the trend in intragenerational mobility, proceeding in the same way but regarding first job, rather than father's occupation, as the origin status.[29]

29 *Ibid.*

INTERCOHORT COMPARISONS IN MOBILITY TO FIRST JOB

One resource remains for the discernment of trends, if we are willing to take a foreshortened perspective on intergenerational mobility, following the OCG cohorts from father's occupation only as far as the respondent's first job. Intergenerational mobility to 1962 occupation yields only equivocal intercohort comparisons, since the older men have lengthier labor-force experience than the younger. This difficulty does not apply when first job is taken as the terminus of intergenerational mobility. Here the four groups of birth cohorts provide us with a genuine time series, on the assumption that the retrospective data are accurate. The time series, moreover, begins at a fairly distant date in the past, since the men aged 55 to 64 in 1962 were 16 years old in 1913 to 1922, and the great majority of them probably entered upon their first jobs during, say, 1911 to 1926.

Inspection of Table 3.8 reveals that there have not been monotonic

TABLE 3.8. OUTFLOW PERCENTAGES, INTERGENERATIONAL MOBILITY FROM FATHER'S OCCUPATION TO FIRST JOB, BROAD OCCUPATION GROUPS, FOR FOUR OCG COHORTS

Cohort (Year Attained Age 16) and Father's Occupation[a]	Total	Respondent's First Job [a]		
		White Collar	Manual	Farm
1943–52				
White-collar	100.0	57.6	40.6	1.8
Manual	100.0	24.7	71.6	3.7
Farm	100.0	15.1	45.6	39.3
1933–42				
White-collar	100.0	54.4	43.1	2.5
Manual	100.0	22.6	72.5	4.9
Farm	100.0	10.5	41.6	47.9
1923–32				
White-collar	100.0	54.5	42.6	2.9
Manual	100.0	25.5	69.2	5.3
Farm	100.0	9.1	36.1	54.8
1913–22				
White-collar	100.0	58.3	38.4	3.3
Manual	100.0	27.5	66.3	6.2
Farm	100.0	10.0	33.8	56.2

[a] Omits cases not reporting one or both occupations.

trends in respect to all of the nine origin-destination combinations. There is, however, unequivocal indication of the declining attraction of farm jobs, irrespective of origin. Although 56 per cent of the oldest cohort originating on the farm found their first jobs in that sector, this was true of only 39 per cent of the most recent cohort. Increasing proportions of men with farm origins have found their first employment at both the manual and the white-collar levels.

From the earliest to the latest cohort, there was a rise (though not an uninterrupted one) in the proportion remaining at the manual level, of those originating there. This was accompanied, up to the 1933 to 1942 cohort, by declining proportions of upward mobility from manual origins to white-collar first jobs. However, in the experience of the most recent cohort, there was a recovery so that the percentage of such upward mobility was hardly less than it had been 20 years earlier.

The pattern of mobility from white-collar origin hardly suggests a trend. The probabilities were very similar for the two middle cohorts. The earliest and the latest cohorts resemble each other more closely than either resembles one of the middle cohorts. There was slightly more downward mobility to manual jobs around the end of World War II than during the corresponding period around World War I, but less than had occurred in the intervening period.

Although it is tempting to associate some of the short-run fluctuations with the historical circumstances of war, prosperity, and depression, it is doubtful that these data can sustain so close an analysis. Each cohort covers a 10-year period of birth dates. But the age at entering first job is somewhat variable, so that the actual experience of each cohort, as recorded in these tables, spans a period of 15 years or more. The successive cohorts had temporally overlapping experience.

Table 3.9 (top half) records the summary measures of mobility suggested by Jackson and Crockett. We note utterly insignificant changes in the over-all volume of movement, but a decline in net (minimum) mobility and a corresponding decline in the amount of movement required by the perfect mobility model. Hence the observed mobility exceeded the minimum by a margin that widened with the passage of time. Simultaneously, it approached more closely the amount expected on the supposition that all three sets of outflow percentages are the same. In terms of sheer volume of movement, then, there was no change. But by comparison with either of these alternative norms there was a relative increase in the amount of movement. The contingency coefficient, V, yields a conclusion consistent with

TABLE 3.9. SUMMARY MEASURES OF MOBILITY IN TABLES OF INTER-GENERATIONAL MOBILITY FROM FATHER'S OCCUPATION TO FIRST JOB, FOR FOUR OCG COHORTS, BY LEVEL OF DETAIL IN OCCUPATION CLASSIFICATION

Occ. Classification and Measure of Mobility	Cohort (Year Attained Age 16)			
	1943–52	1933–42	1923–32	1913–22
THREE BROAD CATEGORIES				
Per cent mobile				
Observed	39.5	39.1	39.0	39.5
Minimum	11.3	12.5	12.7	15.0
Observed minus minimum	28.2	26.6	26.3	24.5
Expected, assuming independence	60.1	62.4	64.1	65.8
Contingency coefficient				
Cramer's V	.405	.434	.454	.453
TEN MAJOR GROUPS				
Per cent mobile [a]				
Observed	78.6	79.2	78.9	79.2
Minimum	38.2	42.5	47.6	52.1
Observed minus minimum	40.4	36.7	31.3	27.1
Expected, assuming independence	89.3	89.9	90.8	91.4
Contingency coefficient				
Pearson's C	.547	.564	.594	.595

[a] These data are reported in U.S. Bureau of the Census, "Lifetime Occupational Mobility of Adult Males: March 1962," Current Population Reports, Series P-23, No. 11 (May 12, 1964), Table B.

the latter observation: the extent of association between origin and destination has been less recently than at an earlier date.

We may interpolate here the observation, supported by the lower half of Table 3.9, that exactly the same summary of trends applies when the data are looked at in terms of movement among 10 major occupation groups, rather than the three broad categories. Increasing the number of classes, of course, increases the amount of movement observed. Very nearly four out of five men in each cohort found first jobs in a different major occupation group from that of their fathers.

The preceding discussion has relied largely on the measures of mobility proposed by Jackson and Crockett, so that our analysis of mobility trends via OCG intercohort comparisons would be parallel to the trend comparisons presented earlier. We may, however, raise the question of what inferences about trends emerge when occupations are scored on status rather than grouped into more or less broad categories. Table 3.10 presents the relevant statistics.

TABLE 3.10. SUMMARY MEASURES OF INTERGENERATIONAL MOBILITY FROM FATHER'S OCCUPATION TO FIRST JOB, IN TERMS OF OCCUPATIONAL STATUS SCORES, FOR FOUR OCG COHORTS, EXCLUDING MEN WITH FARM BACKGROUND

Measure	Cohort (Year Attained Age 16)			
	1943–52	1933–42	1923–32	1913–22
Mean of W (first job status)	30.7	28.8	27.2	28.3
Mean of X (father's status)	33.3	33.1	31.8	32.5
Difference between means, $\overline{W} - \overline{X}$	-2.6	-4.3	-4.6	-4.2
Per cent nonmobile (W = X)	9.2	8.7	11.8	12.3
Correlation, W with X	.380	.377	.388	.384

These data pertain to men with nonfarm background; that is, those whose fathers were farmers or farm laborers are omitted. For several reasons this may be an interesting restriction to entertain. We already know from the study of mobility by major occupation groups that a large part of mobility to first job has consisted in the employment of farmers' sons as farm laborers. Because the farm sector has declined over time this source of mobility has diminished. There is no need to review this fact with a more precise technique. Moreover, now that the farm sector is becoming so small, in future an overwhelming majority of men will come from nonfarm origins. Hence, one may argue, OCG historical data on men from such origins are more comparable to the current and prospective situation than would be the data on all men. Finally, in omitting men with farm background we largely circumvent the question of whether farm occupations as scored on the status scale are truly comparable with nonfarm occupations.

The first measure of mobility in Table 3.10 is the difference in mean status score between the first jobs (W) and father's occupations (X). In all four cohorts there was a net downward movement to first job, as reflected in the negative sign of this difference. The drop was not quite so large, however, for the most recent cohort—entering the labor market in the years toward the end of and just after World War II—as for the three preceding ones. As an aside we might note that the favorable labor market for young men during this period has been held partly responsible for the drop in marriage age and the acceleration of childbearing resulting in the "baby boom."[30]

The second measure of mobility, or rather immobility, is simply the proportion of men whose first job had exactly the same two-digit status score as that of the father's occupation. This need not mean, of course, that the two specific occupations were the same. The respondent's first job may have been as a newsboy, scored 27, whereas his father may have been a tile setter, likewise scored 27. In terms of major occupation groups, this combination would represent mobility from craft to sales worker, or manual to white collar. In the present treatment, however, it is a case of no mobility. Clearly, if we compared specific occupation titles of father and son we should arrive at still lower estimates of immobility or "inheritance." The point of interest here, however, is the decrease in proportion nonmobile (in terms of status scores) from 12 to 9 per cent, comparing the most recent cohorts with the two older ones.

Finally, we consider the coefficient of correlation between the scores of respondent's first job and father's occupation. As explained in Chapter 4, we regard this coefficient as a measure of the extent to which the first job depends on father's occupation—a measure that does not reflect solely the frequency with which the two are identical. In this respect the correlation resembles the contingency coefficients cited earlier, though the two kinds of coefficient may not be compared as to magnitude. Examining the correlations in the last row of Table 3.10, we are hard put to detect any intercohort difference at all, except such as may readily be attributed to sampling error and approximations used in computing. If anything, the correlations are lower for the two youngest than for the two earlier cohorts.

Perhaps the most important comment to make after studying the status scores is that the patterns for the four cohorts are remarkably similar, even though their experience spans a period of 40 years. At least as far as career beginnings are concerned, the influence of social origins has remained constant since before World War I. There is absolutely no evidence of "rigidification."

NET IMPRESSIONS

Anyone who is familiar with the pronounced transformation of the American occupational structure during the twentieth century is likely to suppose that this change has entailed a considerable amount

---

[30] Richard A. Easterlin, "The American Baby Boom in Historical Perspective," *American Economic Review*, 51(1961), 869-911.

of intergenerational mobility. Lenski, for example, when he observed "the marked difference between the occupational distributions of the two generations" in the SRC 1952 mobility table, commented: "These differences clearly reflect the changing occupational structure of American society."[31] His comment would have been more plausible had he written "ambiguously" for "clearly." Intuitively, there is little reason to doubt that rapid changes in the occupational structure will be accompanied by considerable intergenerational mobility, but it is by no means "clear" how this occurs. We have seen that even *net* intergenerational mobility to the occupations held by OCG men in 1962 cannot be closely estimated from the amount of occupational change revealed by aggregate trends. Even the *direction* of intergenerational mobility to first jobs or of intragenerational mobility from first jobs to 1962 may not be the same as the aggregate trends. Our juxtaposition of aggregate trend data and mobility data has highlighted a complex problem in the theory of demographic replacement—or "social metabolism"—for which a solution is not now available. Aside from pointing to a need for additional inquiry, this disconcerting circumstance means that we cannot derive from trend data cogent explanations of changes in the amounts or patterns of mobility.

We may, nevertheless, proceed to study these historical changes in a descriptive fashion on the grounds of their intrinsic interest, essentially deferring the problem of explanation. This kind of study, however, poses some pitfalls of its own, and we have found it necessary first to remove some conceptual confusion surrounding the use of a well-known tool, the "social distance mobility ratio" or "index of association." Even with the conceptual problem of measuring mobility trends resolved, there remain serious difficulties occasioned by sampling and systematic errors in the available data. Our conclusions must, indeed, be stated with caution.

Bringing together the postwar national surveys of intergenerational mobility in the United States, including the OCG study as the latest in a series of four, we find no reason to dissent from the earlier conclusion of Jackson and Crockett that there has been no "rigidification" of the system in this period. An indirect approach to the ascertainment of trends, via intercohort comparisons from the OCG data, sustains this conclusion. It reveals, moreover, that the enhanced opportunity for upward mobility enjoyed by the more recent cohorts has been due primarily to movement into the rapidly expanding higher salaried positions—not especially to mobility into self-employment or lower white-collar jobs.

31 Lenski, *op. cit.*, p. 515.

Finally, intercohort comparisons of mobility to first job, derived from the OCG data, yield somewhat equivocal indications of trends, but certainly no evidence of "rigidification." What is most striking in a regression framework is the essential invariance of the father-son correlation over a period of nearly 40 years. Evidently the fears current in the sociological fraternity a decade or two ago—that the "land of opportunity" was giving way to a society with rigid classes—were ill-founded, or at least premature. Sibley had argued that the decline of immigration would result in a decrease in the pressure for upward movement due to an influx at the bottom of the occupational scale. He failed to note that the domestic movement off farms might assume a similar role, as it appears to have done. If this, indeed, was the source of sustained (if not rising) rates of mobility, then his prognostication may still prove ultimately to be correct, as the farm population no longer is large enough to provide vast numbers of recruits to the non-farm labor force.

We may conjecture, too, that the role of education in engendering movement was inadequately appreciated two decades ago, even though a number of thoughtful writers had identified the school as an institution intimately involved in the process of social selection. The rising trend of educational attainment has continued with little abatement. We are in no position to offer a formal model of how this trend may be reflected in a time series of mobility tables, but the conjecture that there is a relationship may be offered as a basis for further research.

The limitation of our inquiry to the fortunes of men, though a legitimate preliminary simplification, reckons without the impact of the influx of women into the labor force on men's chances of mobility. Women do not offer competition to men in all occupations, but the supply of openings available to men can hardly be independent of the number of women ready and trained to work at a variety of skill levels.

Commonplace observations, therefore, suggest a number of possible factors that must play a role in determining the amount and pattern of mobility observed at different times. Yet we are so far from understanding how these factors combine that our conjectures are virtually gratuitous. One thing seems clear: while there is need for continuing efforts to measure the trend of mobility, we shall ultimately not be satisfied with less than a comprehensive dynamic model of structural change in which mobility is involved as one among several inputs, mechanisms, or outputs. This book can hope at best to suggest some directions in which work on such a model may begin.

CHAPTER 4

Ascribed and Achieved Status: Techniques of Measurement and Analysis

The classic concern with patterns of gross and net occupational mobility, exemplified in the last two chapters, affords a background for the analysis of ways in which other factors influence occupational achievement. We are not interested only in patterns of occupational mobility per se; our primary concern is with the factors affecting these patterns and the individual's chances of success. The prototypical question we ask is how the various ascribed statuses that a man brings to his career affect his achieved status in the occupational structure. To answer questions of this type, the following chapters rely heavily on procedures for analyzing interrelations of several statuses. We insert here a fairly extensive discussion of technical problems that arise when this strategy is adopted. Although this chapter is primarily devoted to methodological problems, we also take this occasion to set out several of the more important empirical results of the study. In particular, the role of education as an intervening link between ascribed status (or social origins) and occupational achievement is treated rather extensively. These results are taken for granted in the subsequent chapters. As a preliminary, however, it is necessary to explain how occupational status itself is measured and to consider an important problem of interpretation that arises in connection with the measurement of occupational status when such a measure is used in multivariable analyses.

In regard to the discussion of methods, the reader is invited to share two of our dilemmas. The first is a problem in presentation. If we explain our methods in sufficient detail to allow the statistician to evaluate them carefully, the text will be burdened with methodological digressions distracting to the reader interested only in findings and interpretations. If we show our results in such a form that the reader could try alternative modes of analysis, the tables would be far too voluminous to publish. (Well over 5,000 tables were run off for the study, though we have by no means fully analyzed all of them in preparing the present report.) The inevitable compromise requires us to ask the reader to take some things on faith (though his suspicions may well be aroused) and to accept our pattern of analysis however much he would have preferred another.

The more basic dilemma had to be confronted near the beginning of our planning for the study. We wanted to examine a significant number of possible determinants of status achievement and not merely to describe patterns of occupational mobility. Further, we wished to consider several such determinants simultaneously, that is, examine the influence on occupational success of entire sets of variables. We could not go very far in this direction using classical methods of multivariate analysis through cross-tabulations. Even with drastic collapsing of categories and class intervals—a procedure introducing errors of its own peculiar type—simultaneous cross-tabulations of several factors would yield tables in which many cells are too small for statistical reliability.

Thus we had to consider statistical techniques making stronger *a priori* assumptions than those underlying conventional cross-tabulation analysis. Unfortunately, the counterpart of such assumptions is the possibility that they do not apply to the data at hand. If a relationship is truly linear, two parameters—an intercept and a slope coefficient—suffice to describe it. If it is not linear, then a straight line is only a more or less adequate approximation. As is the case with the assumption of linearity, we may for most assumptions adopt the pragmatic attitude that some departure from their literal truth may be tolerated if the assumptions facilitate an analytical objective. Yet it is often difficult to know if one has exceeded a legitimate level of tolerance and, especially, to comprehend what the consequences of sizable violations of assumptions may be.

We have sought a way out of this dilemma that will put some burden upon the reader. Instead of using only one or two techniques, with attendant greater or lesser severity of assumptions, we have varied the techniques and consequently the assumptions. With some techniques we clearly go well beyond the point where the requisite assumptions can be at all rigorously justified. This venture, however, will—to the extent possible—be counterpoised by alternative treatments of the same data, avoiding at least some of the questionable assumptions.

A number of our analytical procedures are so simple and conventional that no separate methodological discussion is required. We have used some techniques that are not so conventional, but they are most readily explained at the point where they are required. In this chapter, following the discussion of a problem in measurement, we are concerned with standard techniques applied to problems involving interrelations of three or more variables: multiple classification, regression, and covariance. Each of these is well known, but our particular applications raise some issues needing explicit discussion for the benefit of the reader interested in methodological problems of the study. Finally, we present a technique for analyzing mobility distributions that avoids certain assumptions of the foregoing procedures.

MEASURING THE STATUS OF OCCUPATIONS

In this research we have followed a well-established sociological tradition: the concern with the "vertical" aspect of occupational mobility. This preoccupation is so commonplace one sometimes forgets that it involves a rather drastic abstraction. Although the matter has not been adequately studied, there surely are characteristics of occupations affecting the interchange between them quite apart from their relative position in a hierarchy of prestige or socioeconomic status. The OCG tables show, for example, that a man whose first job is laborer in a manufacturing industry is more likely to move to a craft occupation in manufacturing than to an operative job in a nonmanufacturing industry, though the former move involves a greater "social distance" on a prestige or status scale. The occupation structure intersects with other structures, such as industry, and is differentiated by a variety of factors, such as region, locality, and ethnic group. Hence there are "channels" of mobility—or factors governing access to occupational roles—that complicate the patterns of movement as compared to what can be expected on the simple metaphor of a social elevator going up or down.

If the focus on vertical mobility, therefore, involves a simplification of the actual process by which individuals find their way into occupational roles, it is nonetheless a justifiable simplification. To study one aspect of a complex phenomenon is not to deny that other aspects exist. The sociologist has an ulterior aim in directing his attention to the status hierarchy of occupations. He assumes not only that performance of an occupational role confers occupational status, but also that the latter interacts with other status attributes that in their overall configuration amount to a system of social stratification. A rather special saliency, moreover, is assumed to characterize occupational status, by comparison with other status attributes.

A partial justification of these several assumptions emerged from results using the Guttman-Lingoes program reported in Chapter 2, which showed that the major dimension underlying the social distance between occupations (as manifest in movements) is their relative status. We are encouraged to proceed with a more systematic method of assessing occupational status. In certain earlier studies of occupational mobility the research workers faced the preliminary task of establishing an occupational scale before they could undertake the main task of measuring movement along that scale.[1] We were in a more fortunate position in the OCG study, since some substantial work on occupational status had been completed before we commenced the survey.

Two approaches have dominated the investigations of occupational hierarchy carried out by students of social stratification. One is the effort to develop a socioeconomic classification scheme for occupations. Perhaps the most influential work here was that of the census statistician Alba M. Edwards.[2] His "social-economic grouping" of occupations has been widely used in studies of occupational stratification and mobility. With certain modifications it led to the "major occupation groups" used by the Bureau of the Census since 1940. These groups (or condensations or expansions of them) appear in various sections of the present study. To suggest that his grouping supplied a "scale," Edwards contented himself with showing differences in average or typical levels of education and income of the workers included in the several categories: "Education is a very large factor in the social status of workers, and wage or salary income is a very large factor in their economic status."[3]

A more recent development is the derivation of scores for *detailed* census occupation titles representing a composite index of education and income levels of workers in each such occupation. Priority for this specific technique probably belongs to social scientists in Canada,[4]

---

[1] D. V. Glass (Ed.), *Social Mobility in Britain*, Glencoe: Free Press, 1954; Kaare Svalastoga, *Prestige, Class, and Mobility*, Copenhagen: Gyldendal, 1959.

[2] Alba M. Edwards, *Comparative Occupation Statistics for the United States, 1870 to 1940*, Washington: Government Printing Office, 1943.

[3] *Ibid.*, p. 180.

[4] Enid Charles, *The Changing Size of the Family in Canada*, Census Monograph No. One, Eighth Census of Canada, 1941, Ottawa: The Kings Printer and Controller

with a similar approach being taken in this country by both a private research worker[5] and, lately, in official publications of the U. S. Bureau of the Census.[6]

The second approach to occupational stratification is to secure, from samples more or less representative of the general public, ratings of the "general standing" or "prestige" of selected occupations. Such ratings have been shown to be remarkably close to invariant with respect to (a) the composition and size of the sample of raters; (b) the specific instructions or form of the rating scale; (c) the interpretation given by respondents to the notion of "general standing"; and (d) the passage of time.[7] The high order of reliability and stability evidenced by prestige ratings would commend their use in problems requiring social distance scaling of the occupations pursued by a general sample of the working force, but for one fact: ratings have hitherto been available only for relatively small numbers of occupation titles. Many research workers have resorted to ingenious schemes for splicing *ad hoc* judgments into the series of rated occupations, but no general solution to the problem has been widely accepted.

Work currently in progress at the National Opinion Research Center promises to overcome this difficulty by supplying prestige ratings for a comprehensive list of occupations. In the absence of such ratings at the time of the OCG survey we fell back on the idea of a socioeconomic index of occupational status. The particular index we used, however, was one designed to give near-optimal reproduction of a set of prestige ratings. A full account of the construction of this index is given elsewhere,[8] and only a few general points need to be made before presenting some illustrations of the scale values assigned to occupations.

In the derivation of the socioeconomic index of occupational status, prestige ratings obtained from a sizable sample of the U. S. population

of Stationery, 1948; Bernard R. Blishen, "The Construction and Use of an Occupational Class Scale," *Canadian Journal of Economics and Political Science*, 24(1958), 519-531.

5 Donald J. Bogue, *Skid Row in American Cities*, Chicago: Community and Family Study Center, University of Chicago, 1963, Chapter 14 and Appendix B.

6 U. S. Bureau of the Census, *Methodology and Scores of Socioeconomic Status*, Working Paper, No. 15 (1963); U. S. Bureau of the Census, "Socioeconomic Characteristics of the Population: 1960," *Current Population Reports*, Series P-23, No. 12 (July 31, 1964).

7 Albert J. Reiss, Jr., *et al.*, *Occupations and Social Status*, New York: Free Press of Glencoe, 1961; Robert W. Hodge, Paul M. Siegel, and Peter H. Rossi, "Occupational Prestige in the United States, 1925-63," *American Journal of Sociology*, 70 (1964), 286-302.

8 Otis Dudley Duncan, "A Socioeconomic Index for All Occupations," in Reiss, *op. cit.*, pp. 109-138.

in 1947 were taken as the criterion. These were available for 45 occupations whose titles closely matched those in the census detailed list. Data in the 1950 Census of Population were converted to two summary measures: per cent of male workers with four years of high school or a higher level of educational attainment, and per cent with incomes of $3,500 or more in 1949 (both variables being age-standardized). The multiple regression of per cent "excellent" or "good" prestige ratings on the education and income measures was calculated. The multiple correlation, with the 45 occupations as units of observation, came out as .91, implying that five-sixths of the variation in aggregate prestige ratings was taken into account by the combination of the two socioeconomic variables. Using the regression weights obtained in this calculation, all census occupations were assigned scores on the basis of their education and income distributions. Such scores may be interpreted either as estimates of (unknown) prestige ratings or simply as values on a scale of occupational socioeconomic status ("occupational status" for short). The scale is represented by two-digit numbers ranging from 0 to 96. It closely resembles the scales of Blishen, Bogue, and the U. S. Bureau of the Census mentioned earlier, although there are various differences in detail among the four sets of scores.

One of the most serious issues in using any index of occupational status in the study of mobility has to do with the problem of temporal stability. For the oldest cohorts in the OCG study, we were asking about a father's occupation and a first job that may have been pursued as long ago as before World War I. We know that the occupational structure—in the sense of the relative numbers working in the several occupations—has undergone pronounced change since that time. Many new occupations have risen to prominence, whereas old ones have diminished to virtual insignificance. Granted that the OCG respondents could be accurately graded by occupational status as of 1962 and the preceding few years, can we assume that the status scale is valid for much more remote periods?

Fortunately, we now have a detailed study of temporal stability in occupational prestige ratings. The results are astonishing to most sociologists who have given the matter only casual thought. A set of ratings obtained as long ago as 1925 is correlated to the extent of .93 with the latest set available, obtained in 1963. The analysts conclude, "There have been no substantial changes in occupational prestige in the United States since 1925."[9] Less complete evidence is available for

9 Hodge, Siegel, and Rossi, *op. cit.*, p. 296.

the socioeconomic components of our index, but information available in the Censuses of 1940, 1950, and 1960 points to a comparably high order of temporal stability,[10] despite major changes in the value of the dollar and the generally rising levels of educational attainment.

Like previous investigators,[11] we have assumed, *faute de mieux,* that the scale of occupational status remained fixed over the half-century spanned by our current and retrospective data. Unlike such investigators, we have been able to point to some bodies of evidence supporting the approximate validity of this assumption. As compared with the unreliability in the basic reports on occupation itself, the error induced by historical variation in relative status of the occupations is likely to be minor.

Two-digit status scores are available for 446 detailed occupation titles. Of these, 270 are specific occupation categories; the remainder are subgroupings, based on industry or class of worker, of 13 general occupation categories. The reader may consult the source publication for the scores of particular occupations of interest.[12] Here we shall only illustrate the variation of the scores by citing illustrative occupations, not always those of the greatest numerical importance (see Table 4.1). In most of the OCG tabulations scores were grouped into five-point intervals, and the interval midpoints were used in computing summary statistics.

Table 4.1 makes it clear that occupations of very different character may have similar status scores. In particular, there is considerable overlap of scores of occupations in distinct major occupation groups. Indeed, only five points separate the lowest occupation in the "professional, technical, and kindred workers" group from the highest among "laborers, except farm and mine." Nevertheless, the major occupation group classification accounts for three-fourths of the variation in scores among detailed occupations. The status scores offer a useful refinement of the coarser classification but not a radically different pattern of grading.

Table 4.1 probably does not illustrate adequately the variation by industry subclass of such occupation categories as "operatives, not elsewhere classified" and "laborers, not elsewhere classified." Such variation is fairly substantial. It must be understood, however, that particularly at these levels of the census classification scheme the oc-

10 Reiss, *op. cit.,* p. 152. (Work in progress by Hodge and Treiman further supports this point.)

11 Glass, *op. cit.,* p. 178.

12 Duncan, *op. cit.,* Table B-1, pp. 263-275.

TABLE 4.1.   OCCUPATIONS ILLUSTRATING VARIOUS

Score Interval	Title of Occupation (Frequency per 10,000 Males in 1960 Experienced Civilian Labor Force in Parentheses)
90 to 96	Architects (7); dentists (18); chemical engineers (9); lawyers and judges (45); physicians and surgeons (47)
85 to 89	Aeronautical engineers (11); industrial engineers (21); salaried managers, banking and finance (30); self-employed proprietors, banking and finance (5)
80 to 84	College presidents, professors and instructors (31); editors and reporters (14); electrical engineers (40); pharmacists (19); officials, federal public administration and postal service (13); salaried managers, business services (11)
75 to 79	Accountants and auditors (87); chemists (17); veterinarians (3); salaried managers, manufacturing (133); self-employed proprietors, insurance and real estate (9)
70 to 74	Designers (12); teachers (105); store buyers and department heads (40); credit men (8); salaried managers, wholesale trade (41); self-employed proprietors, motor vehicles and accessories retailing (12); stock and bond salesmen (6)
65 to 69	Artists and art teachers (15); draftsmen (45); salaried managers, motor vehicles and accessories retailing (18); self-employed proprietors, apparel and accessories retail stores (8); agents, n.e.c. (29); advertising agents and salesmen (7); salesmen, manufacturing (93); foremen, transportation equipment manufacturing (18)
60 to 64	Librarians (3); sports instructors and officials (12); postmasters (5); salaried managers, construction (31); self-employed proprietors, manufacturing (35); stenographers, typists, and secretaries (18); ticket, station, and express agents (12); real estate agents and brokers (33); salesmen, wholesale trade (106); foremen, machinery manufacturing (28); photoengravers and lithographers (5)
55 to 59	Funeral directors and embalmers (8); railroad conductors (10); self-employed proprietors, wholesale trade (28); electrotypers and stereotypers (2); foremen, communications, utilities, and sanitary services (12); locomotive engineers (13)
50 to 54	Clergymen (43); musicians and music teachers (19); officials and administrators, local public administration (15); salaried managers, food and dairy products stores (21); self-employed proprietors, construction (50); bookkeepers (33); mail carriers (43); foremen, metal industries (28); toolmakers, and die-makers and setters (41)
45 to 49	Surveyors (10); salaried managers, automobile repair services and garages (4); office machine operators (18); linemen and servicemen, telephone, telegraph and power (60); locomotive firemen (9); airplane mechanics and repairmen (26); stationary engineers (60)
40 to 44	Self-employed proprietors, transportation (8); self-employed proprietors, personal services (19); cashiers (23); clerical and kindred workers, n.e.c. (269); electricians (77); construction foremen (22); motion picture projectionists (4); photographic process workers (5); railroad switchmen (13); policemen and detectives, government (51)

cupation-industry categories represent groups of jobs with quite heterogeneous specifications, although the groups are thought to be somewhat homogeneous as to the degree of skill and experience required for their performance. No one has yet faced the question of what a

SCORES ON THE INDEX OF OCCUPATIONAL STATUS*

Score Interval	Title of Occupation (Frequency per 10,000 Males in 1960 Experienced Civilian Labor Force in Parentheses)
35 to 39	Salaried and self-employed managers and proprietors, eating and drinking places (43); salesmen and sales clerks, retail trade (274); bookbinders (3); radio and television repairmen (23); firemen, fire protection (30); policemen and detectives, private (3)
30 to 34	Building managers and superintendents (7); self-employed proprietors, gasoline service stations (32); boilermakers (6); machinists (111); millwrights (15); plumbers and pipe fitters (72); structural metal workers (14); tinsmiths, coppersmiths, and sheet metal workers (31); deliverymen and routemen (93); operatives, printing, publishing and allied industries (13); sheriffs and bailiffs (5)
25 to 29	Messengers and office boys (11); newsboys (41); brickmasons, stonemasons, and tile setters (45); mechanics and repairmen, n.e.c. (266); plasterers (12); operatives, drugs and medicine manufacturing (2); ushers, recreation and amusement (2); laborers, petroleum refining (3)
20 to 24	Telegraph messengers (1); shipping and receiving clerks (59); bakers (21); cabinetmakers (15); excavating, grading, and road machine operators (49); railroad and car shop mechanics and repairmen (9); tailors (7); upholsterers (12); bus drivers (36); filers, grinders, and polishers, metal (33); welders and flame-cutters (81)
15 to 19	Blacksmiths (5); carpenters (202); automobile mechanics and repairmen (153); painters (118) attendants, auto service and parking (81); laundry and dry cleaning operatives (25); truck and tractor drivers (362); stationary firemen (20); operatives, metal industries (103); operatives, wholesale and retail trade (35); barbers (38); bartenders (36); cooks, except private household (47)
10 to 14	Farmers (owners and tenants)(521); shoemakers and repairers, except factory (8); dyers (4); taxicab drivers and chauffeurs (36); attendants, hospital and other institution (24); elevator operators (11); fishermen and oystermen (9); gardeners, except farm, and groundskeepers (46); longshoremen and stevedores (13); laborers, machinery manufacturing (10)
5 to 9	Hucksters and peddlers (5); sawyers (20); weavers, textile (8); operatives, footwear, except rubber, manufacturing (16); janitors and sextons (118); farm laborers, wage workers (241); laborers, blast furnaces, steel works, and rolling mills (26); construction laborers (163)
0 to 4	Coal mine operatives and laborers (31); operatives, yarn, thread and fabric mills (30); porters (33); laborers, saw mills, planing mills, and millwork (21)

*n.e.c. means "not elsewhere classified"

SOURCES: Reiss, op. cit., Table B-1; and U.S. Bureau of the Census, 1960 Census of Population, Final Report, PC(1)-1D, Table 201.

study of occupational mobility would look like if all the 20,000 or more detailed titles in the *Dictionary of Occupational Titles* were coded without prior grouping.

The use of occupational status scores carries a theoretical implication. We are assuming, in effect, that the occupation structure is more or less continuously graded in regard to status rather than being a set of discrete status classes. The justification of such an assumption is not difficult. One needs only to look at any tabulation of social and economic characteristics of persons engaged in each specific occupation (whatever the level of refinement in the system of occupational nomenclature). We discover that the occupations overlap—to a greater or lesser degree, to be sure—in their distributions of income, educational attainment, consumer expenditures, measured intelligence, political orientations, and residential locations (to mention but a few items). One may sometimes find evidence supporting the interpretation that there are "natural breaks" in such distributions. Interpretations of this kind were advanced in Chapter 2 in respect to the dividing line between farm and nonfarm and between white-collar and manual occupations. The evidence did not permit the conclusion that such occupation categories are entirely disjunct. The analysis in the last two chapters, while it suggests that boundaries may be discerned between the three broad groups, also shows that these are by no means sharp lines without any overlap.

If we choose to think of occupational status as exhibiting continuous variation, the appropriate analytical model is one that treats status as a quantitative variable. This point of view has far-reaching implications for the conceptualization of the process of mobility as well as for the analysis and manipulation of data purporting to describe the process. The repertory of statistical techniques on which we shall draw in this study, therefore, differs somewhat from the set that is conventional in mobility studies, although the techniques are quite standard in other contexts.

When deciding to work with the status index in the OCG study we were aware of one apparent source of spurious results, pointed out (in private communications) by friendly critics of an earlier regression analysis of social mobility.[13] This has to do with the fact that educational attainment is a component of the index used to measure occupational achievement, whereas education appears as an independent variable in the regression equation used to predict occupational achievement. Is not a high correlation between occupation and education built into the status index, and is not the regression analysis producing findings based on circular reasoning? The criticism is

[13] Otis Dudley Duncan and Robert W. Hodge, "Education and Occupational Mobility," *American Journal of Sociology,* **68**(1963), 629-644.

germane, and the critics' point must somehow be met.

We recall that the status index is based on the empirical regression formula

$$\hat{X}_1 = 0.59 \, X_2 + 0.55 \, X_3 - 6.0,$$

where X_1 is the percentage of "excellent" or "good" ratings received by an occupation in the prestige survey, X_2 the proportion of men in the occupation with 1949 incomes of \$3,500 or more, and X_3 the proportion of men in the occupation with four years of high school or higher educational attainment. The coefficient of determination for the 45 occupations is $R^2_{1(23)} = .83$. Using these weights for X_2 and X_3 it was possible to assign a status score (or estimated prestige score) to each occupation for which census data were available.

In the regression analysis of factors affecting individual occupational achievement, each occupation (respondent's and father's) was first coded in terms of the census detailed code, and then recoded to the two-digit status score. Thenceforth the score was treated as a number measuring the individual's occupational socioeconomic status. Note that the occupational status scores were *derived* from *aggregate* data on all males in each occupation category, but *applied* as scores characterizing *individuals*.

The first response to the critics, then, might be that the status score, interpreted as an estimate of occupational prestige, should legitimately reflect the fact that one determinant of an occupation's prestige is, in fact, the educational level of its incumbents. But because not all persons in an occupation have the same educational attainment, the formula for the status score does not by any means produce a perfect correlation between the estimated prestige of the *individual's* occupation and his educational attainment. On the other hand, in the light of our rather full knowledge of occupational prestige,[14] no acceptable estimate of occupational prestige could fail to show *some* appreciable correlation between an individual's education and the prestige of the occupation in which he is engaged. It could be argued, in other words, that the apparent circularity of the procedure that was followed is simply a realistic reflection of the fact that high-prestige occupations do recruit men with superior education whereas low-prestige occupations recruit men with inferior schooling, by and large.

---

14 Reiss, *op. cit.;* Hodge, Siegel, and Rossi, *loc. cit.*

Another approach was taken, however, to ascertain what difference it would make in the results of a mobility study if an alternative index of occupational status were used—one not explicitly including an educational component. Instead of educational level the alternative index uses a dummy variable, Z, that refers to whether an occupation is white-collar ($Z = 1$) or manual ($Z = 0$). Prestige rating (X_1) was estimated from two variables: income level of the occupation as defined above (X_2); and the nonmanual-manual dichotomy (Z), for the same criterion group of 45 occupations. The following empirical formula was obtained:

$$\hat{X}_1 = 0.79\,X_2 + 19.8\,Z + 3.9 \qquad (R^2_{1(2Z)} = .76).$$

Note that the formula attributes a "bonus" of about 20 points for being in the white-collar group. In effect, we have two distinct formulas:

$$\hat{X}_1 = 0.79\,X_2 + 23.7, \qquad \text{for white-collar occupations;}$$

$$\hat{X}_1 = 0.79\,X_2 + 3.9, \qquad \text{for manual occupations.}$$

For any close student of occupational characteristics it will be no surprise to learn that the correlation between the original and the alternative formula, over the 45 occupations, is as high as .96. Yet the alternative formula does not include education as a predictor. Hence if occupational status were scored according to the alternative formula and the scores were employed in a regression analysis of occupational mobility no possible suspicion of circularity could be attached to a correlation between the occupational statuses of individuals and their educational attainment.

How much difference would it have made in the findings, had the alternative procedure been employed? To answer this question a portion of the data used by Duncan and Hodge[15] were recoded, using the alternative scoring of occupational status.

The original results, in slightly altered form, are shown alongside the revised results in Table 4.2. (The letter symbols here have different meanings than in the preceding discussion of index construction.) The reader should evaluate the comparison for himself. It appears that no important substantive conclusions in the original report would require change if the alternative results were accepted. In the revised results the estimated direct effect of father's occupation (X) on respondent's occupation in 1950 (Y_2) falls below twice its standard

[15] Duncan and Hodge, *loc. cit.*

TABLE 4.2. REGRESSION ANALYSIS: RESPONDENT'S OCC. ON EDUCATION AND FATHER'S OCC, WITH OCC. STATUS SCORED BY ALTERNATIVE FORMULAS, FOR 381 WHITE MALES WITH NONFARM BACKGROUND, 35 TO 44 YEARS OLD, IN THE CHICAGO LABOR MOBILITY SAMPLE, 1951

	Published Results[a]				Revised Results		
		Correlation Matrix					
	U	Y_1	Y_2		U	Y_1	Y_2
X	.4285	.3470	.3145	X	.4200	.2972	.2835
U	....	.4270	.5335	U	....	.3749	.5155
Y_1	....	....	.5517	Y_1	....	....	.5113

	Regression Coefficients in Standard Form[b]								
Dep. Var.	Coefficient of --			R^2	Dep. Var.	Coefficient of --			R^2
	X	U	Y_1			X	U	Y_1	
Y_2	.105	.488	...	.29	Y_2	.082	.481	...	.27
Y_1	.201	.341	...	.22	Y_1	.170	.304	...	.16
Y_2	.027	.355	.391	.41	Y_2	.019	.370	.367	.38

	Path Decomposition[c] of Effect of X						
	Total	Direct	Indirect		Total	Direct	Indirect
for Y_2	.314	.105	.209	for Y_2	.284	.082	.202
for Y_1	.347	.201	.146	for Y_1	.297	.170	.127

[a]Duncan and Hodge, loc. cit.
[b]Standard error for each coefficient is approximately .05.
[c]Slight variation from published figures is due to omission of squared term for education.

NOTE: Variables are defined as follows:
   Y_2: Respondent's occ. status, 1950.
   Y_1: Respondent's occ. status, 1940.
   U : Respondent's educational attainment.
   X : Father's occ. status.

error, whereas the original results clearly warranted rejection of the null hypothesis of no net effect for X. The revised results therefore support, even more strongly than the initial ones, the original conclusion that the major influence of father's occupation on respondent's occupation is exerted indirectly, via its influence on respondent's education. Indeed, the revised results imply that its only significant influence is the indirect one via education. The revision certainly does not point to a lesser role of education in the process of occupational mobility than had been estimated previously. In view of the general similarity of the two sets of results we proceed on the assumption that a comparable alteration of the occupational status index used in the OCG analysis would also leave the main results intact.

MULTIPLE-CLASSIFICATION ANALYSIS

This technique was used whenever the problem was in the following form: one dependent variable, regarded as quantitative (i.e., measured on an interval scale), and two or more independent variables, each regarded as qualitative or classificatory. (Any quantitative variable can, of course, be transformed into such a classificatory one.) In the case of the classificatory variables no assumption is made about the order of the several categories comprising the classification. If the categories are taken to be in some order the information about order is not used in obtaining the solution, though it may be considered in interpreting the result. It follows that the technique makes no prior assumption as to the form of the relationship of the dependent variable to any of the classificatory variables or of the classificatory variables with one another. Hence there is no assumption of linearity or even monotonicity.

The basic idea behind the method is essentially that of comparing a set of means. Suppose Y is the (quantitative) dependent variable, $\overline{Y}$ is the grand mean for the entire sample, and $\overline{Y}_h$ is the mean for that part of the sample falling in category h of a classificatory variable, say W. Then the *nature* of the relationship between Y and W is specified by exhibiting the variation in $\overline{Y}_h$ as h ranges over all the categories of W. The *degree* of the relationship has to do with the amount of variation noted in the category means, $\overline{Y}_h$. Ordinarily we compute the between-class sum of squares, $\sum_h n_h (\overline{Y}_h - \overline{Y})^2$, where n_h is the number of cases in category h, and relate it to the total sum of squares, $\sum (Y - \overline{Y})^2$, where the summation is over all cases in the sample. The ratio, between-class/total, is referred to as the proportion of total sum of squares in Y accounted for by W. The square root of this proportion is termed the correlation ratio, symbolized by η_{YW}.

Clearly, we could carry out a parallel analysis for another classificatory variable, say U, where $\overline{Y}_i$ is the mean of the dependent variable for category i of U. We should then have as a summary of the degree of relationship the proportion of total sum of squares in Y accounted for by U, or η^2_{YU}.

Now, suppose we wish to make some statement about the relationship of Y to both W and U, considering the two classificatory variables simultaneously. One way to proceed would be to form a new classificatory variable, say T, with a category for each cell of the cross-classification, W-by-U. As before, we may examine the category means $\overline{Y}_{hi}$ and compare their variation $\Sigma n_{hi}(\overline{Y}_{hi} - \overline{Y})^2$ with the total sum of squares in Y. Note that the number of categories in T is equal to the *product* of the number in W and the number in U. Hence, if we extend the analysis to further classificatory variables, all considered simultaneously, this method demands that the data be available in complete cross-classifications. Moreover, the geometric increase in number of cells as variables are added implies that the number of observations per cell diminishes rapidly and hence that our description of the nature of the multiple relationship becomes quite complex while the individual cell means become less and less reliable (in terms of sampling variation).

We are, therefore, motivated to consider a procedure that does not use up the data in quite so prodigal a fashion. Such a procedure is available, although its use exacts a price: we must make an assumption about the nature of the *multiple* relationship that may be contrary to fact. Even so, we may tolerate the assumption inasmuch as it permits us to deal with several classifications simultaneously, a possibility that is virtually foreclosed on practical grounds if we insist on getting along without any assumptions as to the nature of the relationship.

Suppose it is true that the nature of the multiple relationship of Y to W and U is like this: If we look at the variation of the means $\overline{Y}_{hi}$ we find the same *pattern* as h varies, whatever value of i we specify, and the same pattern as i varies, whatever value of h we fix upon. Algebraically, this says that the cell means of Y in the cross-classification of W by U can be written as follows:

$$\overline{Y}_{hi} = m + w_h + u_i,$$

where m is a constant that applies in all cells; w_h is a constant that applies when we are in row h of the cross-classification; and u_i is a constant that applies when we are in column i. This, therefore, is an additive model, which says that we are dealing with a set of row effects (one for each value of h) and a set of column effects (one for each value of i), but that we need not posit any cell effects apart from those given by the sum of the particular row and column effects for the designated cell. In brief, the model assumes no interaction. The simplification obtained, if this model is satisfactory, is obviously a considerable one. The procedure first described required us to recognize as many different cell effects as there are cells in the cross-classification of W by U, that is, as many as the *product* of the number of rows times the number of columns. The additive model says that the number of distinct effects is only as great as the *sum* of the number of rows and the number of columns in the cross-classification. In view of the obvious economy of the additive model we might well be prepared to accept it as a sufficiently precise description of the data, even if we know that it is not literally correct.

But whence come the additive effects that are posited in this model? We began by describing how one might examine the sets of $\overline{Y}_h$ and $\overline{Y}_i$, studying the relationship, respectively, of Y to W and to U, each without regard to the other. One might suspect that the additive effects in the multiple relationship are some simple function of these category-specific means. This is indeed the case, *if* it happens to be true that W and U are statistically independent, that is, that $n_{hi} = n_h n_i / N$ for all values of h and i. In observational (as opposed to experimental) data, however, we are unlikely to encounter cases of this kind. If W and U are associated rather than independent, we must take account of that association in estimating their respective additive effects. In doing so we are, as it were, adjusting the observed means for each classification in the light of the association (or "correlation") of the classifications.

There are several ways to describe the rationale on which we obtain estimates of the "adjusted," "additive," or "net" effects of the classificatory variables. The reader who wishes to secure a full understanding of the properties of the model and the estimation procedure can only be advised to consult several expositions written from slightly different points of view.[16] Here we must be satisfied with an abbreviated illustration.

Suppose, concretely, that there are just three categories of W and three of U; that is, that $h = 1, 2, 3$ and $i = 1, 2, 3$. We have, then, to obtain the general constant of the model (m), three net effects for W (w_1, w_2, w_3) and three for U (u_1, u_2, u_3). Actually, we shall obtain the solution in a form that requires that the general constant is simply the grand mean: $m = \overline{Y}$. We have to solve the following set of equations:

[16] T. P. Hill, "An Analysis of the Distribution of Wages and Salaries in Great Britain," *Econometrica*, **27**(1959), 355-381; D. B. Suits, "Use of Dummy Variables in Regression Equations," *Journal of the American Statistical Association*, **52**(1957), 548-551; J. N. Morgan, *et al.*, *Income and Welfare in the United States*, New York: McGraw-Hill, 1962, Appendix E; Walter R. Harvey, *Least Squares Analysis of Data with Unequal Subclass Numbers*, ARS-20-8 (Washington: U. S. Department of Agriculture, Agricultural Research Service, July 1960); Emanuel Melichar, "Least-Squares Analysis of Economic Survey Data," *1965 Proceedings of the Business and Economic Statistics Section, American Statistical Association*, Washington: American Statistical Association (1966), pp. 373-385.

$$n_{1.}w_1 + 0 + 0 + n_{11}u_1 + n_{12}u_2 + n_{13}u_3 = n_{1.}(\overline{Y}_{1.} - \overline{Y})$$

$$0 + n_{2.}w_2 + 0 + n_{21}u_1 + n_{22}u_2 + n_{23}u_3 = n_{2.}(\overline{Y}_{2.} - \overline{Y})$$

$$0 + 0 + n_{3.}w_3 + n_{31}u_1 + n_{32}u_2 + n_{33}u_3 = n_{3.}(\overline{Y}_{3.} - \overline{Y})$$

$$n_{11}w_1 + n_{21}w_2 + n_{31}w_3 + n_{.1}u_1 + 0 + 0 = n_{.1}(\overline{Y}_{.1} - \overline{Y})$$

$$n_{12}w_1 + n_{22}w_2 + n_{32}w_3 + 0 + n_{.2}u_2 + 0 = n_{.2}(\overline{Y}_{.2} - \overline{Y})$$

$$n_{13}w_1 + n_{23}w_2 + n_{33}w_3 + 0 + 0 + n_{.3}u_3 = n_{.3}(\overline{Y}_{.3} - \overline{Y})$$

We are here using the conventional notation for a cross-classification table: n_{23} stands for the frequency in the second row, third column; $n_{2.}$ is the (marginal) frequency for row 2. The three means in the set $\overline{Y}_h$ are $\overline{Y}_{1.}$, $\overline{Y}_{2.}$, and $\overline{Y}_{3.}$ and the three in the set $\overline{Y}_i$ are $\overline{Y}_{.1}$, $\overline{Y}_{.2}$, $\overline{Y}_{.3}$. The reader may observe that we have six unknowns (the w's and u's) but not six independent equations. The sum of the first three equations is equal to the sum of the last three. We require additional conditions for a solution. For convenience (and it is no more than that) we specify that the weighted sum of the net effects for W shall be zero, and the same for the net effects for U:

$$n_{1.}w_1 + n_{2.}w_2 + n_{3.}w_3 = 0; \quad n_{.1}u_1 + n_{.2}u_2 + n_{.3}u_3 = 0.$$

On these conventions we force the general constant m to equal the grand mean $\overline{Y}$, and can interpret the net effects as deviations from the grand mean.

A study of the normal equations will disclose why the multiple-classification solution is referred to as an adjustment of the observed means that go with the W and U classifications. If $n_{hi} = n_h.n_{.i}/N$ (the condition of statistical independence), then in the first equation, for example, the sum of the terms in u_i would vanish, by virtue of the condition stated at the end of the preceding paragraph. Then $w_1 = \overline{Y}_{1.} - \overline{Y}$, and the additive effect is merely the deviation of the Y-mean for the first category of W from the grand mean of Y. Because the condition of independence does not hold, the additive effect will not, in general, be the same as the observed or "gross" deviation.

To summarize, although we have made no assumption about the relationship of Y to W and Y to U, individually, we do assume that the combination of their respective effects is additive. If the analyst is worried by this assumption, he can test its adequacy for a given set of data. Let the actual mean for cell (h, i) in the cross-classification of W by U be $\overline{Y}_{hi}$. Let the corresponding value estimated from the additive model be $\hat{Y}_{hi}$. We may then compare the sum of squares accounted for: $\Sigma n_{hi}(\overline{Y}_{hi} - \overline{Y})^2$ with $\Sigma n_{hi}(\hat{Y}_{hi} - \overline{Y})^2$. The former is necessarily larger, but not necessarily *significantly* larger. It may be that the departure from the additive model, or interaction, is readily attributed to random sampling variation of the individual cell means. The statistical technique of analysis of variance—where its assumptions are met—furnishes a test of this hypothesis.[17] In some investigations, where we are specifically concerned with theories that posit an appreciable interaction, we have carried out such tests. In most instances we have not done so, on the supposition that interactions could be neglected when they were not explicit in the formation of the classificatory variables themselves.

We shall not go into details on the matter of how to compute the sum of squares attributed to the combination of classifications in an additive model. The calculation can be carried out in a simpler fashion than is suggested by the definition $\Sigma n_{hi}(\hat{Y}_{hi} - \bar{Y})^2$. In particular, it is not necessary actually to compute the $\hat{Y}_{hi}$ to obtain the sum of squares due to the multiple classification. We shall, however, indicate some guides to interpretation of such sums of squares, since we shall be using them extensively as measures of the degree of relationship.

Although our illustration and discussion to this point have dealt with only two classificatory variables, the same sort of additive model can be developed for three or more classifications. If, for example, X is a third classification and x_j the net effect for its jth category, the additive model is:

$$\bar{Y}_{hij} = \bar{Y} + w_h + u_i + x_j + e_{hij},$$

where $e_{hij} = \bar{Y}_{hij} - \hat{Y}_{hij}$ is the difference between the actual mean of Y for cell (h, i, j) in the three-way cross-classification and the mean imputed on the basis of the additive model. The conditions given above for the solution guarantee that the weighted sum of such differences in any direction parallel to an axis of the three-dimensional classification is zero:

$$\sum_h n_{hij} e_{hij} = \sum_i n_{hij} e_{hij} = \sum_j n_{hij} e_{hij} = 0$$

ILLUSTRATION OF MULTIPLE-CLASSIFICATION ANALYSIS

Let us now turn to results of some actual calculation. The sample is all OCG respondents (20 to 64 years old). Y is the variable assumed to be measured on an interval scale: the status score for respondent's

[17] K. A. Brownlee, *Statistical Theory and Methodology in Science and Engineering*, New York: Wiley, 1960, pp. 515-521.

occupation in March 1962. W is first job, treated as a classificatory variable with 20 categories: 19 intervals of the occupation status score, plus a residual class of persons not stating first job. X is father's occupation, treated in the same way. U is respondent's educational attainment, in nine class intervals according to number of years of school completed. We have deliberately taken an example in which all three of the classificatory variables can be regarded as quantitative, so that a comparison can later be made between the results of linear-regression analysis and multiple-classification analysis.

In this example we examine the gross effects for each classification by itself, the net effects for each combination of two classifications, and the net effects for the combination of all three. Here is a summary, expressed in terms of percentage of total sum of squares (SS) in Y attributed to each classification or combination of classifications:

Independent Variables	Per Cent of Total SS(Y)
X, U, W	41.93
X, U	37.59
W, U	40.93
X, W	31.57
X	15.05
U	35.48
W	27.40

Listed first, because some readers will be anxious to know how much variation is "explained," is the proportion of total sum of squares attributed to the additive combination of the three classifications. It comes to nearly 42 per cent, not a trivial magnitude surely, but considerably short of exhausting the variation in the dependent variable.

Let us note first that this total is rather less than the total of the three sums of squares for the gross effects of the three classifications taken individually, which would be nearly 78 per cent of total SS(Y). This sum, however, has no meaning, except to show that there is, indeed, a good deal of "positive overlap" of the three classifications. The total of the three sums of squares for gross effects would exactly equal the sum of squares for the additive model in the event of statistical independence of the classificatory factors, or it could be less, in the event of "negative overlap." The latter eventuality, however, is somewhat rare, and is not to be expected in most of our analysis.

We may next study the differences between the per cent of total SS(Y) for the three-factor combination and that for the several two-factor combinations. For the combination (X, U, W) less the combination (X, U) we have $41.93 - 37.59 = 4.34$, termed the sum of squares for "direct" or "net effects" of W. Similarly, we find:

Net Effects of:	Per Cent of Total SS(Y)
X	1.00
U	10.36
W	4.34

The sum of these, 15.70, is far less than the percentage of total SS(Y) for the combination as such. This reveals, again, the extent of positive overlap of the classifications. In the event of no overlap, or statistical independence, the two sums would be equal (whereas negative overlap could render the sum of net effects greater than the per cent of total SS(Y) for the combination). Because the net effects do not sum up to the latter, there really is no way to say how much of the 42 per cent for the combination is due to each component classification. We may, if we like, say that 16 per cent is due to their respective net effects and 26 per cent to their overlapping, or correlated effects.

Still other ways of expressing the results may be useful in reaching an interpretation. If we look at W alone we have 27.40 per cent of total SS(Y) for its gross effects. Comparing this with the combination (W, U), we find an increment for U of 13.53 ($40.93 - 27.40$). Comparing (W, U) with (W, U, X), we obtain an increment for X in the latter combination of $41.93 - 40.93 = 1.00$ per cent of total SS(Y). In summary:[18]

Variables	Per Cent of Total SS(Y)
W, others ignored	27.40
U, with W fixed	13.53
X, with U and W fixed	1.00
Sum	41.93

This, however, is not a unique decomposition of the "explained" sum of squares. As a matter of fact it may be more plausible to compute the values in opposite sequence, in chronological order.

Variables	Per Cent of Total SS(Y)
X, others ignored	15.05
U, with X fixed	22.54
W, with U and X fixed	4.34
Sum	41.93

[18] Cf. L. N. Hazel, "The Covariance Analysis of Multiple Classification Tables with Unequal Subclass Numbers," *Biometrics Bulletin*, **2**(1946), 21-25.

Other such breakdowns can be worked out, but these seem to be the most interesting ones, if we assume a temporal or causal ordering of the variables $X—U—W—Y$. In the first decomposition we gave maximum importance to the most recent cause, so that (gross) per cent of total SS(Y) for W represents the direct effects of W plus all the effects of the other two variables that overlap with effects of W. We then divided the remainder so that we added to the direct effects of U, the next most recent cause, the effects due to its overlap with X (but not W). Finally, we attributed to X only its direct effects.

In the second partitioning, of course, we moved through the sequence in the opposite direction. Here, presumably, we are interested in knowing how much of the total variation in Y is attributable to the earliest cause, both directly and via its overlap with subsequent causes. Then, we ask, how much predictability of the dependent variable is gained from adding the second cause, irrespective of whether it works directly or via the third intervening variable. The figures reveal that occupational origins account, directly or indirectly, for 15 per cent of the variation in occupational achievement, education for an additional 23 per cent, and first jobs for another 4 per cent.

This sort of analysis is useful in demonstrating that there is no unique answer to the question of how important a particular variable is in a set of intercorrelated independent variables. The answer depends in part on point of view and the perspective from which we wish to venture an interpretation. The material for many such interpretations (in addition to the ones discussed in subsequent chapters) is given in Appendix H, "Summary of Results of Multiple-Classification Analysis."

All the discussion to this point has been in terms of *degree* of relationship, treated in terms of magnitude of variation to be attributed to single classificatory factors or combinations thereof. We turn to the question of the *nature* of the relationships.

Table 4.3 displays a summary of relevant information for one of the variables, U. Column 1 shows the estimated population (inflated sample) in each category of U. It is well to have this information, for two reasons: First, the weighted sum of both gross effects and net effects is zero. We sometimes see a set of effects in which only one category has a small positive deviation (observed or adjusted), whereas several others have large negative deviations. It is the weighting that makes this apparently anomalous result reasonable. Second, the contribution a category can make to a sum of squares depends on its size. In the example we would not change the sum of squares due to U very much by giving the "none" category any value it could

TABLE 4.3.   EFFECTS OF EDUCATIONAL ATTAINMENT ON OCC. STATUS IN 1962

Years of School Completed	Estimated Population (in Thousands) (1)	1962 Occ. (Means of Y) (2)	Observed Deviations (Gross Effects) (3)	Net Effects (Adjusted Deviations) Net of X[a] (4)	Net of W[a] (5)	Net of W,X (6)
Total	44,984	36.3	.0	.0	.0	.0
None	562	18.2	-18.1	-15.6	-13.8	-12.5
Elementary						
1 to 4 years	1,901	19.6	-16.7	-14.1	-12.7	-11.3
5 to 7 years	4,317	21.4	-14.9	-12.9	-11.7	-10.6
8 years	6,128	25.1	-11.2	- 9.5	- 8.4	- 7.5
High school						
1 to 3 years	8,478	28.8	- 7.5	- 7.0	- 5.9	- 5.6
4 years	12,788	37.6	1.3	1.0	1.2	1.0
College						
1 to 3 years	5,277	46.3	10.1	8.1	8.2	7.1
4 years	3,256	63.7	27.4	24.7	21.0	19.7
5 or more years	2,276	71.2	34.9	32.0	24.9	23.5

[a] X: Father's occupational status
   W: Status of first job.

possibly take, because 1 per cent of the population falls into this category. It may, of course, be a particularly interesting category for theoretical reasons, or because it is subject to special kinds of response error, and so on. These sorts of importance should not necessarily be taken to be identical with importance in producing variation on the dependent variable in the whole population.

In column 2 we have the observed mean of Y for each category of U. This is expressed as a deviation from the grand mean in the third column, which we shall take to represent the pattern or nature of the gross effects (as distinct from their degree of importance). Here, of course, it is natural to consider the order of the classes of U, though the order is not mathematically relevant to the proportion of sum of squares accounted for, nor to the values of the additive effects estimated from the multiple-classification model. Given the order, it is evident that Y is monotonically related to U: the higher a man's education, the higher, on the average, is his occupational status.

Finally, we have three sets of net effects, according to whether U is combined with X, with W, or with W and X in an additive model. The pattern of relationship of Y to U (that is, its monotonic form) remains intact when the other variables are taken into account. The individual net effects, however, tend to converge toward zero when one or both of the other classifications are fixed. Hence we see again that part of the gross influence of U on Y is due to overlap of effects of U with those of W and X. The analysis of sums of squares already

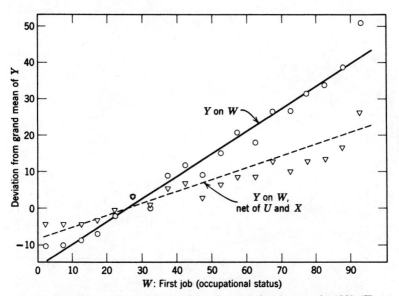

Figure 4.1. Gross and net relationship of occupational status in 1962 (Y) to occupational status of first job (W), based on multiple-classification and regression analysis.

given assures us that the net effects, though generally slighter than the gross effects of U, are nevertheless appreciable.

Turning to the other two independent variables, we depict the nature of the gross and net relationship of Y to X and W by means of graphic presentation. This will help to show the advisability of keeping in mind the order of categories (when there is a natural order), even though the information on order is not used in arriving at the statistical measures.

Figure 4.1 shows gross effects on Y for the W classification and net effects of W in the combination (W, U, X). These are analogous to columns 3 and 6 of Table 4.3. The straight lines are derived from linear regression calculations and will be discussed subsequently. For the moment they serve merely as guidelines for discerning the pattern of gross and net effects.

When the W classification is given in as much detail as is used here, there are apparently some fluctuations of the gross and net effects that cannot readily be interpreted. Despite these fluctuations the over-all drift of the data is clearly toward a monotonic relationship when the order of the W-classes is taken into account. Indeed, if these classes are assumed to be arrayed on an interval scale (as plotted), the relation-

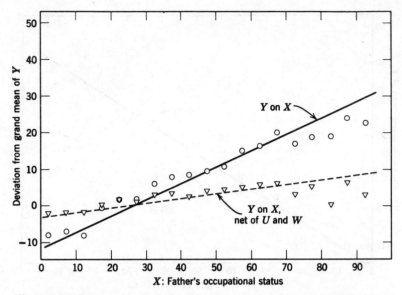

Figure 4.2. Gross and net relationship of occupational status in 1962 (Y) to father's occupational status (X), based on multiple-classification and regression analysis.

ship is not badly approximated by a straight line, although a slight tendency toward curvilinearity might be detected.

Much the same set of remarks applies to Figure 4.2, showing gross and net effects of the X-classification. Comparison of the two figures reveals the steeper slope for W, in conformity with the conclusions already reached from studying sums of squares, that occupational status is more influenced by early career than by social origins.

A few other points need to be remembered in studying Figures 4.1 and 4.2. Unlike Table 4.3, the graphic display does not call attention to variation in the population size of categories of the independent variables. At the upper end of the scale of both W and X there are several categories containing relatively small frequencies. We should, in consequence, expect greater random fluctuation of gross and net effects in this region of the chart. Also missing from the figure are gross and net effects for the NA category (men not answering the question on first job or father's occupation, respectively). As we mentioned, in obtaining the multiple-classification solution NA is simply treated as a category of the independent variable. When there is an NA category of the dependent variable it is given the mean value for all cases reporting. In the case of Y, NA actually refers to men not in the experienced civilian labor force; these men are all assumed to have an occupational status just equal to the average for all men in the civilian labor force. In the regression calculations NA cases on either the independent or the dependent variable were simply omitted from the calculation. This is a source of minor discrepancies between the regression results and those obtained in the multiple-classification analysis.

A number of other points enter into the interpretation of a set of results from an analysis of multiple classifications. It seems best, however, to take these up when they occur in connection with particular examples. In conclusion, it seems desirable to mention the problem of statistical inference. For the most part, we make little use of the formal apparatus of analysis of variance, including the several F-tests that are available for interactions, net effects, and so on. In part this represents our intuitive reliance on the supposition that we are in the realm of "large samples," where most effects that are large and consistent enough to be substantively interesting or interpretable are likely to show up as significant in terms of the conventions of statistical inference.

A second consideration is a suspicion that our data do not meet all the specifications for valid calculation of F-tests. The analysis-of-variance model assumes, in particular, that the individual observations on the dependent variable are independently and normally distributed with constant variance around the means estimated by the additive model. We have no way of checking the assumption that the data approximate this condition, since the detailed cross-classifications needed to test it simply were not run.

In this connection, however, we should like to call attention to an experiment reported by Hill, who analyzed a body of survey data somewhat resembling ours. The dependent variable was income, which, like our occupational status variables, has a highly skewed distribution. He used multiple-classification analysis with independent variables such as occupation, industry, age, town size, and region. A study of the distribution of residuals showed that "residuals from the additive model are obviously wildly heteroscedastic." Hill had, however, carried out a parallel analysis with a multiplicative model involving the same multiple classification. That is, he used the logarithm of income as the dependent variable. Here he found that "the variance of the logarithmic residuals is fairly stable."[19] Perhaps we may assume that the logarithmic transformation—which is, in fact, a

[19] Hill, *op. cit.*, p. 374.

rather drastic transformation—yielded a superior analysis from the standpoint of statistical inference. If so, it is interesting that the two models yielded quite comparable results from the descriptive standpoint. The patterns of gross and net effects for most of the classifications were much alike. The additive model for all classifications in combination accounted for 49 per cent of total sum of squares of the dependent variable, the multiplicative model for 47 per cent. (Hill does not report sums of squares for gross and net effects of the individual classificatory variables.)

The method of multiple classification as employed in this study is no doubt crude in several respects. Yet it serves to reduce a very considerable quantity of data in what we believe is basically a sound framework, if regarded as a first approximation. Moreover, we have supplemented the results obtained with it by using other methods in particular instances. We have not aimed at the ultimate of elegance in statistical analysis but at a useful summary of a number of interesting relationships that had not hitherto been described.

REGRESSION ANALYSIS

When we are prepared to regard all the variables, dependent and independent, entering into an analysis as quantitative (measured on an interval scale), then our preferred procedure is regression analysis. It is possible to construct regression models that incorporate curvilinear relationships. We found no occasion to use such models; hence the present discussion is confined to linear regression.

The topic has been adumbrated in the previous section, and some results of regression calculations were shown in Figures 4.1 and 4.2. The two-variable regression case, for example, involves ascertaining the best-fitting or "least-squares" line passing through the means of Y corresponding to class intervals of X. In Figure 4.2, the (total) regression of Y on X is shown as having a slope of .46. That is, for every increase of 10 points in father's occupational status we raise our estimate of son's occupational status by 4.6 points. The regression line is constrained to pass through the point $(\overline{Y}, \overline{X})$, the plot of the grand means of the two variables.

The other statistic, in addition to the slope and the two means, that is usually cited in connection with a regression analysis is the coefficient of correlation—in this example, .405. From one point of view this coefficient is a measure of the goodness of fit of the regression line. Its square, .164, represents the proportion of total sum of squares in Y accounted for by the linear part of the relationship of Y to X. It is thus comparable to the sum of squares for gross effects of X cited in connection with the multiple-classification analysis, which was given as .1505 or 15.05 per cent. Actually, when computed from the same data the squared correlation coefficient, r_{YX}^2, must be less than, or at most equal to η_{YX}^2. But, as was pointed out, in our multiple-classification work we included NA cases, while excluding them in computing linear-regression statistics. This gives rise to minor statistical discrepancies that make it impossible to compare closely the results from the regression and the multiple-classification analyses. It is, however, clear from the graphic display that a straight line does not exactly describe the progression of means although it comes very close to doing so.

Another point of view for interpreting the correlation coefficient is that it is identical with the regression coefficient when both variables are expressed in standard form, that is, in units of their respective standard deviations (usually after having been coded into deviations from the respective means). Thus we might write the regression equation as simply $\hat{y} = r_{yx}x$, where $y = (Y - \overline{Y})/\sigma_Y$ and $x = (X - \overline{X})/\sigma_X$. In the example at hand, $\hat{y} = .405x$, so that if a respondent were one standard deviation above the mean in the distribution of respondents by father's occupational status (X) we should estimate that he stands about four-tenths of a standard deviation above the mean in the distribution of respondents' occupational status (Y). When we make use of correlations we have in mind this interpretation of r as a "standardized regression coefficient."

A third interpretation of the correlation coefficient is that it is an estimate of a certain parameter of a bivariate normal frequency distribution. We do not have any occasion to make use of this interpretation, as we do not require the assumption of bivariate normality and should be hard put to justify that assumption in any event.

The reader unaccustomed to working with regression statistics will want to have some guidelines for their interpretation. Is a correlation such as $r_{YX} = .40$ a "large" or a "small" value? One standard, of course, is the maximum value of the coefficient, 1.00 (or —1.00 in the case of an inverse relationship). If $r_{YX} = 1.00$, this means that we can estimate perfectly the respondent's occupational status, knowing his father's status. In a completely rigid society, in which every son follows his father's occupation, this is the value we should observe. Now, from previous studies of occupational mobility, as well as from everyday life, we are aware that not all sons take up their fathers' occupations. Yet it is generally supposed that the proportion who do so is substantial. This supposition derives from studies showing mobility tables in which occupations are grouped into quite broad classes. The OCG data permit us to make a more refined estimate of the frequency of occupational inheritance. Just over 10 per cent of the OCG respondents have two-digit occupational status scores identical with those of their fathers. Moreover, identity of status score does not imply that father and son were in the same occupation. (The father may have been an electrician, scored 44, and the son a cashier, likewise scored 44.) Hence the figure given here is a *maximum* estimate of the extent of occupational inheritance, if defined as *identity* of specific occupations in a detailed classification, in the OCG population. What is the implication for the father-son correlation of 10 per cent occupational inheritance? Let us make some simplifying assumptions in order to deduce a definite answer. Suppose the population consists of two groups. The means of Y and X and the respective standard deviations are the same in the two groups. The first group consists of those "inheriting" their fathers' occupations; within this group, of course, $r_{YX} = 1.00$. In the other group, where there is no inheritance, assume $r_{YX} = .00$. Then in the whole population—the composite of these two groups—the correlation r_{YX} will be exactly equal to the proportion who "inherit" their father's status, or, in the present example, .10. The observed correlation, $r_{YX} = .40$, evidently exceeds by a substantial margin the hypothetical value due solely to occupational "inheritance," narrowly construed. This is true even though the actual proportion of "inheritance" is rather greater than its hypothetical chance magnitude.

Perhaps the foregoing argument will lend some perspective to the finding that $r_{YX} = .40$. Though far below the maximum, this degree of relationship is well above the value that could be induced by the specific mechanism of the father training the son in his own line of work. If we are to argue for a causal interpretation of r_{YX}, we shall have to posit a somewhat more complex sort of causation than mere apprenticeship or strict occupational inheritance. Economic resources and socialization processes are probably the major factors underlying this correlation.

Another perspective on the intergenerational correlation is afforded by data and theory from other fields. A classic result obtained by Karl Pearson is a father-son correlation of .51 with respect to stature (adult height in inches).[20] If stature were wholly determined genetically, and on certain assumptions about the specific genetic mechanism, including a lack of assortative mating, a correlation of precisely .5 would be predicted on theoretical grounds. A recent review of an even dozen

    [20] Cf. G. U. Yule and M. G. Kendall, *An Introduction to the Theory of Statistics* (13th ed.), London: Griffin, 1947, Chapter 11.

studies on the subject[21] indicates that the median value of the parent-child correlations in test intelligence obtained in the 12 investigations is .50. This is again an interesting coincidence with the value predicted on a simplified genetic model of transmission of intelligence. However, we do not wish to go into the question of genetic versus environmental determinants here.

Although nothing is proved by the comparison—at least in the absence of additional explicit premises—it is at least curious that the father-son correlation in respect to occupational status is comparable in order of magnitude to the correlation obtained for a character, like stature, for which genetic transmission is strongly indicated and for a psychological trait, like intelligence, whose mode of transmission is unknown. If we reasoned that stature (certainly) and intelligence (probably) are measured with greater reliability than occupational status, we should assume the correlation for the latter to be more highly attenuated by random measurement errors than the others. If so, the similarity of the three coefficients of parent-child resemblance might be assumed to be even closer than has been indicated.

From this perspective the value of the correlation r_{YX} seems neither unusually low nor inexplicably high. On the basis of its magnitude, one can argue that there is a definite and discernible influence of the father's status on the son's occupational achievement, but that the latter is affected by various other factors that operate like "chance" insofar as their connection with father's status is concerned. In this problem, of course, we lack any definite conception of a chance mechanism that would correspond to random segregation of genes in genetic theory. On the other hand, we shall be able to be somewhat more specific as to certain factors in occupational achievement that operate —at least in part—independently of the factor of father's status.

The prime requirement for linear-regression analysis is, of course, that the relationship actually be linear, at least to an acceptable degree of approximation. Figures 4.1 and 4.2 exhibit the sorts of variation from strict linearity that we typically find in the OCG data. Inspection of a large number of similar data plots satisfies us that the assumption of linearity is usually close enough to the truth, where we require it, to make regression analysis worthwhile.

The relationship that probably shows the most definite pattern of curvilinearity is the one summarized in Table 4.3, occupational status (Y) in relation to educational attainment (U). We shall consider this relationship further, for it affords an opportunity to illustrate some

21 L. Erlenmeyer-Kimling and Lissy F. Jarvik, "Genetics and Intelligence," *Science*, 142(1963), 1477-1479.

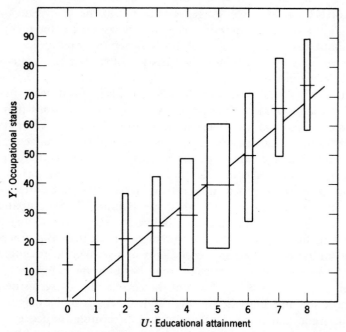

Figure 4.3. Mean of $Y \pm$ one standard deviation for each category of educational attainment (U) with linear regression computed on the assumption of interval measurement of U, for males 20 to 64 years old with nonfarm background.

limitations of the regression analysis in addition to departure from linearity. Figure 4.3 is a graph of this relationship, but for a different sample, that is, the one representing the subpopulation of OCG respondents 20 to 64 years old whose fathers were not in farm occupations. (We shall make a number of our subsequent calculations for this nonfarm-background group.)

Educational attainment, U, is represented here by an arbitrary scoring system: 0 for no schooling, 1 for one to four years elementary, 2 for five to seven years elementary, 3 for eight years of elementary, 4 for one to three years of high school, 5 for high-school graduation, 6 for one to three years of college, 7 for college graduation, and 8 for five or more years of college. The bar for each value of U represents the mean value of Y for men with the specified amount of schooling plus or minus one standard deviation of the Y scores observed in that educational category. The width of the bar is roughly proportional to the number of men in the population at the given educational level.

Finally, the least-squares regression line is plotted so that we may judge the degree of conformity of the relationship to linearity. The diagram brings out several points pertinent to an interpretation of the regression statistics.

First, the progression of Y means obviously is not perfectly linear. The greatest departures from linearity are, however, in the two very thinly populated intervals at the bottom of the U-scale. It evidently would have been desirable to compress the scale in this region in order to improve the approximation to linearity. Yet, because of the small numbers involved, this would have made very little difference in the correlation coefficient. In fact, for these data we find the (linear) correlation $r_{YU} = .595$ as compared to the η_{YU} of .619. The proportion of variation accounted for by the linear part of the relationship is, therefore, 35 per cent, whereas the actual between-mean sum of squares is 38 per cent of the total sum of squares.

Second, the data are evidently heteroscedastic. That is, the dispersion of Y scores is not constant. Indeed, there is a rather clear pattern of variation in the standard deviations: they are low at both extremes of the education scale and high in the intermediate intervals (scores 5 and 6).

Finally, as can be deduced from the diagram and confirmed upon inspection of the original data, the Y scores are not symmetrically, let alone normally, distributed around the U-specific means. When U is low, the Y distribution is positively skewed. Y can go no lower than zero, but even at the lowest level of education some men have quite high occupational status. Conversely, when U is high, the Y distribution is negatively skewed. For men with college degrees, there is a low ceiling—that is, from the mean performance to the top is a rather short interval—but it is a long distance to the floor. Yet some college graduates—if their reports on educational attainment and occupation are to be believed—are found in occupations scored below 10.

In the light of these observations on the statistical misbehavior of the data, can we still justify the use of regression statistics? We shall, indeed, proceed to use these statistics, but with the recognition that they cannot disclose everything one might like to know about the nature of the relationships under study. The fact is that, in a situation where we encounter curvilinearity, heteroscedasticity, and skewed distributions of residuals, no set of second-degree statistics (such as variances and covariances, or standard deviations and linear-regression coefficients) can summarize all the information in the data. We can claim that our measures give a partial and approximate reduction of the data, but that is all. As long as we are in the two-variable case we can supplement the regression statistics with other kinds of description. When we get into problems involving several variables we can compare the regression approach with the multiple-classification approach. The latter, as we have seen, copes with the problem of curvilinearity, though not with the other two problems mentioned. No doubt more sophisticated procedures could be invoked to provide greater analytical precision. But such procedures would doubtlessly require much more complicated cross-tabulations than we could afford to procure or analyze.

The problems being discussed here are not problems of statistical inference in the sense of reckoning with sampling variation. We are working with large samples and our problem is one of adequate data reduction or statistical description, not of determining whether the data exhibit "significant differences." We shall occasionally cite crude estimates of standard errors of correlation coefficients. On any reasonable estimate of such standard errors it is clear that the principal variations in size of correlations that we note cannot be accidents of sampling.

The discussion to this point has been limited to the two-variable regression problem. Actually, the principal motivation for regression techniques is not their convenience as a summary of the two-variable relationship but their power in expressing the essential facts of multivariable relationships. If the requisite assumptions hold, all the information needed for an adequate description of a k variable system is contained in the $k(k-1)/2$ distinct two-variable relationships included in the set.

From this standpoint, the motivation for multiple regression is just like that for multiple classification. Moreover, the essential assumption (in addition to those of linearity and constancy of residual variation) is also the same, namely, that net relationships are additive. On this assumption, one may not only take advantage of multiple regression as an exceedingly compact summary of relationships. One can construct, on the basis of the regression statistics, a systematic causal interpretation, using the technique of path analysis. We shall postpone a discussion of path coefficients to the next chapter, where they are actually used. Here we simply note that the path technique involves some substantive or theoretical assumptions, but that its statistical basis is essentially the same as that of multiple regression. On the specific problem of additivity of net relationships, a partial check on the assumption of additivity is provided by the technique of covariance analysis, to be discussed in the next section.

A number of detailed points of interpretation arise in applying multiple-regression procedures. It will be best to take these up in the context of the exposition of substantive findings. We may conclude the present discussion by calling attention once more to Figures 4.1 and 4.2. In addition to the total regressions already discussed, these figures show two of the net relationships estimated from the multiple regression of Y on W, U, and X. We also have the comparison with the net relationships obtained in the multiple-classification analysis. The main thing to observe is that the general impression to be gained is much the same, whichever technique is used. The departures from linearity in the net relationships are much like those occurring in the gross relationships. In Figure 4.2 the slope of the net regression of Y on W, U and X being fixed, may seem a little too steep by comparison with the general "drift" of the adjusted deviations. Such a discrepancy is quite possible, since the multiple-classification procedure partials out not only the linear effects of U and X, but all their additive effects irrespective of form. The remarkable thing, then, is that the net linear relationship does so well as a summary of the net relationship estimated by a technique that makes no assumption of linearity. We have here another bit of evidence that the moderate departures from linearity observed in these data are hardly the major stumbling block to a straightforward interpretation of regression results. We need only add that we have inspected many other comparisons like those given in Figures 4.1 and 4.2, and most of them yield much the same impression that the linear assumption is a fair approximation.

COVARIANCE ANALYSIS

This technique is applicable when the dependent variable is quantitative, one independent variable likewise is quantitative and another is classificatory. (There are extensions to multiple covariance, with more than one quantitative covariable, but we have not employed them.) No assumptions are made about the nature of the relationship of either quantitative variable to the classificatory variable. In this respect the technique resembles multiple classification. We do assume that the relationship of the measured dependent variable to the quantitative independent variable is linear, *within* each category of the classificatory variable. (Extensions to curvilinear within-group relationships are available, but we have not considered them.) We do not, however, assume initially that the slope of this linear relationship is constant. Indeed, the primary objective of our use of covariance is to investigate whether the several slopes are in fact the same, or nearly so. When the slopes are distinctly different we have an interaction of the quantitative with the classificatory independent variable

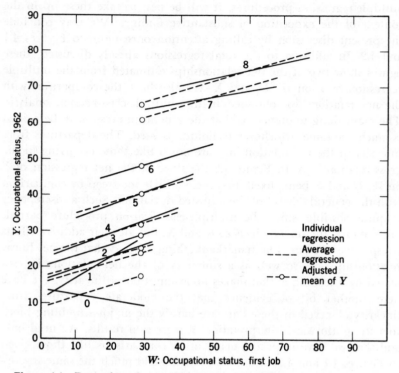

Figure 4.4. Regression of occupational status in 1962 on occupational status of first job, within categories of educational attainment (0, 1, ..., 8), for males 20 to 64 years old with nonfarm background.

with respect to their effects on the dependent variable. In other words, the net effects of the two independent variables are nonadditive. In still a different phrasing, interaction in this context means that the nature of the effects of either independent variable depends on the level or class of the other independent variable.

To proceed at once to an illustration, Figure 4.4 portrays some results of a covariance analysis of the relationship of Y to W and U, the latter being regarded here as a classificatory variable. Essentially what we have are nine different two-variable regression calculations, one for each category of education (U). The outcomes of these nine calculations are represented by the solid lines denoted "individual regression." Each line, of course, passes through the means ($\overline{W}$, $\overline{Y}$) for the appropriate category of educational attainment.

The other result of a covariance calculation is an "average within-group regression." This is obtained by pooling the within-group sums of squares and products, in the process automatically taking account of the numbers in the respective groups. In the figure a line having this average slope is plotted through the means for each group, except in the case of groups 3 and 6, where the average is so close to the individual regression that the two cannot be distinguished graphically. A significance test is available for testing whether it is reasonable to suppose that the departures of the individual from the average regressions are simply due to sampling variation.[22] We have not relied heavily on such tests, on the supposition that differences large enough to be interesting would most likely turn out to be significant.

In the illustrative data the average regression is .29, and for five of the education categories the individual regressions fall in a fairly small range from .29 to .36. These are, in fact, the groups of intermediate educational attainment, categories 2 to 6. At the low end of the education scale we find two slopes deviating markedly from the average. It will be recalled that these two categories are thinly populated, so we might expect substantial sampling variation here. Because one of the two slopes is negative and the other is decidedly positive, it seems difficult to venture any substantive interpretation.

At the other end of the education scale, looking at college graduates and those with postgraduate experience, we find the individual slopes are somewhat lower than the average. For the college graduate, apparently, the status of the first job is not so important a determinant of subsequent occupational status as for, say, the high-school graduate. We should also consider the possibility of a "ceiling effect" that flattens the regression of Y on W for a group in which W is very high to begin with. It would seem that we can get a mildly interesting substantive interpretation of the interaction observed here. However, it also appears that no great violence is done if we accept the average regression as representative of the net relationship of Y to W, U being fixed.

In the multiple-regression analysis of these same data we obtain a net coefficient of .34 for Y on W, with U (treated as a quantitative variable linearly related to the others) held constant. This is comparable in concept with the average regression of .29 estimated from the covariance results. In the latter case, of course, we are not only holding constant the linear effect of U, but its entire additive effect.

Another set of results in the covariance analysis is the adjusted Y means, which we may compute if we accept the assumption of a uniform within-group regression equal to the computed average. Here we are interested in estimating the net effects of the classificatory

22 Helen M. Walker and Joseph Lev, *Statistical Inference*, New York: Holt, 1953, Chapter 15.

TABLE 4.4. EFFECTS OF EDUCATIONAL ATTAINMENT ON OCC. STATUS IN 1962, COMPUTED BY TWO METHODS, FOR MEN WITH NONFARM BACKGROUND

Educational Attainment	Estimated Population (in Thousands) (1)	Covariance Analysis[a]		Multiple Classification[a]	
		Gross Effects[b] (2)	Net of W[c] (3)	Gross Effects[b] (4)	Net of W[c] (5)
All men	32,879	.0	.0	.0	.0
(0) No school years	287	-27.9	-22.7	-19.3	-14.4
Elementary					
(1) 1 to 4 years	824	-20.5	-15.8	-17.2	-12.7
(2) 5 to 7 years	2,363	-18.7	-15.0	-16.6	-13.2
(3) 8 years	3,474	-14.7	-11.6	-13.7	-10.8
High school					
(4) 1 to 3 years	6,364	-10.5	- 8.1	- 9.8	- 7.7
(5) 4 years	10,050	- .5	- .1	- .4	- .1
College					
(6) 1 to 3 years	4,556	9.7	8.0	8.2	7.0
(7) 4 years	2,890	26.6	20.7	24.6	19.4
(8) 5 or more years	2,072	34.3	25.0	31.5	22.2

[a]In covariance calculations, men not in the experienced civilian labor force (NA on Y) are omitted.   In multiple classification they are assigned a score equal to the grand mean of Y.
[b]Deviations from grand mean of Y, 40.1.
[c]W: Status of first job.

variable on the dependent variable, with the quantitative covariate held constant. As is suggested by Figure 4.4, the adjusted Y means are obtained by equalizing the education groups with respect to W—specifically, by computing what the mean of Y would be if all groups had the same mean on W with the average regression line passing through that mean. Deviations of the adjusted Y means from the grand mean of Y are comparable in concept with the adjusted deviations (net effects) obtained in the multiple-classification analysis. In both procedures we assume additive net effects. In the covariance method we require one of the relationships to take a linear form (here, Y on W), whereas this restriction does not apply in the multiple-classification procedure.

Table 4.4 compares the findings obtained on the two approaches. The reader will note that the covariance analysis yields a wider spread of both gross and net effects than does the multiple-classification analysis. This is *not,* however, a function of the difference between the two analytical models but an artifact arising from a circumstance of the way the data were tabulated. In the covariance analysis, we ignored the NA category, whereas in the multiple-classification work we had to assign it an arbitrary score. This has the effect of attenuating the effects estimated by the multiple-classification procedure. The extent of this discrepancy is indicated by the per cent of total sum of squares in Y attributed to gross effects of U. This comes out as 38.6 per cent for the covariance calculation, 34.9 per cent for the multiple-classification calculation.

Despite this discrepancy the reader may note that the consequences of the adjustment for W are much the same in the two calculations. That is, the differences between corresponding gross and net effects in the two sets are much the same in the two series: compare column 2 minus column 3 with column 4 minus column 5. Here is a summary, of the kind suggested in a previous section for the multiple-classification results, illustrating the discrepancies between the two calculations:

	Per Cent of Total SS(Y)	
Variables	Multiple Classification	Covariance
U	34.91	38.58
W	26.25	27.48
U, W	40.26	42.87
U, net	14.01	15.39
W, net	5.35	4.29

Except when otherwise specified, the multiple-classification procedure is used for all calculations of per cent of total sums of squares in the following chapters.

We must mention still another source of possible inconsistency in the covariance results. Although the NA category was disregarded for both the quantitative variables, the cases excluded were not necessarily the same for the two variables. This difficulty arises from the form of the tabulations. We have, for example, a distribution of Y scores, a distribution of W scores, and a distribution of the differences $(Y - W)$, each given in class intervals. From the three distributions we compute, within categories of the classificatory variables,

$$\Sigma Y, \Sigma Y^2, \Sigma W, \Sigma W^2, \quad \text{and} \quad \Sigma(Y - W)^2 = \Sigma(Y^2 - 2YW + W^2).$$

We are thus able to obtain ΣYW as

$$[\Sigma Y^2 + \Sigma W^2 - \Sigma(Y - W)^2]/2.$$

Given these quantities, we can secure the variances and covariances required for the remaining calculations. It was possible to adjust for the fact that the three distributions, Y, W, and $(Y - W)$, were based on somewhat different total numbers (NA's having been excluded from each), but this would not remove any inconsistency that would arise, say, if the NA's on W were not representative with respect to Y. Besides this problem there is the comparatively minor one of approximations introduced in the groupings of the data into class intervals.

The reader will perhaps appreciate that errors from these sources arose from the necessity of working with multipurpose tabulations that had to be designed in as simple a form as possible for reasons of economy—and designed, moreover, before any information was available from the OCG survey itself on the one-way or two-way distributions of variables and the relative frequency of NA's. We are forced, in effect, to tolerate some approximations in computing, just as we must tolerate sampling variation and largely unknown errors of response and data processing. As we are well aware of the different kinds of computing errors to which the several kinds of analysis are subject, we do not, of course, attempt inferences based on precise comparisons of results between kinds of analysis.

With specific reference to the covariance calculations, we believe these are useful in detecting any major patterns of interaction present in three-variable problems. We recognize, however, that small differences in the individual regression coefficients are not to be regarded as accurate and reliable.

ANALYZING MOBILITY DISTRIBUTIONS: THE CASE OF EDUCATION

Three measures of the respondent's occupational mobility are provided by the OCG study: (1) intergenerational mobility, father's occupation to respondent's occupation in 1962; (2) initial intergenerational mobility, father's occupation to respondent's first job; and (3) intragenerational mobility, first job to 1962 occupation. All three occupations are scored on the status index. Hence, when we want a measure of "distance" moved, it is natural simply to use the difference in status scores of the two occupations, movement between which constitutes mobility. Thus if father's occupational status score is designated as X, first job status as W, and 1962 status as Y, the distance measures for the three foregoing types of mobility are simply (1) $Y - X$; (2) $W - X$; and (3) $Y - W$. Any of these mobility scores can be positive (connoting upward mobility), negative (indicating downward mobility) or zero (corresponding to immobility in terms of occupational status, though not necessarily in terms of specific occupation). In principle the mobility score may be as high as $+96$ or as low as -96, though such extremes are unlikely in fact to occur.

For theoretical purposes, when one tries to establish either causes or consequences of mobility it is *not* generally desirable to attempt to use the mobility score as a variable in a straightforward statistical analysis. The reasons for this are detailed in Chapter 5. The essential consideration is that the phenomenon of "mobility" is not causally homogeneous. What determines where a person starts (his initial or origin status) may be different from what determines where he goes (his terminal or destination status). Moreover, owing to the universally observed pattern of regression toward the mean, mobility (in a specified direction) from one starting point may be easier or more likely than from another. Hence the origin status is part of the causal configuration determining destination status. To manipulate a mobility score statistically is to run the risk of confounding cause and effect.

By the same token, when studying hypothesized consequences of mobility there is the distinct possibility that the effect of the origin status is not the same as that of the destination status. The two are mixed, in unknown quantities, in a mobility score. The same limitations of a mobility measure apply even if no formal scoring device is used as, for example, when research workers simply classify persons as upwardly, downwardly, or not mobile.

Despite the hazards to correct interpretation, we have examined mobility score distributions for two reasons: First, there is a certain curiosity about what segments of the population experience greater or lesser amounts of mobility. The data have a descriptive interest. Yet, in trying to satisfy this curiosity, we must warn the reader not to venture unwarranted inferences from the observed variation in mobility distributions. If he is tempted to infer some consequence from the fact that a certain group experiences a greater or lesser amount of mobility than the average, then he should resort to a method of analysis suited to the test of such an inference.

Second, by employing a correct, though apparently circuitous, method of analyzing mobility distributions it is possible to reach interesting and valid characterizations of the mobility process. The method illustrated here yields a useful summary statement—one that does not differ qualitatively from conclusions reached by regression, covariance, and multiple-classification procedures, but one that is free of some of the assumptions of those techniques and takes into account the actual form of the score distributions in a way that they do not. Hence, analysis of mobility distributions along the lines set forth here is useful in checking conclusions reached by other means and possibly in expressing those conclusions in a fashion that some readers may find more interesting.

In order to put the least strain on the assumption that social distance

TABLE 4.5.   PERCENTAGE DISTRIBUTION OF MEN BY INTERGENERATIONAL OCC.
MOBILITY SCORES (Y-X), OBSERVED AND EXPECTED ON TWO HYPOTHESES

Mobility Score	Observed	Expected[a]		Observed Minus A	Observed Minus B
		A	B		
26 to 96 (long distance upward)	24.9	30.7	27.6	-5.8	-2.7
6 to 25 (short distance upward)	24.7	21.2	25.1	3.5	-0.4
-5 to 5 (relatively stable)	28.1	18.5	20.7	9.6	7.4
-25 to -6 (short distance downward)	15.5	15.6	16.2	-.1	-0.7
-96 to -26 (long distance downward)	6.8	14.0	10.4	-7.2	-3.6
Total	100.0	100.0	100.0	0.0	0.0

[a]A: Expected on the hypothesis that Y and X are statistically independent in the whole population.
B: Expected on the hypothesis that Y and X are statistically independent within categories of education.

is measured on an interval scale we have drastically collapsed the mobility distributions. Five categories of mobility are recognized, and their definition in terms of score intervals is given in Table 4.5. Because the categories are arbitrarily delimited, there is no meaning in the absolute distribution of scores. Had we been a little more liberal in our definition of "relative stability," for example, that category would have claimed larger numbers, at the expense of the categories of "short-distance mobility."

There is meaning, however, in the observation that in the "observed" column of Table 4.5 there is more upward than downward mobility—which is just another way of stating that respondents' own occupational statuses in 1962 are higher on the average than their social origins as defined by father's status.

We get more information from the distribution of mobility scores when we compare it with a distribution generated on a specific hypothesis about how mobility takes place. One such hypothesis frequently examined is that there is "perfect mobility," that is, respondent's status is statistically independent of father's status. Expected distribution A in Table 4.5 is obtained on this hypothesis, given the marginal distributions of Y and X. Comparing the observed with the expected A distribution, we see that there is considerably more relative stability in actual fact than the hypothesis of perfect mobility predicts, and also somewhat more short-distance upward mobility, though just about the same amount of short-distance downward mobility as the hypothesis suggests. The observed mobility distribution falls measurably short of the expected distribution in regard to long-distance mobility, either upward or downward.

The reader must understand that there is an unknown error of computation in the expected distribution, both the one just discussed and all others considered in our analyses of mobility distributions. Our marginal distributions of status scores are tabulated in class intervals and our mobility score distributions are also available in class intervals. To calculate an expected distribution of mobility scores so that it can be presented in the same class intervals as the observed distribution requires an interpolation within class intervals,[23] which can only yield approximate results. Hence it is easily possible for our calculation of an expected percentage of, say, short-distance upward mobility to differ by one or two percentage points from what we would have obtained with our marginal distributions tabulated in greater detail. Besides, the problem of sampling fluctuations must also be kept in mind.

The reader may wonder why there should be a peculiar departure of the observed mobility distribution from that expected (in *A*) on the supposition of perfect mobility, such that there is an excess of short-distance upward but not of short-distance downward mobility over expectation. We cannot give a straightforward and demonstrable answer, but we can exhibit another set of results in which this peculiarity—if it is such—disappears and hence, in a sense, is explained. The premise, hardly a startling one, of the calculation is that education is a major factor intervening between occupational status of origin and achieved occupational status. Although the amount of education attained depends in part on level of origin, it also depends on other factors. It is quite possible, therefore, that a substantial number of men receive enough education to insure a moderate amount of upward mobility, taking into account the levels at which they start.

To make this interpretation operational consider a model, not of perfect mobility in the population at large, but of a restricted kind of perfect mobility in which respondent's occupational status is statistically independent of father's occupational status *within categories* of respondents having the same amount of education. The mobility distribution obtained on this hypothesis is presented as "Expected *B*" in Table 4.5. Operationally the calculation proceeds by grouping respondents into nine categories of educational attainment. We first calculate the expected mobility score distribution (in terms of population frequencies) for each education category, assuming independence of *Y* and *X*. Then we sum up the nine expected distributions into a single distribution for the whole population. The latter is then reduced to percentages. The mobility distribution obtained on this hypothesis—which may be termed that of conditional

---

[23] A computer program to carry out this otherwise extremely tedious calculation was specially written by J. Michael Coble.

perfect mobility with respect to education—is compared with the observed distribution in the last column of Table 4.5, "Observed minus B."

Here we still find an excess of relatively stable men in actuality, compensated by deficiencies of long-distance mobility, both upward and downward. The observed proportions of short-distance mobility are close to the expected, and the discrepancy hardly varies by direction of mobility, contrary to what was found for hypothesis A.

Here we have looked at the partial relationship of son's status to father's status, holding constant educational attainment. As in other analyses in which this same partial association is studied by different techniques, we find that there is a definite net effect of father's on son's status, independent of education. The present set of results indicates, specifically, that this net relationship consists in the respondent's being somewhat more likely to have an occupation closely similar in status to his father's than would be the case if education were the only factor through which father's status influences son's achievement.

The technique for analyzing mobility distributions illustrated here may be a useful supplement to analyses based on least-squares procedures (regression, covariance, multiple-classification). It makes no assumption of linearity or additivity of relationships and it takes into account any peculiar features of score distributions as well as ceiling and floor effects. Its limitation, as we have used it, is that it is suitable only for problems in which the dependent variable is an occupational status, one independent variable is another occupational status, and a second independent variable is classificatory. Some caution is necessary in aggregating expected distributions over all categories of the classificatory variable. In the example above this seemed justifiable, because the deviations of observed from expected frequencies fell into a similar pattern in all education categories. When this is not true it may be best to refrain from this aggregation, leaving the analysis in the extended form presented below.

The results displayed in summary form in Table 4.5 include some interesting details that merit a more elaborate presentation. We have so far used the technique to give an answer to the question of how education influences occupational achievement. It also permits us to respond circumspectly to the question of how education affects men's chances of experiencing intergenerational mobility, that is, the likelihood that they move up from their social origins, remain on about the same level as their fathers', or move down to lower levels.

The chances of upward mobility are directly related to education,

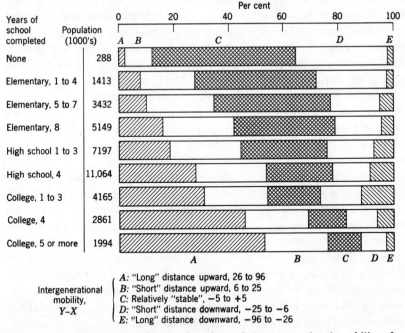

Figure 4.5. Percentage distribution by observed intergenerational mobility, for men in each category of educational attainment (based on data in Table J4.1).

as Figure 4.5 shows. (For the data see Table J4.1 in the Appendix.) The proportion of men who experience some upward mobility increases steadily with education from a low of 12 per cent for those reporting no schooling to a high of 76 per cent for those who have gone beyond college. The proportion who have moved up a long distance from their social origins increases in the same regular fashion from under 8 per cent for those with less than five years of schooling to 53 per cent for those with some postgraduate work. The proportion of immobile reveals a complementary decrease with advancing education, with close to one-half of the men with less than five years of education experiencing hardly any change from the occupational level of their fathers, in contrast to only one-eighth of those who have gone beyond college. Downward mobility, however, does not exhibit a corresponding linear association with education.

Men who started but did not complete college are more likely to experience downward mobility not only than those with more education but also than most of those with less education. By and large, to be sure, downward mobility is inversely related to education, ranging from more than one-quarter of those with less than five years of school-ing to one-eighth of the most educated. But the relationship is not monotonic; men who interrupted high school and those who inter-rupted college deviate from the trend by having disproportionately high downward mobility. Indeed, the trend becomes partly reversed and assumes the shape of an inverted U for the data on long-distance movement down from social origins. The likelihood that a man experi-ences much downward mobility increases from 2 per cent for the least educated regularly to a high of 12 per cent for those with one to three years of college, and then decreases to 2.5 per cent for the most educated.

Men with an intermediate amount of education—those who have gone beyond the compulsory eight grades but have not finished col-lege—are most likely to experience considerable downward mobility from their social origins. The reason that the less-educated are not as likely to move down from the level of their fathers may well be that most of them come from families with low socioeconomic status from which a man cannot easily drop very much lower. The reason that the college graduates are less likely to experience downward mobility may well be that they are a select group, as evidenced by their ability to complete college. Such *ad hoc* explanations, however, are unsatisfac-tory, and ways must be found to ascertain whether, for example, the inverse ceiling effect or other correlates of the educational differences can account for the observed pattern. Whatever the underlying ex-planation, however, the fact remains that men with a medium amount of education are most likely to suffer the presumably depriving ex-perience of having to move down a long way from the socioeconomic level on which they were raised. This greater risk of serious loss of status and relative deprivation of men who did not quite attain a higher education might help explain why, as has often been alleged, the lower middle class generally, and the downwardly mobile among them particularly, are especially susceptible to authoritarian and totalitarian ideologies and to prejudice of various kinds.[24] Clearly, it is important to keep distinct the issues of what causes differential mobility by education categories and what effects may flow from such differentials; only the former problem is systematically analyzed here.

The model tests the assumption that the occupational attainments

[24] Seymour M. Lipset, *Political Man*, New York: Doubleday, 1959, pp. 134ff.; Rudolph Heberle, *From Democracy to Nazism*, Baton Rouge: Louisiana State Univer. Press, 1945, pp. 10ff.; Bruno Bettelheim and Morris Janowitz, *Dynamics of Prejudice*, New York: Harper, 1950, pp. 58ff.; Samuel A. Stouffer, *Communism, Conformity and Civil Liberties*, New York: Doubleday, 1955, pp. 26-57, 139.

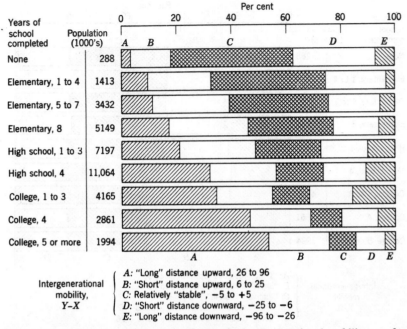

Figure 4.6. Expected percentage distribution by intergenerational mobility, on the hypothesis of independence within educational categories, for men in each category of educational attainment (based on data in Table J4.2).

of men depend on their education and that education depends on their father's socioeconomic status, but that the combination of education and father's status does not interact in affecting occupational mobility. In other words, the mobility experienced by men is simply a function of their education and their social origins, and there are no further conditions that affect the mobility chances of the various educational groups. The calculated values obtained when testing this assumption are presented in Figure 4.6 (and Table J4.2 in the Appendix). These expected values reproduce the observed ones quite closely. Upward mobility is expected to increase with increasing levels of education, and immobility is expected to decrease in complementary fashion. Even the U-shaped curve for long-distance downward mobility is replicated in the calculated values.

What does it mean to say that men with some college education are *expected* to be much downwardly mobile in greater numbers than either better-educated or less-educated men? It implies that the social origins of these men are considerably higher than of those with less

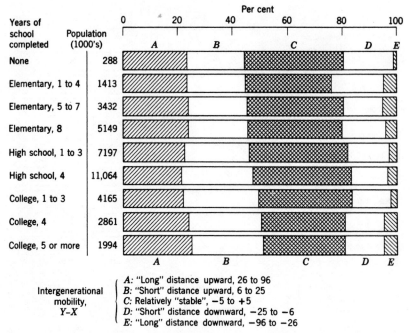

Figure 4.7. **Standardized percentage distribution by intergenerational mobility for men in each category of educational attainment (based on data in Table J4.3).**

education, and that their education is not quite commensurate with these high social origins to overcome the danger of downward mobility inherent in a high starting point, unless this danger is neutralized by superior education. The best-educated have the qualifications to live up to their social origins, and the less-educated have less high origins to live up to. But the college dropout is a man whose not-quite-good-enough educational qualifications enhance the risk of downward mobility from the high socioeconomic level his father typically occupied, as implied by the father's ability to send him to college.

The model of independence within educational levels predicts the observed values quite accurately, though not perfectly. Figure 4.7, as well as Appendix Table J4.3, shows the standardized residuals (the differences between observed and calculated percentages added to the distribution for all men, the latter being the value in the "Total" column of Table J4.1). These vary little among educational categories. There is some variation left, however, in respect to long-distance downward mobility, although it reveals the opposite trend from that apparent in the observed frequencies. In terms of these standardized values, men who went beyond grammar school but did not complete college are less likely to move far down from the level of their fathers than either less educated or more educated men. In short, although the men with an intermediate amount of education actually move down far below their social origins in disproportionate numbers, given their social origins they experience such serious loss of status less frequently than might be expected. The differences are small, however, and well within the range of the errors discussed earlier.

It is worth repeating that the finding that men who do not quite achieve a higher education are more likely than either better-educated or less-well-educated men to experience considerable downward mobility is not spurious but reflects a real state of affairs. To be sure, the analysis has demonstrated that it is the social composition of men on this educational level that accounts for their downward mobility. But showing what accounts for it is not to deny the reality of the experience. Men who started college without finishing it and, to a lesser extent, those with one to four years of high school actually are in greater danger of serious downward mobility than either the educated elite or the uneducated mass who did not go to high school. The relative deprivation of social status implicit in downward mobility is suffered most often by men in the intermediate educational brackets, and their exposure to this greater risk of deprivation may well make them a potentially explosive force in periods of economic crisis.

CHAPTER 5

The Process of Stratification

Stratification systems may be characterized in various ways. Surely one of the most important has to do with the processes by which individuals become located, or locate themselves, in positions in the hierarchy comprising the system. At one extreme we can imagine that the circumstances of a person's birth—including the person's sex and the perfectly predictable sequence of age levels through which he is destined to pass—suffice to assign him unequivocally to a ranked status in a hierarchical system. At the opposite extreme his prospective adult status would be wholly problematic and contingent at the time of birth. Such status would become entirely determinate only as adulthood was reached, and solely as a consequence of his own actions taken freely—that is, in the absence of any constraint deriving from the circumstances of his birth or rearing. Such a pure achievement system is, of course, hypothetical, in much the same way that motion without friction is a purely hypothetical possibility in the physical world. Whenever the stratification system of any moderately large and complex society is described, it is seen to involve both ascriptive and achievement principles.

In a liberal democratic society we think of the more basic principle as being that of achievement. Some ascriptive features of the system may be regarded as vestiges of an earlier epoch, to be extirpated as rapidly as possible. Public policy may emphasize measures designed to enhance or to equalize opportunity—hopefully, to overcome ascriptive obstacles to the full exercise of the achievement principle.

The question of how far a society may realistically aspire to go in this direction is hotly debated, not only in the ideological arena but in the academic forum as well. Our contribution, if any, to the debate will consist largely in submitting measurements and estimates of the strength of ascriptive forces and of the scope of opportunities in a large contemporary society. The problem of the relative importance of the two principles in a given system is ultimately a quantitative one. We have pushed our ingenuity to its limit in seeking to contrive relevant quantifications.

The governing conceptual scheme in the analysis is quite a commonplace one. We think of the individual's life cycle as a sequence in time that can be described, however partially and crudely, by a set of classificatory or quantitative measurements taken at successive stages. Ideally we should like to have under observation a cohort of births, following the individuals who make up the cohort as they pass through life. As a practical matter we resorted to retrospective questions put to a representative sample of several adjacent cohorts so as to ascertain those facts about their life histories that we assumed were both relevant to our problem and accessible by this means of observation.

Given this scheme, the questions we are continually raising in one form or another are: how and to what degree do the circumstances of birth condition subsequent status? and, how does status attained (whether by ascription or achievement) at one stage of the life cycle affect the prospects for a subsequent stage? The questions are neither idle nor idiosyncratic ones. Current policy discussion and action come to a focus in a vaguely explicated notion of the "inheritance of poverty." Thus a spokesman for the Social Security Administration writes:

It would be one thing if poverty hit at random and no one group were singled out. It is another thing to realize that some seem destined to poverty almost from birth—by their color or by the economic status or occupation of their parents.[1]

Another officially sanctioned concept is that of the "dropout," the person who fails to graduate from high school. Here the emphasis is not so much on circumstances operative at birth but on the presumed effect of early achievement on subsequent opportunities. Thus the "dropout" is seen as facing "a lifetime of uncertain employment,"[2] probable assignment to jobs of inferior status, reduced earning power, and vulnerability to various forms of social pathology.

[1] Mollie Orshansky, "Children of the Poor," *Social Security Bulletin*, 26(July 1963).

[2] Forrest A. Bogan, "Employment of High School Graduates and Dropouts in 1964," *Special Labor Force Report*, No. 54 (U. S. Bureau of Labor Statistics, June 1965), p. 643.

In this study we do not have measurements on all the factors implicit in a full-blown conception of the "cycle of poverty" nor all those variables conceivably responding unfavorably to the achievement of "dropout" status. For practical reasons, as explained in Chapter 1, we were severely limited in the amount of information to be collected. For theoretical reasons—also spelled out more fully in Chapter 1—and in conformity with the tradition of studies in social mobility, we chose to emphasize occupation as a measure both of origin status and of status achievement. The present chapter is even more strictly limited to variables we think can be treated meaningfully as quantitative and therefore are suited to analysis by the regression technique described in Chapter 4. This limitation, however, is not merely an analytical convenience. We think of the selected quantitative variables as being sufficient to describe the major outlines of status changes in the life cycle of a cohort. Thus a study of the relationships among these variables leads to a formulation of a basic model of the process of stratification. In this chapter we consider also certain extensions of this model. Subsequent chapters provide, in effect, a number of additional detailed extensions, although these are secured only by giving up some of the elegance and convenience of the particular analytical procedures employed here.

A BASIC MODEL

To begin with, we examine only five variables. For expository convenience, when it is necessary to resort to symbols, we shall designate them by arbitrary letters but try to remind the reader from time to time of what the letters stand for. These variables are:

V: Father's educational attainment
X: Father's occupational status
U: Respondent's educational attainment
W: Status of respondent's first job
Y: Status of respondent's occupation in 1962

Each of the three occupational statuses is scaled by the index described in Chapter 4, ranging from 0 to 96. The two education variables are scored on the following arbitrary scale of values ("rungs" on the "educational ladder") corresponding to specified numbers of years of formal schooling completed:

0: No school
1: Elementary, one to four years
2: Elementary, five to seven years

3: Elementary, eight years
4: High school, one to three years
5: High school, four years
6: College, one to three years
7: College, four years
8: College, five years or more (i.e., one or more years of postgraduate study)

Actually, this scoring system hardly differs from a simple linear transformation, or "coding," of the exact number of years of school completed. In retrospect, for reasons given in Chapter 4, we feel that the score implies too great a distance between intervals at the lower end of the scale; but the resultant distortion is minor in view of the very small proportions scored 0 or 1.

A basic assumption in our interpretation of regression statistics—though not in their calculation as such—has to do with the causal or temporal ordering of these variables. In terms of the father's career we should naturally assume precedence of V (education) with respect to X (occupation when his son was 16 years old). We are not concerned with the father's career, however, but only with his statuses that comprised a configuration of background circumstances or origin conditions for the cohorts of sons who were respondents in the OCG study. Hence we generally make no assumption as to the priority of V with respect to X; in effect, we assume the measurements on these variables to be contemporaneous from the son's viewpoint. The respondent's education, U, is supposed to follow in time—and thus to be susceptible to causal influence from—the two measures of father's status. Because we ascertained X as of respondent's age 16, it is true that some respondents may have completed school before the age to which X pertains. Such cases were doubtlessly a small minority and in only a minor proportion of them could the father (or other family head) have changed status radically in the two or three years before the respondent reached 16.

The next step in the sequence is more problematic. We assume that W (first job status) follows U (education). The assumption conforms to the wording of the questionnaire (see Appendix B), which stipulated "the first full-time job you had after you left school." In the years since the OCG study was designed we have been made aware of a fact that should have been considered more carefully in the design. Many students leave school more or less definitively, only to return, perhaps to a different school, some years later, whereupon they often finish a degree program.[3] The OCG questionnaire contained information relevant to this problem, namely the item on age at first job. Through an oversight no tabulations of this item were made for the present study. Tables prepared for another study[4] using the OCG data, however, suggest that approximately one-eighth of the respondents report a combination of age at first job and education that would be very improbable unless (a) they violated instructions by reporting a part-time or school-vacation job as the first job, or (b) they did, in fact, interrupt their schooling to enter regular employment. (These "inconsistent" responses include men giving 19 as their age at first job and college graduation or more as their education; 17 or 18 with some college or more; 14, 15, or 16 with high-school graduation or more; and under 14 with some high school or more.) When the two variables are studied in combination with occupation of first job, a very clear effect is evident. Men with a given amount of education beginning their first jobs early held lower occupational statuses than those beginning at a normal or advanced age for the specified amount of education.

Despite the strong probability that the U-W sequence is reversed for an appreciable minority of respondents, we have hardly any alternative to the assumption made here. If the bulk of the men who interrupted schooling to take their first jobs were among those ultimately securing relatively advanced education, then our variable W is downwardly biased, no doubt, as a measure of their occupational status immediately after they finally left school for good. In this sense, the correlations between U and W and between W and Y are probably attenuated. Thus, if we had really measured "job after completing education" instead of "first job," the former would in all likelihood have loomed somewhat larger as a variable intervening between education and 1962 occupational status. We do not wish to argue that our respondents erred in their reports on first job. We are inclined to conclude that their reports were realistic enough, and that it was our assumption about the meaning of the responses that proved to be fallible.

The fundamental difficulty here is conceptual. If we insist on *any* uniform sequence of the events involved in accomplishing the transi-

---

[3] Bruce K. Eckland, "College Dropouts Who Came Back," *Harvard Educational Review*, 34(1964), 402-420.

[4] Beverly Duncan, *Family Factors and School Dropout: 1920–1960*, U. S. Office of Education, Cooperative Research Project No. 2258, Ann Arbor: Univers. of Michigan, 1965.

tion to independent adult status, we do violence to reality. Completion of schooling, departure from the parental home, entry into the labor market, and contracting of a first marriage are crucial steps in this transition, which all normally occur within a few short years. Yet they occur at no fixed ages nor in any fixed order. As soon as we aggregate individual data for analytical purposes we are forced into the use of simplifying assumptions. Our assumption here is, in effect, that "first job" has a uniform significance for all men in terms of its temporal relationship to educational preparation and subsequent work experience. If this assumption is not strictly correct, we doubt that it could be improved by substituting any other *single* measure of initial occupational status. (In designing the OCG questionnaire, the alternative of "job at the time of first marriage" was entertained briefly but dropped for the reason, among others, that unmarried men would be excluded thereby.)

One other problem with the U-W transition should be mentioned. Among the younger men in the study, 20 to 24 years old, are many who have yet to finish their schooling or to take up their first jobs or both —not to mention the men in this age group missed by the survey on account of their military service (see Appendix C). Unfortunately, an early decision on tabulation plans resulted in the inclusion of the 20 to 24 group with the older men in aggregate tables for men 20 to 64 years old. We have ascertained that this results in only minor distortions by comparing a variety of data for men 20 to 64 and for those 25 to 64 years of age. Once over the U-W hurdle, we see no serious objection to our assumption that both U and W precede Y, except in regard to some fraction of the very young men just mentioned.

In summary, then, we take the somewhat idealized assumption of temporal order to represent an order of priority in a causal or processual sequence, which may be stated diagrammatically as follows:

$$(V, X) - (U) - (W) - (Y).$$

In proposing this sequence we do not overlook the possibility of what Carlsson calls "delayed effects,"[5] meaning that an early variable may affect a later one not only via intervening variables but also directly (or perhaps through variables not measured in the study).

In translating this conceptual framework into quantitative estimates the first task is to establish the pattern of associations between the variables in the sequence. This is accomplished with the correlation coefficient, as explained in Chapter 4. Table 5.1 supplies the correla-

[5] Gösta Carlsson, *Social Mobility and Class Structure,* Lund: CWK Gleerup, 1958, p. 124.

TABLE 5.1. SIMPLE CORRELATIONS FOR FIVE STATUS VARIABLES

Variable	Variable				
	Y	W	U	X	V
Y: 1962 occ. status	...	.541	.596	.405	.322
W: First-job status		...	.538	.417	.332
U: Education			...	.438	.453
X: Father's occ. status				...	.516
V: Father's education					...

tion matrix on which much of the subsequent analysis is based. In discussing causal interpretations of these correlations, we shall have to be clear about the distinction between two points of view. On the one hand, the simple correlation—given our assumption as to direction of causation—measures the gross magnitude of the effect of the antecedent upon the consequent variable. Thus, if $r_{YW} = .541$, we can say that an increment of one standard deviation in first job status produces (whether directly or indirectly) an increment of just over half of one standard deviation in 1962 occupational status. From another point of view we are more concerned with net effects. If both first job and 1962 status have a common antecedent cause—say, father's occupation—we may want to state what part of the effect of W on Y consists in a transmission of the prior influence of X. Or, thinking of X as the initial cause, we may focus on the extent to which its influence on Y is transmitted by way of its prior influence on W.

We may, then, devote a few remarks to the pattern of gross effects before presenting the apparatus that yields estimates of net direct and indirect effects. Since we do not require a causal ordering of father's education with respect to his occupation, we may be content simply to note that $r_{XV} = .516$ is somewhat lower than the corresponding correlation, $r_{YU} = .596$, observed for the respondents themselves. The difference suggests a heightening of the effect of education on occupational status between the fathers' and the sons' generations. Before stressing this interpretation, however, we must remember that the measurements of V and X do not pertain to some actual cohort of men, here designated "fathers." Each "father" is represented in the data in proportion to the number of his sons who were 20 to 64 years old in March 1962.

The first recorded status of the son himself is education (U). We note that r_{UV} is just slightly greater than r_{UX}. Apparently both measures on the father represent factors that may influence the son's education.

In terms of gross effects there is a clear ordering of influences on first job. Thus $r_{WU} > r_{WX} > r_{WV}$. Education is most strongly corre-

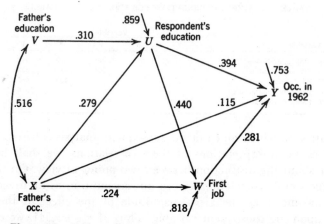

Figure 5.1. Path coefficients in basic model of the process of stratification.

lated with first job, followed by father's occupation, and then by father's education.

Occupational status in 1962 (Y) apparently is influenced more strongly by education than by first job; but our earlier discussion of the first-job measure suggests we should not overemphasize the difference between r_{YW} and r_{YU}. Each, however, is substantially greater than r_{YX}, which in turn is rather more impressive than r_{YV}.

Figure 5.1 is a graphic representation of the system of relationships among the five variables that we propose as our basic model. The numbers entered on the diagram, with the exception of r_{XV}, are path coefficients, the estimation of which will be explained shortly. First we must become familiar with the conventions followed in constructing this kind of diagram. The link between V and X is shown as a curved line with an arrowhead at both ends. This is to distinguish it from the other lines, which are taken to be paths of influence. In the case of V and X we may suspect an influence running from the former to the latter. But if the diagram is logical for the respondent's generation, we should have to assume that for the fathers, likewise, education and occupation are correlated not only because one affects the other but also because common causes lie behind both, which we have not measured. The bidirectional arrow merely serves to sum up all sources of correlation between V and X and to indicate that the explanation thereof is not part of the problem at hand.

The straight lines running from one measured variable to another represent *direct* (or net) influences. The symbol for the path coefficient, such as p_{YW}, carries a double subscript. The first subscript is the variable at the head of the path, or the effect; the second is the causal variable. (This resembles the convention for regression coefficients, where the first subscript refers to the "dependent" variable, the second to the "independent" variable.)

Finally, we see lines with no source indicated carrying arrows to each of the effect variables. These represent the residual paths, standing for all other influences on the variable in question, including causes not recognized or measured, errors of measurement, and departures of the true relationships from additivity and linearity, properties that are assumed throughout the analysis (as explained in the section on regression in Chapter 4).

An important feature of this kind of causal scheme is that variables recognized as effects of certain antecedent factors may, in turn, serve as causes for subsequent variables. For example, U is caused by V and X, but it in turn influences W and Y. The algebraic representation of the scheme is a system of equations, rather than the single equation more often employed in multiple regression analysis. This feature permits a flexible conceptualization of the *modus operandi* of the causal network. Note that Y is shown here as being influenced directly by W, U, and X, but not by V (an assumption that will be justified shortly). But this does not imply that V has no influence on Y. V affects U, which does affect Y both directly and indirectly (via W). Moreover, V is correlated with X, and thus shares in the gross effect of X on Y, which is partly direct and partly indirect. Hence the gross effect of V on Y, previously described in terms of the correlation r_{YV}, is here interpreted as being entirely indirect, in consequence of V's effect on intervening variables and its correlation with another cause of Y.

PATH COEFFICIENTS

Whether a path diagram, or the causal scheme it represents, is adequate depends on both theoretical and empirical considerations. At a minimum, before constructing the diagram we must know, or be willing to assume, a causal ordering of the observed variables (hence the lengthy discussion of this matter earlier in this chapter). This information is external or *a priori* with respect to the data, which merely describe associations or correlations. Moreover, the causal scheme must be complete, in the sense that all causes are accounted for. Here, as in most problems involving analysis of observational data, we achieve a formal completeness of the scheme by representing unmeasured causes as a residual factor, presumed to be uncorrelated with the remaining factors lying behind the variable in question. If any factor is known or presumed to operate in some other way it must be represented in the diagram in accordance with its causal role, even though it is not measured. Sometimes it is possible to deduce interesting implications from the inclusion of such a variable and to secure useful estimates of certain paths in the absence of measurements on it, but this is not always so. A partial exception to the rule that all causes must be explicitly represented in the diagram is the unmeasured variable that can be assumed to operate strictly as an intervening variable. Its inclusion would enrich our understanding of a causal system without invalidating the causal scheme that omits it. Sociologists have only recently begun to appreciate how stringent are the logical requirements that must be met if discussion of causal processes is to go beyond mere impressionism and vague verbal formulations.[6] We are a long way from being able to make causal inferences with confidence, and schemes of the kind presented here had best be regarded as crude first approximations to adequate causal models.

On the empirical side, a minimum test of the adequacy of a causal diagram is whether it satisfactorily accounts for the observed correlations among the measured variables. In making such a test we employ the fundamental theorem in path analysis, which shows how to obtain the correlation between any two variables in the system, given the path coefficients and correlations entered on the diagram.[7] Without stating this theorem in general form we may illustrate its application here. For example,

$$r_{YX} = p_{YX} + p_{YU}r_{UX} + p_{YW}r_{WX};$$

and

$$r_{WX} = p_{WX} + p_{WU}r_{UX}.$$

We make use of each path leading to a given variable (such as Y in the first example) and the correlations of each of its causes with all other variables in the system. The latter correlations, in turn, may be analyzed; for example, r_{WX}, which appeared as such in the first equation, is broken down into two parts in the second. A complete expansion along these lines is required to trace out all the indirect connections between variables; thus,

$$r_{YX} = p_{YX} + p_{YU}p_{UX} + p_{YU}p_{UV}r_{VX} + p_{YW}p_{WX} + p_{YW}p_{WU}p_{UX} + p_{YW}p_{WU}p_{UV}r_{VX}.$$

[6] H. M. Blalock, Jr., *Causal Inferences in Nonexperimental Research*, Chapel Hill: Univer. of North Carolina Press, 1964.

[7] Sewall Wright, "Path Coefficients and Path Regressions," *Biometrics*, **16** (1960), 189–202; Otis Dudley Duncan, "Path Analysis," *American Journal of Sociology*, **72**(1966), 1-16.

Now, if the path coefficients are properly estimated, and if there is no inconsistency in the diagram, the correlations calculated by a formula like the foregoing must equal the observed correlations. Let us compare the values computed from such a formula with the corresponding observed correlations:

$$r_{WV} = p_{WX}r_{XV} + p_{WU}r_{UV}$$
$$= (.224)(.516) + (.440)(.453)$$
$$= .116 + .199 = .315$$

which compares with the observed value of .332; and

$$r_{YV} = p_{YU}r_{UV} + p_{YX}r_{XV} + p_{YW}r_{WV}$$
$$= (.394)(.453) + (.115)(.516) + (.281)(.315) = .326$$

(using here the calculated rather than the observed value of r_{WV}), which resembles the actual value, .322. Other such comparisons—for r_{YX}, for example—reveal, at most, trivial discrepancies (no larger than .001).

We arrive, by this roundabout journey, at the problem of getting numerical values for the path coefficients in the first place. This involves using equations of the foregoing type inversely. We have illustrated how to obtain correlations if the path coefficients are known, but in the typical empirical problem we know the correlations (or at least some of them) and have to estimate the paths. For a diagram of the type of Figure 5.1 the solution involves equations of the same form as those of linear multiple regression, except that we work with a recursive system of regression equations[8] rather than a single regression equation.

Table 5.2 records the results of the regression calculations. It can be seen that some alternative combinations of independent variables were studied. It turned out that the net regressions of both W and Y on V were so small as to be negligible. Hence V could be disregarded as a direct influence on these variables without loss of information. The net regression of Y on X was likewise small but, as it appears, not entirely negligible. Curiously, this net regression is of the same order of magnitude as the proportion of occupational inheritance in this population—about 10 per cent, as discussed in Chapter 4. We might speculate that the direct effect of father's occupation on the occupational status of a mature man consists of this modest amount of strict occupational inheritance. The remainder of the effect of X on Y is indirect, inasmuch as X has previously influenced U and W, the son's education and the occupational level at which he got his start. For reasons noted in Chapter 3 we do not assume that the full impact of

[8] Blalock, *op. cit.*, pp. 54ff.

TABLE 5.2. PARTIAL REGRESSION COEFFICIENTS IN STANDARD FORM (BETA COEFFICIENTS) AND COEFFICIENTS OF DETERMINATION, FOR SPECIFIED COMBINATIONS OF VARIABLES

Dependent Variable[a]	Independent Variables[a]				Coefficient of Determination (R^2)
	W	U	X	V	
U[b]	...	...	.279	.310	.26
W	...	.433	.214	.026	.33
W[b]	...	.440	.224	...	.33
Y	.282	.397	.120	-.014	.43
Y[b]	.281	.394	.115	...	.43
Y	.311	.428	...	...	.42

[a]V: Father's education.
  X: Father's occ. status.
  U: Respondent's education.
  W: First-job status.
  Y: 1962 occ. status.
[b]Beta coefficients in these sets taken as estimates of path coefficients for Figure 5.1.

the tendency to take up the father's occupation is registered in the choice of first job.

With the formal properties of the model in mind we may turn to some general problems confronting this kind of interpretation of our results. One of the first impressions gained from Figure 5.1 is that the largest path coefficients in the diagram are those for residual factors, that is, variables not measured. The residual path is merely a convenient representation of the extent to which measured causes in the system fail to account for the variation in the effect variables. (The residual is obtained from the coefficient of determination; if $R^2_{Y(WUX)}$ is the squared multiple correlation of Y on the three independent variables, then the residual for Y is $\sqrt{1 - R^2_{Y(WUX)}}$.) Sociologists are often disappointed in the size of the residual, assuming that this is a measure of their success in "explaining" the phenomenon under study. They seldom reflect on what it would mean to live in a society where nearly perfect explanation of the dependent variable could be secured by studying causal variables like father's occupation or respondent's education. In such a society it would indeed be true that some are "destined to poverty almost from birth . . . by the economic status or occupation of their parents" (in the words of the reference cited in footnote 1). Others, of course, would be "destined" to affluence or to modest circumstances. By no effort of their own could they materially alter the course of destiny, nor could any stroke of fortune, good or ill, lead to an outcome not already in the cards.

Thinking of the residual as an index of the adequacy of an explanation gives rise to a serious misconception. It is thought that a high multiple correlation is presumptive evidence that an explanation is correct or nearly so, whereas a low percentage of determination means that a causal interpretation is almost certainly wrong. The fact is that the size of the residual (or, if one prefers, the proportion of variation "explained") is *no* guide whatever to the validity of a causal interpretation. The best-known cases of "spurious correlation"—a correlation leading to an egregiously wrong interpretation—are those in which the coefficient of determination is quite high.

The relevant question about the residual is not really its size at all, but whether the unobserved factors it stands for are properly represented as being uncorrelated with the measured antecedent variables. We shall entertain subsequently some conjectures about unmeasured variables that clearly are not uncorrelated with the causes depicted in Figure 5.1. It turns out that these require us to acknowledge certain possible modifications of the diagram, whereas other features of it remain more or less intact. A delicate question in this regard is that of the burden of proof. It is all too easy to make a formidable list of unmeasured variables that someone has alleged to be crucial to the process under study. But the mere existence of such variables is already acknowledged by the very presence of the residual. It would seem to be part of the task of the critic to *show*, if only hypothetically, but *specifically*, how the modification of the causal scheme to include a new variable would disrupt or alter the relationships in the original diagram. His argument to this effect could then be examined for plausibility and his evidence, if any, studied in terms of the empirical possibilities it suggests.

Our supposition is that the scheme in Figure 5.1 is most easily subject to modification by introducing additional measures of the same kind as those used here. If indexes relating to socioeconomic background other than V and X are inserted we will almost certainly estimate differently the direct effects of these particular variables. If occupational statuses of the respondent intervening between W and Y were known we should have to modify more or less radically the right-hand portion of the diagram, as will be shown in the next section. Yet we should argue that such modifications may amount to an enrichment or extension of the basic model rather than an invalidation of it. The same may be said of other variables that function as intervening causes. In theory, it should be possible to specify these in some detail, and a major part of the research worker's task is properly defined as an attempt at such specification. In the course of such work, to be sure, there is always the possibility of a discovery that would require a fundamental reformulation, making the present model obsolete. Discarding the model would be a cost gladly paid for the prize of such a discovery.

Postponing the confrontation with an altered model, the one at hand is not lacking in interest. An instructive exercise is to compare the magnitudes of gross and net relationships. Here we make use of the fact that the correlation coefficient and the path coefficient have the same dimensionality. The correlation $r_{YX} = .405$ (Table 5.1) means that a unit change (one standard deviation) in X produces a change of 0.4 unit in Y, in gross terms. The path coefficient, $p_{YX} = .115$ (Figure 5.1), tells us that about one-fourth of this gross effect is a result of the direct influence of X on Y. (We speculated above on the role of occupational inheritance in this connection.) The remainder ($.405 - .115 = .29$) is indirect, via U and W. The sum of all indirect effects, therefore, is given by the difference between the simple correlation and the path coefficient connecting two variables. We note that the indirect effects on Y are generally substantial, relative to the direct. Even the variable temporally closest (we assume) to Y has "indirect effects"—actually, common antecedent causes—nearly as large as the direct. Thus $r_{YW} = .541$ and $p_{YW} = .281$, so that the aggregate of "indirect effects" is .26, which in this case are common determinants of Y and W that spuriously inflate the correlation between them.

To ascertain the indirect effects along a given chain of causation we must multiply the path coefficients along the chain. The procedure is to locate on the diagram the dependent variable of interest, and then trace back along the paths linking it to its immediate and remote causes. In such a tracing we may reverse direction once but only once, following the rule "first back, then forward." Any bidirectional correlation may be traced in either direction. If the diagram contains more than one such correlation, however, only one may be used in a given compound path. In tracing the indirect connections no variable may be intersected more than once in one compound path. Having traced all such possible compound paths, we obtain the entirety of indirect effects as their sum.

Let us consider the example of effects of education on first job, U on W. The gross or total effect is $r_{WU} = .538$. The direct path is $p_{WU} = .440$. There are two indirect connections or compound paths: from W back to X then forward to U; and from W back to X, then back to V, and then forward to U. Hence we have:

$$r_{WU} = p_{WU} + \underbrace{p_{WX}p_{UX} + p_{WX}r_{XV}p_{UV}}$$

(gross)   (direct)   (indirect)

or, numerically,

$$.538 = .440 + (.224)(.279) + (.224)(.516)(.310)$$
$$= .440 + .062 + .036$$
$$= .440 + .098.$$

In this case all the indirect effect of U on W derives from the fact that both U and W have X (plus V) as a common cause. In other instances, when more than one common cause is involved and these causes are themselves interrelated, the complexity is too great to permit a succinct verbal summary.

A final stipulation about the scheme had best be stated, though it is implicit in all the previous discussion. The form of the model itself, but most particularly the numerical estimates accompanying it, are submitted as valid only for the population under study. No claim is made that an equally cogent account of the process of stratification in another society could be rendered in terms of this scheme. For other populations, or even for subpopulations within the United States, the magnitudes would almost certainly be different, although we have some basis for supposing them to have been fairly constant over the last few decades in this country. The technique of path analysis is not a method for discovering causal laws but a procedure for giving a quantitative interpretation to the manifestations of a known or assumed causal system as it operates in a particular population. When the same interpretive structure is appropriate for two or more populations there is something to be learned by comparing their respective path coefficients and correlation patterns. We have not yet reached the stage at which such comparative study of stratification systems is feasible.

AGE GROUPS: THE LIFE CYCLE OF A SYNTHETIC COHORT

For simplicity, the preceding analysis has ignored differences among age groups. Our present task is to venture some interpretation of such differences. The raw material for the analysis is presented in Table 5.3 in the form of simple correlations between pairs of the five status variables under study. For the reasons mentioned in Chapter 3, this analysis is confined to men with nonfarm background.

We must consider immediately what kinds of inferences or interpretations are allowed by comparisons among the four cohorts. Three of the variables are specified as of a more or less uniform stage of the respondent's life cycle: father's occupation (X), respondent's education (U), and first job (W). Father's education (V), on the other hand, was presumably determinate in the father's youth; the time interval between V and any of the former variables would be determined in large part by father's age at respondent's birth. This interval is variable in length. We might, however, assume that the time interval from V to X, though highly variable within each cohort of respondents, has a similar average and dispersion from one cohort to another. If father's education is taken as a fixed status once the father has completed his

TABLE 5.3.   SIMPLE CORRELATIONS BETWEEN STATUS VARIABLES, FOR FOUR AGE
GROUPS OF MEN WITH NONFARM BACKGROUND

Age Group and Variable	Variable			
	W	U	X	V
25 to 34 (age 16 in 1943 to 1952)				
Y: 1962 occ. status	.584	.657	.366	.350
W: Status of first job	...	.574	.380	...[a]
U: Education		...	.411	.416
X: Father's occ. status			...	.488
V: Father's education				...
35 to 44 (age 16 in 1933 to 1942)				
Y: 1962 occ. status	.492	.637	.400	.336
W: Status of first job	...	.532	.377	...[a]
U: Education		...	.440	.424
X: Father's occ. status			...	.535
45 to 54 (age 16 in 1923 to 1932)				
Y: 1962 occ. status	.514	.593	.383	.261
W: Status of first job	...	.554	.388	...[a]
U: Education		...	.428	.373
X: Father's occ. status			...	.481
55 to 64 (age 16 in 1913 to 1922)				
Y: 1962 occ. status	.513	.576	.340	.311
W: Status of first job	...	.557	.384	...[a]
U: Education		...	.392	.409
X: Father's occ. status			...	.530

[a]Not computed because requisite tabulation was not available.

schooling, then the temporal proximity of V to respondent's education (U) and first job (W) is about the same from one cohort to another.

Tentatively, therefore, we might assume that intercohort comparisons with respect to V, X, U, and W, and their interrelations, are
tantamount to a historical time series, such as might have been
observed had we surveyed men 25 to 34 years old not only in 1962
but also in 1952, 1942, and 1932. This assumption, of course, entails
some corollary premises: most particularly, the reliability of retrospective data and the representativeness of the survivors to 1962 of
the cohort membership at earlier dates. If these assumptions are accepted, we may inspect Table 5.3 in a straightforward manner for
historical trends. The correlation between W and X was studied in
just this way in Chapter 3.

The correlation between father's education and his occupation, r_{XV},
fluctuates between cohorts without showing a unidirectional trend.
We are somewhat reluctant to give an interpretation to these fluctua-

tions, in view of the fact that both variables place a heavy requirement on the respondent's knowledge and memory. The proportion of NA's for this combination of variables is relatively high.

The correlation of respondent's with father's education, r_{UV}, shows one cohort out of line with what is otherwise a nearly constant value. No plausible interpretation of this fluctuation comes to mind. There was an apparent, if slight, increase in r_{UX}—respondent's education with father's occupation—up to 1933 to 1942, dating the cohort by the years in which its members reached age 16. This was followed by a drop to the most recent cohort. It may be sheer coincidence that both r_{UX} and r_{UV} show the highest value for the 1933 to 1942 cohort. This cohort happens to be the one with by far the largest proportion (roughly three-quarters) of its members veterans of World War II. Sociologists have sometimes speculated that the availability of educational benefits in the "G.I. Bill" may have equalized opportunities for men coming from different socioeconomic backgrounds. The present data contain no hint of such an equalization effect, which would reduce r_{UV}, not enhance it.

We have already noted in Chapter 3 that there is hardly a trend worth discussing in r_{WX}, first job with father's occupation. Somewhat greater fluctuations, though no monotonic trend, are observed for r_{WU}, first job with education. The lowest value is for the 1933 to 1942 cohort, many of whom entered the labor market in the depression years. Perhaps the circumstances of that period made education a somewhat less important advantage than in the subsequent period of more nearly full employment.

It is difficult, in summary, to detect any bona fide trends in the correlations just reviewed. There are some intercohort fluctuations possibly too large to attribute to sampling variation alone. Attributing these to particular historical circumstances of the several cohorts involves a large element of conjecture. Indeed, despite the occurrence of some puzzling fluctuations, we get the strong impression of an essentially stable pattern of interrelationships.

When we turn to correlations involving respondent's occupational status in 1962 (Y), the interpretation of intercohort differences as a historical time series is no longer legitimate. The cohorts, observed as a cross-section of age groups in 1962, differed in length of working experience and in time elapsed since leaving their families of orientation. Effects of these differences are inextricably mixed with any differences due to the periods at which the cohorts initiated their careers.

Consider r_{YU}, the correlation of 1962 occupational status with education of respondent. There is a monotonic increase in the magnitude of this correlation, from .576 for the oldest cohort to .657 for the youngest. This could mean either (1) that education has been becoming a more important factor in occupational achievement in recent decades, or (2) that education is most important at the stage of one's career just following the completion of schooling. Whereas it is not possible to distinguish between these two interpretations unequivocally, some data permit us to make plausible inferences in this case. The second interpretation would imply that the correlation between education and first job, r_{WU}, is larger than that between education and 1962 occupation, r_{YU}. In fact, however, r_{WU} is smaller than r_{YU} for all four age cohorts. The probable inference, therefore, is that the first of the two alternatives is the correct interpretation, though the questionable reliability of the data on first jobs would make us reluctant to rest the case on evidence provided by these data alone. But the tentative conclusion is that the influence of education on ultimate occupational achievement, though not on career beginnings, has increased in recent decades. The correlation between education and occupational status is considerably higher for respondents (r_{YU}) than for their fathers (r_{XV}) in all four age groups, and the difference between son's and father's correlation has become more pronounced for the youngest age cohort. Any one of these findings might be explained differently, but all of them together constitute fairly convincing evidence that the influence of education on careers has become more pronounced over time, the most reliable evidence in support of this contention being the difference between fathers and sons.

None of the other three correlations involving Y shows a similar monotonic relationship with age. Making use of the model developed earlier in this chapter, we examine in Table 5.4 the dependence of each of the respondent's achieved statuses on a combination of antecedent statuses. For the moment, each of the four cohorts is regarded as a distinct population, and we shall consider whether the time series interpretation of intercohort differences is informative.

The regression of respondent's education on father's education and occupation (first line in each of the four panels of Table 5.4) shows some variation over cohorts. Father's occupation appears to have the greater relative importance for the two middle cohorts, father's education for the two extreme age groups. It is difficult to suggest an interpretation for this variation, if it is, indeed, a genuine phenomenon. The combined effects of the two background variables, as registered in the coefficients of determination, are just slightly greater for the two most recent cohorts than for the two earlier ones.

In the set of regressions for first job (second line of each panel) there

TABLE 5.4. PARTIAL REGRESSION COEFFICIENTS IN STANDARD FORM (BETA COEFFICIENTS) AND COEFFICIENTS OF DETERMINATION FOR SPECIFIED COMBINATIONS OF VARIABLES, FOR FOUR AGE GROUPS OF MEN WITH NONFARM BACKGROUND

Age Group and Dependent Variable	Independent Variable				Coefficient of determination (R^2)
	Respondent's First Job (W)	Respondent's Education (U)	Father's Occ. (X)	Father's Education (V)	
25 TO 34 (AGE 16 IN 1943 TO 1952)					
Respondent's education (U)	...	...	.273	.283	.23
Respondent's first job (W)	...	.503	.174	...	.36
1962 occ. (Y)	.294	.462	.065	...	.50
35 TO 44 (AGE 16 IN 1933 TO 1942)					
Respondent's education (U)	...	...	.299	.264	.24
Respondent's first job (W)	...	.455	.177	...	.31
1962 occ. (Y)	.191	.485	.115	...	.45
45 TO 54 (AGE 16 IN 1923 TO 1932)					
Respondent's education (U)	...	...	.323	.218	.22
Respondent's first job (W)	...	.474	.186	...	.33
1962 occ. (Y)	.243	.410	.114	...	.41
55 TO 64 (AGE 16 IN 1913 TO 1922)					
Respondent's education (U)	...	...	.244	.280	.21
Respondent's first job (W)	...	.481	.195	...	.34
1962 occ. (Y)	.258	.399	.084	...	.39

is again fluctuation, albeit of modest magnitude, in the size of the net regression coefficients. There is no ambiguity about the relative importance of the two independent variables: education is a much more important influence on first job than is father's occupation. The only noteworthy fluctuation in the coefficients of determination is the relatively low value for the 1933 to 1942 cohort. We have already noted that this cohort may have been especially subject to depression influences. If these are indeed the relevant influences here the finding suggests that the depression lessened the significance of education and background for first jobs. With its heavy quota of World War II veterans, moreover, this cohort may have deviated more widely than others from our idealized assumption about the temporal sequence of the status variables. Despite the fluctuation noted we are inclined to emphasize the intercohort stability of the regression pattern.

With 1962 occupational status as the dependent variable (third line in each panel), we are back in the situation in which intercohort comparisons must involve an inescapable ambiguity. There is, in any case, no monotonic relationship with age for any of the three net regression coefficients. The 1933 to 1942 cohort is distinctive in that the coefficient for first job is the lowest among the four cohorts, whereas the coefficients for education and father's occupation are the highest. It seems that first jobs in the depression were out of line, but that education and social origins made up for their lesser influence on first jobs by influencing later careers more. In addition to the possibly relevant special historical circumstances of this depression cohort, there is another consideration of a different kind. At age 35 to 44 in 1962, this cohort had attained the age probably most typical of fathers of 16-year-old boys. We might suppose that at this age the effect of father's occupation (when the respondent was 16 years old) via occupational "inheritance" would be at a maximum. This interpretation gains no support from a tabulation of the proportions of men in the four cohorts having occupational status scores identical with those of their fathers: 7.3 per cent for men 25 to 34; 7.1 per cent at 35 to 44; 7.0 at 45 to 54; and 7.6 at 55 to 64. (Recall that the data in this section omit men whose fathers were in farm occupations.)

To find a striking monotonic relationship with age we need only inspect the coefficients of determination, $R^2_{Y(WUX)}$. These range from .39 for the oldest cohort to .50 for the youngest. If we were to make the time-series interpretation of the intercohort comparisons we should have to conclude that occupational achievement has been becoming much more closely dependent on antecedent statuses. At this point, however, the completely confounded factor of length of time in the working force presents itself for a rival interpretation. At age 55 to 64 the oldest men are 30 years or more removed from the experiences indexed by variables W, U, and X. Over this span of time many influences on occupational status that are unrelated to background and early experience have had a chance to operate. The youngest men, conversely, are still fairly near the time when their working life actually got under way, and the many contingencies yet to come can be expected to attenuate the initially established relationship of achievement to antecedent statuses.

The final topic of this discussion is the development of the latter interpretation, which rests on the assumption that the cohort differences in Y are due to the individual's age and not to a secular trend, an assumption that cannot be tested with our data. As a vehicle for the interpretation, we treat the observations on the four cohorts as four sets of observations on a single *synthetic* cohort. As will become evident, it is difficult to maintain this fiction with complete consistency, as demographers have found in connection with the synthetic-cohort approach to fertility analysis. Nevertheless, the artifice has considerable didactic value and, at the least, formulates hypotheses that one might hope to check later with more complete data on real cohorts.

As a first step we assume that the intercohort fluctuations in the three intercorrelations among W, U, and X are mere sampling variations. We eliminate these fluctuations by averaging the four sets of correlations. Then we assume that the correlations involving Y (1962 occupational status) represent a time series of observations on a single cohort observed at decade intervals. For notational convenience, let Y_1 stand for occupational status at age 25 to 34, Y_2 at 35 to 44, Y_3 at 45 to 54, and Y_4 at 55 to 64. The variable Y, by virtue of this mental experiment, is thus to be regarded as four different variables, depending on the age at which occupational status is measured. One further simplification is easily justified. We disregard altogether variable V (father's education) in view of the earlier evidence that it affects occupational status almost exclusively via X and U. This allows us to represent the relationship between U and X as merely a bidirectional correlation.

The model suggested for the synthetic cohort interpretation is portrayed in the form of a path diagram in Figure 5.2. This diagram suggests that each achieved occupational status is affected directly by the immediately preceding occupational status (that is, by first job in the case of the men aged 25 to 34, and by status 10 years ago for men at

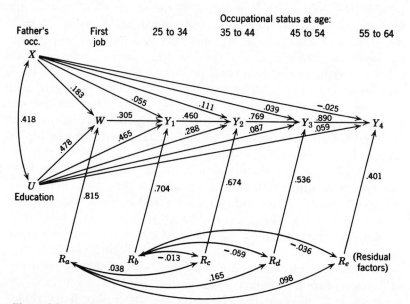

Figure 5.2. Synthetic cohort interpretation of the achievement of occupational status, for men with nonfarm background (numerical values from "Set 4," Appendix Table J5.1).

the more advanced ages). Moreover, each such status is assumed to be subject to direct influence by educational attainment and by father's occupational status.

To obtain a solution for this model we must rely on partial information. Although we have distinguished four occupational statuses subsequent to first job (Y_1, Y_2, Y_3, Y_4) we have no observations in the OCG data from which to estimate the six intercorrelations among these four variables. Nonetheless, if the model were literally correct and if we assumed no intercorrelations among residual factors, we could write just exactly the number of equations required to solve for each path in the diagram. The reason is that the unknown correlations can be expressed as a function of known correlations in the particular causal structure portrayed by this diagram. A first solution was obtained in this way (set 1, Appendix Table J5.1). Unfortunately, it turned out to be an unacceptable solution, for two of the implied values of unknown correlations were required to be above unity, which is algebraically impossible.

To overcome this difficulty, external information was brought to bear on the problem. Two studies in the literature report certain correlations that are lacking in the OCG data: present occupation with occupation 10 years earlier. Both sets of correlations pertain to the 1940 to 1950 decade. Data for a Chicago sample[9] supply the values $r_{21} = .55$, $r_{32} = .77$, and $r_{43} = .87$. Correlations for a Minneapolis sample[10] run appreciably higher: $r_{21} = .83$, $r_{32} = .91$, $r_{43} = .96$. Discounting the likelihood of so great a difference between the two cities, there are at least two reasons why the discrepancy may have occurred. First, the measure of occupational status was not the same. The Chicago study used the same index of occupational status as that employed in the OCG research, whereas the Minneapolis investigators used an "occupational rating" that is not fully described. Second, the Chicago results derive from a detailed investigation of labor mobility in which respondents gave complete work histories for the period 1940 to 1951. The Minneapolis study apparently asked respondents only to report current occupation and occupation 10 years earlier. The approach taken in Chicago may well have elicited a more complete report of actual changes in status during the decade. The Chicago data are presumably, therefore, the more reliable as well as the more nearly comparable, in terms of the concept of occupational status, to the OCG data. Yet there is one respect in which the Minneapolis data may actually be preferable. The OCG questionnaire, like the Minneapolis interview (we assume), asked for only one antecedent occupational status: first job in the case of OCG and occupation ten years ago in the Minneapolis study. If there is a tendency for respondents to err in making retrospective information more compatible with current status than may actually have been the case, then the two studies must have shared a common source of spurious correlation.

Without offering a dogmatic resolution to this dilemma, we simply computed alternative solutions for the diagram in Figure 5.2 using the correlations for Chicago, for Minneapolis, and the average of the two sets in turn (respectively, set 3, set 4, and set 5 in Appendix Table J5.1). The last expedient, in a sense, worked best, and it is the one used in Figure 5.2. It gave results not too dissimilar from still another alternative (set 2). Here we borrowed from the Chicago data not the correlations but the path coefficients, p_{21}, p_{32}, and p_{43}, which had been obtained from a calculation with the Chicago data for a causal diagram much like Figure 5.2.[11]

[9] Otis Dudley Duncan and Robert W. Hodge, "Education and Occupational Mobility," *American Journal of Sociology*, **68**(1963), 629-644. (The correlations appear on p. 641.)

[10] Godfrey Hochbaum, John G. Darley, E. D. Monachesi, and Charles Bird, "Socioeconomic Variables in a Large City," *American Journal of Sociology*, **61** (1955), 31-38. (The correlations are in Table 7.)

[11] Duncan, "Path Analysis," *loc. cit.*

All four alternatives yield results that are not only permissible algebraically but also plausible in a crude quantitative sense. All require that we acknowledge certain intercorrelations among residual factors. No substantive interpretation can be given to these correlations which, fortunately, are almost negligible in size, especially in the set shown in Figure 5.2. The presence of such correlations can suggest three conclusions: (1) The model is not entirely correct; unmeasured variables disturb the relationships portrayed in it in a systematic rather than random fashion. (2) There are real differences in the experience of the four cohorts such that the heuristic fiction of a synthetic cohort recapitulating the pattern of each does not yield a self-consistent set of assumptions. (3) There are correlated errors in the data, as suggested above in regard to the possible distortion of retrospective information.

In all likelihood there is an element of truth in each explanation. Yet we must not exaggerate the possible defects in our interpretation. The intercorrelation of residuals arises from the fact that the model omitting them does not fully account for the observed correlations of Y with W in the three older age groups. We can compute values of r_{YW} assuming the path coefficients shown in Figure 5.2 and neglecting the correlations among the residuals. Here are the computed values (with actual values in parentheses): $r_{Y_2 W} = .471$ (.492); $r_{Y_3 W} = .442$ (.514); $r_{Y_4 W} = .481$ (.513). This is quite a close agreement. Hence the intercorrelations of residuals, though they are required for the sake of consistency, may have little substantive importance.

Despite the extended discussion of technicalities, Figure 5.2 is offered as something more than a methodological *tour de force*. It is a compact representation of our causal interpretation of a vast body of data, an interpretation contrived to take account of and thus help explain the patterns of association revealed by those data. Let us dwell, in conclusion, on some substantive implications of the results.

By showing that we can come close to forcing the data into conformity with the synthetic cohort model, we suggest strongly that there has been a quite stable—though not completely invariant—pattern of occupational status achievement in this country over the past four decades. This suggestion is at least not seriously compromised by our earlier results on trends in occupational mobility. For direct evidence one may compare the average path coefficients p_{WX} and p_{WU} in Figure 5.2 with the corresponding statistics for individual cohorts in Table 5.4. No single set of these coefficients differs from the average by more than a trivial amount.

The model suggests that factors salient at an early stage of a man's career may continue to play a *direct* role as he grows older. But the direct effects of education and father's status are attenuated drastically with the passage of time. A compensatory effect is the increasing relevance of the accumulation of occupational experience as time passes. A striking result is the diminution in importance of unspecified residual factors with aging of a cohort. This is directly opposite to the finding of higher coefficients of determination for the younger cohorts observed in Table 5.4. (The implied coefficients of determination in the model are obtained by subtracting from unity the squared values of the appropriate residual paths. Hence decreasing values of the residual path imply increasing coefficients of determination.) The explanation is, of course, that the synthetic-cohort model takes into account the occupational experience intervening between first job and a given age, allowing such experience to have a cumulative effect as the cohort grows older. The calculations for individual age groups in Table 5.4 do not take this factor of work experience into account in any direct way.

One may properly be skeptical of the precise numerical values in Figure 5.2: they are, in any case, values for an unobservable entity, the synthetic cohort. We could possibly make a case for the realism of the estimate that $p_{Y_2X} > p_{Y_1X}$ in terms of the previously noted delayed impact of background on achievement for the depression cohort, though it seems unwise to press the point. We doubt that the negative value of p_{Y_4X} corresponds to any true effect; the safe conclusion is that this path is essentially zero. There is every reason to suppose that education is, at every stage, a more important influence, both direct and indirect, on occupational achievement than father's occupation.

As a by-product of the solution, we secure values for correlations between occupational statuses held two or three decades ago. Since we know of no published values of such coefficients, there is no way to check the plausibility of these results. The solution shown in Figure 5.2 implies that $r_{Y_3Y_1} = .602$, $r_{Y_4Y_2} = .775$, and $r_{Y_4Y_1} = .565$. These correlations imply a considerable persistence of status over long intervals of time. Yet they do allow some significant amount of status mobility after age 25 to 34 or even 35 to 44, by which time the principal effects of background already have been registered. Although the literature has stressed intergenerational transmission of status and, by implication, the younger ages during which career lines are established, there is room for more careful study of intragenerational transmission from the middle to the later years of the working life cycle.

When and if complete data become available for a real cohort, we shall expect the quantitative relationships to differ somewhat from those estimated here. In the meantime we have a description of the "typical" life cycle of a cohort that is more detailed, precise, and explicit as to causal or sequential relationships than any hitherto available.

CONJECTURES AND ANTICIPATIONS

In an earlier section of this chapter we suggested that the critic might share part of the burden of proof for the proposition that our results are distorted by the omission of important variables. There is, however, evidence at hand, supplemented by judicious conjecture, to show that at least some obvious candidates for crucial omitted variables are not as formidable as might be supposed.

One kind of question has to do with the temporal relevance of our measure of father's status. The OCG questionnaire asked for father's occupation at the time the respondent was about 16 years old. Might we not suppose that father's occupation at an earlier date would have been a better choice, on the theory that occupational ambitions are developed in late childhood and early adolescence, being more or less fixed by the time a boy reaches high school age? Moreover, if the father were mobile during the respondent's youth, the sharing of the experience of mobility may have induced distinctive orientations in the respondent.

A different issue is whether we have overlooked a crucial factor in failing to procure some information about the respondent's mother. Several sociologists have recently emphasized the mother's role in the formation of achievement orientation and have called attention to her educational attainment as an indicator of her possible influence.

We shall discuss these two possibilities together because our approach in both cases is to present hypothetical calculations based on data that are largely conjectural but include a key item of information for which reasonably firm estimates are available.

Suppose the OCG survey had ascertained not only father's occupation at respondent's age 16 (variable X) but also at respondent's age 6 (variable X'). We must make two sorts of assumption. The first assumption is that X' has the same correlation with the other variables, V, U, W, and Y, as that observed for X. There is some support for this assumption. In the son's generation, as shown by the OCG data, r_{UW} is not strikingly different from r_{UY}. This suggests that in the father's generation X and X' might have similar correlations with V. As for the father-son correlations, we assume that the earlier occupation is as highly correlated with son's educational attainment and occupational achievement as is the later occupation of the father; that

TABLE 5.5. HYPOTHETICAL REGRESSION COEFFICIENTS IN STANDARD FORM (BETA COEF-
FICIENTS), FOR SPECIFIED COMBINATIONS OF VARIABLES, FOR MEN WITH NONFARM BACKGROUND,
BASED ON PARTLY CONJECTURAL DATA

Dependent Variable[a]	Independent Variables[a]						Coefficient of Determination (R^2)
	W	U	X'	X	V'	V	
SET 1							
U	...	...	...	.265	...	.285	.23
U	...	...	.183	.183	...	.233	.25
W	...	.450	...	.170	...	.037	.32
W	...	.434	.120	.120	...	.008	.33
Y	.279	.411	...	.103	...	-.019	.43
Y	.271	.405	.074	.074	...	-.037	.43
SET 2							
U	...	...	...	.265	...	.285	.23
U	...	...	...	.209	.196	.196	.25
W	...	.450	...	.170	...	.037	.32
W	...	.446	...	.163	.027	.027	.32
Y	.279	.411	...	.103	...	-.019	.43
Y	.279	.413	...	.107	-.014	-.014	.43

[a]V: Father's education.
V': Mother's education (conjectured).
X: Father's occ. status at respondent's age 16.
X': Father's occ. status at respondent's age 6 (conjectured).
U: Respondent's education.
W: Respondent's first job status.
Y: Respondent's occ. status in 1962.

is, that the correlations of X and X' with U, W, and Y are the same. The second assumption—and this is the crucial one—concerns the correlation of X with X'. Here we can draw on the data given earlier as well as on an OCG finding. The latter, which may be less relevant, is that for men 35 to 44 years old r_{YW} is .492. It will be recalled that there are two sources giving correlations between current occupation and occupation ten years earlier. For men 35 to 44 years old the Chicago data showed this to be .55; in the Minneapolis study it was .83. Our argument will only be weakened if we estimate $r_{XX'}$ on the low side; accordingly, we assign it the low compromise value of .60.

With these assumptions we have enough actual and hypothetical data to enter X' into a regression equation alongside X. Set 1 of Table 5.5 shows the results, in each case the previously calculated regression followed by the new hypothetical calculation in which X' is included as an independent variable. For each dependent variable the two measures of father's occupation split into equal shares the net influence formerly attributed to X alone. This particular result is without interest, as it merely reflects the assumption of equality of the respective correlations, which we assumed. The more important results—those we take to be indicative of what actual data might well show—concern the coefficients of the other variables in the equations and the over-all change in proportion of variation determined. The most substantial change, and it is small enough, is noted with U as the dependent variable. With both occupational variables in the equation, the net influence of father's education is slightly diminished, and R^2 is two percentage points higher than with only X and V in the equation. At the other extreme, with Y as the dependent variable, we find no change in the other coefficients worth reporting and no detectable increase in R^2 due to the addition of X' to the other four variables.

Altogether, these results suggest that having much more detailed information on the father's occupational career would change very little our estimate of the relative importance of this factor as a determinant of the son's occupational achievement. The results leave open, of course, the question of the age at which the influence of father's occupation is most directly relevant to the course of the son's career, as well as the question of the particular influence a rare but extreme change in the father's career may have on that of the son.

In set 2 of Table 5.5 we have carried out the analogous exercise, considering hypothetical variable V' (mother's education) alongside measured variable V (father's education). Again we assume that their respective correlations with other variables in the system are the same. Unpublished data we have seen on educational plans and occupational aspirations of high-school youth suggest that mother's education is, at most, no more highly correlated with such variables than is father's education. Again, the crucial assumption has to do with the intercorrelation of the two key independent variables, V and V'. From the OCG data we can ascertain that there is substantial assortative mating by education in the respondent's generation. For men 45 to 54 years of age, the correlation between husband's and wife's education is .580, and for men 55 to 64 years old it is no less than .632. In 1940 Census tables on fertility we find a tabulation of education of husband by education of wife for parents of children under five years old; this correlation, computed somewhat approximately owing to broad class intervals, is .637. There should, of course, be little difference between this correlation and one computed for parents of boys 16 years old. Evidently we shall not greatly overestimate $r_{VV'}$ in setting it equal to .60.

The reader who has grasped the principle at work here will not be surprised to see in set 2 results much like those obtained in set 1. Mother's education divides with father's education the influence initially attributed to the latter, as a consequence of the assumptions made. With U (respondent's education) as the dependent variable, inclusion of V' results in an appreciable diminution of the net influence attributed to father's occupation and a measurable increase in the proportion of variation in the dependent variable accounted for. For dependent variables W and Y, however, the additional variable contributes no additional information, since the education of neither parent has an appreciable direct effect on respondent's occupational status. It should be reiterated that these calculations do not answer the question of whether mother's or father's education exerts more influence on sons.

It is hardly conjectural to generalize from these two experiments in a certain respect. If we think of additional socioeconomic indicators applying to the respondent's family background it is fairly certain that each of them will correlate moderately highly with the two that we have measured here. We do not know for sure, but it seems rather unlikely that any of them will have a much higher simple correlation with our measures on the respondent than X or V. In this event inclusion of other family background socioeconomic variables may lead to some reinterpretation of how the effect of such variables is transmitted, or of what is their relative importance, but it will not alter greatly our over-all estimate of the importance of variables of this kind. He who thinks differently, of course, has the option of trying to support his opinion with evidence. As far as we can see there is every reason to suppose that we have not appreciably underestimated the role of the socioeconomic status of the family of orientation as an influence upon the respondent's occupational achievement.

Concerning several other omitted variables, we need not resort to conjecture but merely to anticipate a little of the content of subsequent chapters in this volume. These chapters are mainly concerned with qualitative or classificatory factors as possible influences on occupational achievement. This kind of factor is not readily introduced into the kind of causal diagram we have been working with in this chapter. We can, however, inquire whether neglect of such factors may have seriously misled us in regard to the nature of the causal relationships we have assumed. If, for example, a qualitative factor H operates as a determinant of both one (or more) of the independent variables and one (or more) of the dependent variables in our causal model, then the link between the two that we postulate is, in greater or lesser degree, spurious. In the event of this kind of spuriousness, holding the qualitative factor constant should markedly reduce, if not eliminate entirely, the apparent correlation between the two variables.

In Table 5.6 we report the amount of change in the correlation

TABLE 5.6.   EXCESS OF SIMPLE CORRELATION OVER PARTIAL CORRELATION WITH DESIGNATED FACTOR HELD CONSTANT, FOR SELECTED PAIRS OF STATUS VARIABLES, BY FARM BACKGROUND

Background and Factor[a] Held Constant	Pair of Variables[b] Correlated			
	Y and X	W and X	Y and W	U and V
All men				
A	.039	.031	.026	.016
B	.029	.022	.022	.033
C	.002	.001	.002	-.001
D	.066	.071	.045	.037
E	.043	.044	.029	.056
F	.026	.019	.020	.029
G	.000	.002	-.003	.002
Nonfarm background				
A	.010	.008	.010	.007
B	.025	.017	.019	.022
C	.003	.002	.005	-.001
D	.025	.024	.025	.019
E	.034	.034	.025	.048
F	.023	.014	.017	.019
G	.001	.002	-.003	.002
Farm background				
A	...	...	.024	.003
B	...	...	.018	.061
C	...	...	.001	.003
D	...	...	.024	.002
E	...	...	.008	.026
F	...	...	.014	.044
G	...	...	.001	.001

[a]A: Size of place (community of residence in 1962).
 B: Race, nativity, and migration from region of birth.
 C: Presence of parents in family in which respondent grew up.
 D: Geographic mobility since age 16.
 E: Number of siblings and sibling position.
 F: Region by color.
 G: Marital status in 1962.

[b]Y: Respondent's occ. status in 1962.
 W: Respondent's first job status.
 U: Respondent's education.
 X: Father's occ. status.
 V: Father's education.

between two quantitative variables when each of seven qualitative factors is held constant. That is, we compare the simple correlation between, for example, Y and X with the average within-class correlation, holding constant, say, factor A, as derived from covariance statistics. In general, Table 5.6 suggests that any element of spuriousness in the correlations we have been using is rather minor. When there is an appreciable difference between the respective simple and partial correlations, moreover, each of the correlations r_{YX}, r_{WX}, r_{YW}, and r_{UV} is affected in much the same way. Hence the *pattern* of correlations tends to remain intact. If the effects suggested by Table 5.6 are taken as evidence of spuriousness the main conclusion we should draw is that the path coefficients in our causal diagram may all be slightly overestimated, although their relative magnitudes are probably not greatly distorted.

Even this qualification is not unequivocally indicated. It is not clear that all the factors in Table 5.6 may logically be regarded as sources of spurious correlation. We do not wish to enter here upon the question of the correct causal interpretation of each of these factors, since this matter is considered in detail in subsequent chapters. One element of factor E (number of siblings and sibling position), for example, is probably best conceived as an intervening variable, accounting for part of the relationship of X and V to U. As such, its introduction into a causal scheme provides a useful extension or elaboration of the interpretation but does not require us to think of the original relationship as spurious.

We note that the discrepancies between simple and partial correlations are generally reduced when attention is focused on the nonfarm-background population. Several of the factors in Table 5.6 have to do with residence or change of residence—size of place, interregional migration, geographic mobility, and region of residence. Such factors tend to pick up the correlated effect of farm origin. When we eliminate this influence by confining the analysis to men with nonfarm background, the disturbance issuing from these factors is minimized.

We should observe, finally, that the disturbances suggested in Table 5.6 are not additive over the seven factors there listed. These factors, as defined, are in several instances logically redundant. As just noted, residential location is an aspect of four of the classifications; race or color appears in two. Hence simultaneous control of several factors would probably not produce much greater discrepancies between simple and partial correlations than appear in the table.

We must likewise be clear about what is *not* established by this analysis. First, it does not purport to estimate the effects or relative importance of the several classificatory variables; that task is reserved for subsequent chapters. It only shows that, whatever their effects, taking them into account will not require us to modify drastically our previous estimate of relationships among the quantitative variables. Second, this summary does not confront the issue of possible interaction effects. The statistic used here is the average within-class correlation. If there are wide differences between classes in the magnitude of correlations like r_{YX} or r_{UV} we would, indeed, be in serious difficulty. This would mean that the causal relationships hitherto described actually differ from one subpopulation to another. (See the discussion of interaction in Chapter 4.) To anticipate the findings of later chapters, there are in fact some interactions that are sizable enough to be interesting. For most of them, however, it appears that we have not done too great violence to the data in averaging the within-class correlations. A possible exception is the factor of color. Many relationships are different among nonwhites than among whites. This important finding, which merits considerable emphasis, is dealt with at length in Chapter 6. Yet its importance should not be allowed to cloud the issue at hand—whether our analysis to this point is vitiated by the action of color as a disturbing factor. The fact is that nonwhites are a small proportion of the whole population; hence results for the total sample approximate closely results for the white subpopulation.

These observations suggest the appropriate qualifications for the analyses reported in this chapter. The findings are probably most valid for the white population, and particularly for the segment of the white population with nonfarm origins. Extended to persons of farm origin or to nonwhites, the results may require more or less drastic revision to render them applicable, in consequence of disturbances our model has not taken into account. The error to avoid, then, is that of overgeneralization. For particular subpopulations, defined in terms of variables studied here or other variables that might be suggested, our estimates of causal relationships may be more or less wide of the mark. For the bulk of the U. S. population considered in the aggregate, we have no strong evidence that they need major revision.

ISSUES POSED BY MOBILITY VARIABLES

Again, methodology rears its ugly head. We did not begin with the intention of writing a treatise on methodology. Appearances to the contrary notwithstanding, we have tried to limit the presentation of methodological problems to the very minimum necessary for the critical reader to grasp the rationale of our procedures. The truth of the matter is, however, that many an issue ordinarily considered to fall exclusively within the province of theory turns out to hinge on principles of methodology as soon as we consider how the issue could conceivably be resolved by empirical inquiry. We are, therefore, contending for a much more intimate relationship between theory and method than ordinarily has been contemplated, even by writers preoccupied with this particular interface between segments of the scientific quest. Our causal diagram, for example, is not to be regarded as merely a convenient device for summarizing data, although it is at least that. It purports to be a theoretical model—even if the theory is quite tentative and rudimentary and as yet on a rather low level of generality and abstraction—about how a given process works in a particular society.[12] The stance on method taken here has other implications for theory that might go unnoticed unless made explicit. In particular, it has implications for some issues that loom large in the literature on the subject under study.

In most studies and discourses on social mobility it seems to be taken for granted that the phenomenon to be explained is, indeed, "mobility"—either actual movement between positions or intentions, aspirations, and orientations concerning mobility. We have acknowledged the significance of this interest in mobility by describing patterns of movement between occupations in Chapters 2 and 3. Once we go beyond description, however, and seek a conceptual framework with potential explanatory value, the focus on mobility—so we shall argue—becomes a liability. For this reason the present chapter, concerned as it is with the causal interpretation of relationships involved in the process of stratification, has avoided more than incidental reference to the concept of mobility. In effect, the process of stratification has been analyzed by decomposing the concept of occupational mobility into its major components.

An initial simplification will permit us to avoid some cumbersome notation. Assume that all status variables are measured in standard form, and designate such standardized variables by lower-case letters, such as $y = (Y - \overline{Y})/\sigma(Y)$. This implies that mobility has reference to a change in position in a distribution, abstracting from the mean difference between the two status variables. Thus $(y - x)$ could in some cases be negative when $(Y - X)$ is positive. But this does not affect the principles to be stated below.

Let us consider some distinct types of correlation involving mobility variables, thus defined. A Type-1 correlation is a correlation between two mobility variables, involving four distinct status variables in their definition. An example is the correlation between "occupational mobility" and "educational mobility," that is, between $(y - x)$ and $(u - v)$. Without indicating the derivation of the formula, we simply state that

$$r_{(y-x)(u-v)} = \frac{r_{yu} - r_{xu} - r_{yv} + r_{xv}}{2\sqrt{1 - r_{yx}}\sqrt{1 - r_{uv}}}.$$

[12] Herbert L. Costner and Robert K. Leik, "Deductions from 'Axiomatic Theory'," *American Sociological Review*, **29**(1964), 819-835.

From this mathematical identity it is immediately evident that the correlation of mobility variables is nothing more than a tautological rearrangement of the information contained in the six possible correlations of status variables. Such a tautology could, of course, be interesting insofar as it enabled the investigator to perceive a property of the system not otherwise evident to him (see the discussion in the next paragraph). For men 25 to 64 years of age having nonfarm background (taking this population for purposes of illustration), we have the following simple correlations (the correlation between two standardized variables is, of course, the same as the correlation between their raw-score forms):

$$r_{yu} = .611$$
$$r_{xu} = .414$$
$$r_{yv} = .317$$
$$r_{xv} = .505$$
$$r_{yx} = .377$$
$$r_{uv} = .418$$

Substitution in the formula yields $r_{(y-x)(u-v)} = .320$. We conclude that occupational mobility is not strongly related to educational mobility, in conformity with the conclusion reached by the author of "A Skeptical Note on the Relation of Vertical Mobility to Education,"[13] after elaborate manipulations of two-way and three-way tables, presented *in extenso*. His conclusion could have been obtained simply by observing that education and occupation are far from perfectly correlated, either within or between generations.

The finding that the correlation between occupational and educational intergenerational mobility is not very high—lower than most of the correlations between statuses that underlie it—serves to focus attention on the elements contributing to the process of mobility. To simplify the discussion let us look at upward movements from low positions of fathers to higher positions of sons; the principle illustrated here applies to other movements as well. If upward mobility would usually be due to the fact that the fathers are low on both education and occupational status and the sons are high on both, the correlation between educational and occupational mobility would be high. But the facts underlying upward mobility may well be different. Thus an uneducated father may have improved his occupational position, permitting him to provide his sons with a better education, which raises their occupational chances; this would be reflected in a low

[13] C. Arnold Anderson, "A Skeptical Note on the Relation of Vertical Mobility to Education," *American Journal of Sociology*, **66**(1961).

correlation between the mobility measures. Or the sons of an unedu-cated father with low occupational status may themselves receive little education but nevertheless rise above their father in occupational status; this also would be reflected in a low correlation between edu-cational and occupational mobility. These possibilities are by no means purely hypothetical, given the correlations between status variables. The finding that the correlation between educational and occupational mobility is low calls attention to the fact that the process of upward mobility does not necessarily or typically involve a jump from fathers inferior on all dimensions to sons superior on all. *Inter*-generational mobility may result from a variety of combinations of *intra*generational and intergenerational movements, and most of these combinations depress the correlation between different aspects of intergenerational mobility, such as that between educational and occupational mobility.

A Type-2 correlation likewise involves two mobility variables, but the initial status in the definition of one mobility variable is also the terminal status in the definition of the other. This arises, for example, in correlating intergenerational mobility from father's occupation to first job with intragenerational mobility from first job to subsequent occupation. The formula can again be written as an identity in terms of simple correlations among status variables:

$$r_{(y-w)(w-x)} = \frac{r_{yw} - r_{yx} + r_{wx} - 1}{2\sqrt{1 - r_{yw}}\sqrt{1 - r_{wx}}}.$$

To evaluate this correlation in the same population as used for the previous example, we need the additional simple correlations

$$r_{yw} = .529$$
$$r_{wx} = .382.$$

Before peeking at the answer, the reader might make a guess as to how it comes out. It could be reasoned that a man who demonstrated his mobility drive by achieving upward mobility from his origin level to his first job will further express that drive by strong intragenera-tional mobility. Conversely, a man who has already started to "skid" when he takes his first job may persist in the habit, undergoing still further downward mobility. On this argument, early mobility should be prognostic of—that is, positively correlated with—later mobility.

This fine example of deductive reasoning comes to grief when we look at the actual value of $r_{(y-w)(w-x)}$, which turns out to be —.432, modest enough in size but negative in sign. What went wrong? Our point is that the intuition behind such reasoning is sound but leads to a sound conclusion only if the steps in the argument are carried through in terms of status variables, not mobility variables. We see from $r_{yw} = .529$ that a good start on the first job is indeed a favorable sign for later occupational status, in that a man initially high is likely to be high later on. When we try to express the matter in terms of mobility variables, what happens is this. The scale interval from x to y, whatever it may turn out to be, is a distance. If movement from x to w covers most of that interval there is only a short distance left to go from w to y. But if x to w covers only a little of the interval there is a long distance left to go from w to y. For this reason the lengths of the two mobility steps, x to w and w to y, *tend* to be inversely related. Once we have found that r_{yw}, r_{yx}, and r_{wx} all are positive and of a similar order of magnitude, the negative sign for the correlation between mobility variables, $r_{(y-w)(w-x)}$, is a tautological necessity, and not a very illuminating tautology at that. A Type-2 correlation, in fact, is perilously close to being simply a spurious correlation, in the classical sense of that term.

In a Type-3 correlation a mobility variable is correlated with a status variable other than one of the two whose difference is the measure of mobility. Is educational mobility affected by a person's level of origin? Let us consider $r_{(u-v)x}$. It will occasion no surprise to learn that it, too, can be written as a function of simple correlations between status variables:

$$r_{(u-v)x} = \frac{r_{ux} - r_{vx}}{\sqrt{2(1 - r_{uv})}}.$$

With data already given, we obtain —.085. But what has this told us? We could certainly have anticipated that a man's occupation will be more closely related to his own education than to the education of his son, and this information is summarized in straightforward fashion by the two coefficients r_{ux} and r_{xv}. The negative sign for $r_{(u-v)x}$ is then guaranteed. Once we reflect on the matter the more or less mechanical explanation of the negative sign is evident: the higher the father's occupational level, the higher his educational level is likely to be and hence the harder it will be for his son to exceed it. Type-3 correlations are well designed to demonstrate such truisms. Yet they do not, of themselves, give any useful indication of the interesting associations whose magnitudes cannot be foretold. The exercise of computing Type-3 correlations is harmless enough. But if we had *only* such correlations involving mobility variables our interpretation would have to involve exceedingly devious circumlocution to avoid erroneous inferences. At the same time, such correlations would have concealed useful information.

One might be tempted, finally, to consider a Type-4 correlation, relating intergenerational mobility to the level of the origin status. The verbal rationale seems straightforward. We would like to know if "lower-class" people have the same "chance for upward mobility" as "middle-class" people. It is easily shown, however, that

$$r_{(y-x)x} = \frac{r_{yx} - 1}{\sqrt{2(1 - r_{yx})}} = -\frac{\sqrt{1 - r_{yx}}}{\sqrt{2}}.$$

Hence $r_{(y-x)x}$ is merely a simple transformation of r_{yx}. Its algebraically necessary negative sign only serves to express what is obvious from the fact that $r_{yx} < 1$; there is an inescapable "regression toward the mean."[14] Substantively, this says that the higher a man's status, the less are his son's chances of upward mobility.

We have illustrated pitfalls in the study of mobility variables as they are encountered in correlation analysis, but the same logical problems are involved even in such simple procedures as the classification of persons into categories like "upward mobile," "stable," and "downward mobile." Unless we take extraordinary precautions, using such a classification as a dependent variable incurs a serious risk of rediscovering "regression toward the mean" in a variety of disguised forms. How elaborate the precautions must be has been indicated in Chapter 4 (section entitled "Analyzing Mobility Distributions").

THE CONCEPT OF A VICIOUS CIRCLE

The problem just considered is basically one in which there is grave danger of circular reasoning. The other issue on which we have some comments concerns reasoning about circles, specifically the "vicious circle" that is sometimes identified as a crucial feature of stratification processes.

Although the concept of a "cycle of poverty" has a quasi-official sanction in U. S. public policy discussion, it is difficult to locate a systematic explication of the concept. As clear a formulation as any that may be found in academic writing is perhaps the following:[15]

Occupational and social status are to an important extent self-perpetuating. They are associated with many factors which make it difficult for individuals

14 Duncan and Hodge, *op. cit.*, esp. p. 639.
15 Seymour M. Lipset and Reinhard Bendix, *Social Mobility in Industrial Society*, Berkeley: Univer. of California Press, 1959, pp. 198-199.

to modify their status. Position in the social structure is usually associated with a certain level of income, education, family structure, community reputation, and so forth. These become part of a vicious circle in which each factor acts on the other in such a way as to preserve the social structure in its present form, as well as the individual family's position in that structure. . . . The cumulation of disadvantages (or of advantages) affects the individual's entry into the labor market as well as his later opportunities for social mobility.

The suspicion arises that the authors in preparing this summary statement were partly captured by their own rhetoric. Only a few pages earlier they had observed that the "widespread variation of educational attainment within classes suggests that one's family background plays an enabling and motivating rather than a determining role."[16] But is an "enabling and motivating role" log ally adequate to the function of maintaining a "vicious circle"? In focusing closely on the precise wording of the earlier quotation we are not interested in splitting hairs or in generating a polemic. It merely serves as a convenient point of departure for raising the questions of what is specifically meant by "vicious circle," what are the operational criteria for this concept, and what are the limits of its usefulness.

To begin with, there is the question of fact—or, rather, of how the quantitative facts are to be evaluated. How "difficult" is it, in actuality, "for individuals to modify their status" (presumably reference is to the status of the family of orientation)? We have found that the father-son correlation for occupational status is of the order of .4. (Assuming attenuation by errors of measurement, this should perhaps be revised slightly upward.) Approaching the measurement problem in an entirely different way, we find that the amount of intergenerational mobility between census major occupation groups is no less than seven-eighths as much as would occur if there were no statistical association between the two statuses whatsoever, or five-sixths as much as the difference between the "minimum" mobility involved in the intergenerational shift in occupation distributions and the amount required for "perfect" mobility.[17] Evidently a very considerable amount of "status modification" or occupational mobility does occur. (There is nothing in the data exhibited by Lipset and Bendix to indicate the contrary.) If the existing amount of modification of status is insufficient in terms of some functional or normative criterion implicitly employed,

[16] *Ibid.*, p. 190.
[17] U. S. Bureau of the Census, "Lifetime Occupational Mobility of Adult Males: March 1962," *Current Population Reports*, Series P-23, No. 11 (May 12, 1964), Table B.

the precise criterion should be made explicit: *How much mobility must occur to contradict the diagnosis of a "vicious circle"*?

Next, take the postulate that occupational status (of origin) is "associated with many factors" and that "each factor acts on the other" so as "to preserve . . . the individual family's position." Here the exposition virtually cries out for an explicit *quantitative* causal model; if not one of the type set forth in the first section of this chapter, then some other model that also takes into account the way in which several variables combine their effects. Taking our own earlier model, for want of a better alternative, as representative of the situation, what do we learn about the "associated factors"? Family "position" is, indeed, "associated with . . . education," and education in turn makes a sizable difference in early and subsequent occupational achievement. Yet of the total or gross effect of education (U) on Y, occupational status in 1962 $(r_{YU} = .596)$, only a minor part consists in a transmission of the prior influence of "family position," at least as this is indicated by measured variables V (father's education) and X (father's occupation)—and this statement requires little modification on behalf of our conjectured variables V' (mother's education) and X' (father's earlier occupation). A relevant calculation concerns the compound paths through V and X linking Y to U. Using data for men 20 to 64 years old with nonfarm background, we find:

$$p_{YX}p_{UX} = .025$$
$$p_{YX}r_{XV}p_{UV} = .014$$
$$p_{YX}p_{WX}p_{UX} = .014$$
$$p_{YW}p_{WX}r_{XV}p_{UV} = .008$$
$$\text{Sum} = \overline{.061}$$

This is the *entire* part of the effect of education that has to do with "perpetuating" the "family's position." By contrast, the direct effect is $p_{YU} = .407$ and the effect via W (exclusive of prior influence of father's education and occupation on respondent's first job) is $p_{YW}p_{WU} = .128$, for a total of .535. Far from serving in the main as a factor perpetuating initial status, education operates *primarily* to induce variation in occupational status that is independent of initial status. The simple reason is that the large residual factor for U is an indirect cause of Y. But by definition it is quite uncorrelated with X and V. This is not to gainsay the equally cogent point that the degree of "perpetuation" (as measured by r_{YX}) that does occur is mediated in large part by education.

This conclusion is so important that we should not allow it to rest on a single calculation. The reader accustomed to a calculus of "explained variation" may prefer the following. For men 35 to 44 years of age with nonfarm background (a convenient and not unrepresentative illustration), we have these pertinent results: $r_{YX} = .400$; $R_{Y(XV)} = .425$; $R_{Y(UXV)} = .651$. Note that adding the "associated factor" of father's education to father's occupation increases very slightly our estimate of the influence of "family position" on occupational achievement. Including respondent's education, however, makes quite a striking difference. Squaring these coefficients to yield an accounting of the total variation in respondent's 1962 occupational status (Y), we obtain these percentages:

(i)	Gross (or total) effect of father's education and occupation	18.06
(ii)	Education of respondent, independent of (i)	24.32
(iii)	All other factors, independent of (i) and (ii)	57.62
	Total	100.00

An analogous calculation, derived from multiple-classification rather than linear-regression statistics, was offered in Chapter 4. The results are rather similar. Here we have imputed to the measures of "family position," X and V, their *total* influence, including such part of this as works through education; the 24 per cent contribution of respondent's education refers only to the part of the effect of education that is net of the background factors. Still, education has a greater influence, *independent of these factors,* than they have themselves, operating both directly and indirectly. Overshadowing both these components, of course, is the unexplained variation of nearly 58 per cent, which can have nothing to do with "perpetuating status."

Whatever the merit of these observations, they should at least make clear that statistical results do not speak for themselves. Rather, the findings of a statistical analysis must be controlled by an interpretation—one that specifies the form the analysis will take—and be supplemented by further interpretations that (ideally) make explicit the assumptions on which the analyst is proceeding. The form in which our results are presented is dictated by a conception of status achievement as a temporal process in which later statuses depend, in part, on earlier statuses, intervening achievements, and other contingent factors. In such a framework it may not be a meaningful task to evaluate the relative importance of different causal factors. Instead, attention is focused on how the causes combine to produce the end result. From this point of view we can indicate, first, the gross effect of the measured background factors or origin statuses of a cohort of men on their adult achievement. We can then show how and to what extent this effect is transmitted via measured intervening variables and, finally, to what extent such intervening variables contribute to the outcome, independently of their role in transmission of prior statuses. In a balanced interpretation all these questions should be dealt with explicitly.

Our treatment seems to indicate the advisability of keeping in perspective the magnitude of the gross relationship of background factors and status of origin to subsequent achievement. The relationship is not trivial, nor is it, on the other hand, great enough in itself to justify the conception of a system that insures the "inheritance of poverty" or otherwise renders wholly ineffectual the operation of institutions supposedly based on universalistic principles.

Our model also indicates where the "vicious circle" interpretation is vulnerable. In the passage on the vicious circle quoted there seems to be an assumption that because of the substantial intercorrelations between a number of background factors, each of which has a significant relationship to subsequent achievement, the total effect of origin on achievement is materially enhanced. Here, in other words, the concept of "cumulation" appears to refer to the intercorrelations of a collection of independent variables. But the effect of such intercorrelations is quite opposite to what the writers appear to suppose. They are not alone in arguing from a fallacious assumption that was caustically analyzed by Karl Pearson half a century ago.[18] The crucial point is that if the several determinants are indeed substantially intercorrelated with each other, then their combined effect will consist largely in redundancy, not in "cumulation." This circumstance does not relieve us from the necessity of trying to understand better *how* the effects come about (a point also illustrated in a less fortunate way in Pearson's work). It does imply that a refined estimate of how much effect results from a combination of "associated factors" will not differ greatly from a fairly crude estimate based on the two or three most important ones. Sociologists have too long followed the mirage of "increasing the explained variance."

Let us not fall into the trap of supposing that, had we measured more of the "real" background factors, the outcome would have been greatly different. (Had it occurred to the reader, perchance, that background determines the kind of marriage contracted and the latter then plays a crucial role in the subsequent career? Then let him consult Chapter 10, wherein we evaluate the importance of "making a good match.") Either the "real" factors would be associated with the

18 Karl Pearson, "On Certain Errors with Regard to Multiple Correlation Occasionally Made by Those Who Have Not Adequately Studied This Subject," *Biometrika*, 10(1914), 181-187.

measured ones, or they would not. If the former, they would add little to the "explained variation"—as we illustrated, quite cogently though conjecturally, with two "omitted variables." If, on the other hand, the "real" factors are not associated with our measures of "family position," then they would operate independently thereof and *not* to "perpetuate" family position.

We do not wish to imply that the idea of cumulation of influences, or even the particular form of cumulation describable as a "vicious circle," is without merit. Our aim is to call attention to the necessity of specifying the actual mechanism that is only vaguely suggested by such terms. One legitimate meaning of cumulation is illustrated by the model of a synthetic cohort presented earlier in this chapter. In this case what is cumulative is the experience of an individual or a cohort of individuals over the life cycle, so that in the latter part of the life cycle achieved status depends heavily on prior achievements, whatever the factors determining those achievements may have been. The cumulation here consists in large measure of the effects of contingent factors not related to social origins or measured background factors.

The situation of the Negro American, which is analyzed in Chapter 6, exemplifies mechanisms inviting the label of a vicious circle. What is crucial in this case is not merely that Negroes begin life at a disadvantage and that this initial disadvantage, transmitted by intervening conditions, has adverse effects on later careers. Rather, what happens is that, in addition to the initial handicap, the Negro experiences further handicaps at each stage of the life cycle. When Negroes and whites are equated with respect to socioeconomic circumstances of origin and rearing, Negroes secure inferior education. But if we allow for this educational disadvantage as well as the disadvantage of low social origins, Negroes find their way into first jobs of lower status than whites. Again, allowing for the handicap of inferior career beginnings, the handicap of lower education, and the residual effect of low socioeconomic origins—even with all these allowances—Negroes do not enjoy comparable occupational success in adulthood. Indeed, even though we have not carried our own analysis this far, there is good evidence that Negroes and whites do not have equal incomes even after making allowance for the occupational status difference and the educational handicap of Negroes.[19] Thus there surely are disadvantaged minorities in the United States who suffer from a "vicious circle" that is produced by discrimination. But not all background factors that create occupational handicaps are necessarily indicative

[19] See Herman P. Miller, *Rich Man, Poor Man,* New York: Crowell, 1964, pp. 90-96.

of such a vicious circle of *cumulative* disadvantages; the handicaps of the Southern whites, for example, are not cumulative in the same sense, as Chapter 6 will reveal. A vicious circle of cumulative impediments is a distinctive phenomenon that should not be confused with any and all forms of differential occupational achievement.

As noted earlier, the issue of equalitarianism is one that has generally been more productive of debate than of cogent reasoning from systematized experience. Without becoming fully involved in such a debate here, we must at least attempt to avoid having our position misunderstood. We have *not* vouchsafed a "functional interpretation" that asserts that somehow American society has just the right amount of stratification and just the appropriate degree of intergenerational status transmission. We *have* indicated that it is easy to exaggerate the latter and, in particular, that it is possible seriously to misconstrue the nature of the causal relationships in the process that characterizes status transmission between generations.

In conclusion, one question of policy may be briefly mentioned, which pertains to the distinction between the plight of the minorities who do suffer disadvantages due to their ascribed status and the influence of ascribed factors on occupational life in general. To help such minorities to break out of the vicious circle resulting from discrimination and poverty is a challenge a democratic society must face, in our opinion. To advocate this policy, however, is not the same as claiming that *all* ascriptive constraints on opportunities and achievements could or should be eliminated. To eliminate all *dis*advantages that flow from membership in a family of orientation—with its particular structure of interpersonal relationships, socioeconomic level, community and regional location, and so on—would by the same token entail eliminating any *advantages* the family can confer or provide. If parents, having achieved a desirable status, can *ipso facto* do nothing to make comparable achievement easier for their offspring, we may have "equal opportunity." But we will no longer have a family system—at least not in the present understanding of the term. (This point has not been misunderstood in radical, particularly Marxist, ideologies.)

We do not contemplate an effortless equilibrium at some optimum condition where the claims of egalitarian values and the forces of family attachment are neatly balanced to the satisfaction of all. A continuing tension between these ultimately incompatible tendencies may, indeed, be a requisite for social progress. We do contend that both equity and effectiveness in the policy realm call for a deeper understanding of the process of stratification than social science and politics yet can claim.

CHAPTER 6

Inequality of Opportunity

Equality of opportunity is an ideal in the United States, not an accomplished fact. The chances of occupational achievement are limited by the status ascribed to a man as the result of the family into which he was born. Indeed, a stable society is hardly conceivable that does not ascribe to every child a status in some kinship group, which is responsible for rearing and socializing him, and which, therefore, strongly influences his motivation to achieve, his qualifications for achievement, and hence his chances for success. The limitations on the opportunity to achieve imposed by ascribed status, however, are due not only to differences in acquired orientations and abilities but also to discrimination. This is particularly so for the ethnic status that a man's parental family bestows upon him—whether he is Negro or white, Southerner or Northerner, a son of immigrants or of native Americans.

This chapter is concerned with such ethnic variations in occupational achievement. Three sets of comparisons will be made. First, the basic inequalities of occupational chances between Negroes and whites are revealed by the contrast between whites and nonwhites, 94 per cent of whom are Negroes. Second, Southerners and Northerners (all non-Southerners) are compared in respect to both place of birth and place of residence, separately for whites and Negroes. Third, three broad white ethnic groupings are compared to white men of native parentage: the foreign-born, American-born men whose parents were born in northern or western Europe or in Canada, and American-born men whose parents were born elsewhere. To be sure, whether observed differences in occupational achievement are results of discrimination, ability, or motivation can only be inferred from the data at hand. These inferences can be rendered more plausible, however, by taking into account intervening variables, such as first job and, particularly, education, and by controlling the influence of correlated factors, such as father's occupational status. The analysis suggests that the handicap of Negroes is, at least in part, a result of discrimination, that the handicap of Southerners is largely produced by inadequate occupational preparation, and that the minor differences among white ethnic groupings probably rest on selective experience and motivation.

NEGROES AND WHITES

Negroes have, of course, far less educational opportunity than do whites in the United States. The first two columns of Table 6.1 show that whites are much more likely than nonwhites to attain higher edu-

TABLE 6.1.   EFFECTS OF COLOR AND EDUCATION ON OCC. STATUS

Education	Population (in Thousands)		Mean 1962 Occ. Status (Y)			Deviation from Mean[a], Controlling X and W[b]	
	White[c] (1)	Nonwhite (2)	White[c] (3)	Nonwhite (4)	Difference (5)	White[c] (6)	Nonwhite (7)
0 to 8 years	7,286	2,243	23.6	16.8	6.8	-8.1	-14.0
High School 1 to 3 years	5,420	1,032	29.7	18.6	11.1	-4.3	-13.1
High School 4 years	8,855	827	37.8	22.8	15.0	1.7	-10.5
College, 1 or more years	7,534	477	56.8	41.1	15.7	13.4	3.0

[a]Deviations from the total population mean, not just that portion of it treated in this table (which excludes men of foreign parentage).
[b]X: Father's occ. status.
   W: Status of first job.
[c]Native whites of native parentage.

cational levels. Among native whites there are as many men with some college experience as there are men without any high school (column 1), but Negroes without high school outnumber the college-educated nearly five to one (column 2). About one-half of the Negroes in contrast to one-quarter of the native whites have only eight or fewer years of schooling. (The same differences are found in the better-educated nonfarm population, which shows that they are not simply due to the poorly educated Negro sharecropper and migrant laborer. Here the ratio of men with some college experience to men without any high school is two to one for whites and two to five for Negroes.[1])

It is interesting that educational attainment varies by age to an even greater extent than by race. Among the native whites with native parents, merely 9 per cent of the 20- to 24-year-olds have no more than

[1] For complete data on the occupational achievement of the four major ethnic groups, controlling education and farm background, see Table J6.1 in the Appendix.

eight years of education, but 49 per cent of the 55- to 64-year-olds do. Among Negroes, similarly, 27 per cent of the youngest but fully 79 per cent of the oldest age group have not gone beyond elementary school. Discrimination notwithstanding, the tremendous expansion of education in the United States has had the result that young Negroes today are better educated than older whites are. Negroes, nevertheless, continue to suffer serious educational handicaps, and these are not the only handicaps that impede their occupational opportunities.

Negroes are disadvantaged relative to whites not only educationally but also in respect to all other career contingencies. Columns 3 and 4 of Table 6.1 show that the mean occupational status of nonwhites is lower than that of whites at all educational levels. Similarly, the occupational status of the fathers of nonwhites is consistently lower than that of the fathers of whites; the same is true for status of first job. The important fact is that even when the lower social origin, education, and first occupation of Negroes have been taken into account, their occupational achievement is still far inferior to that of whites. The net effects of race on occupational status within educational categories with father's occupation and first job controlled are presented, in terms equivalent to deviations from the mean, in columns 6 and 7 of Table 6.1. The average difference in ultimate occupational status when social origins, career beginnings, and education are held constant remains fully 9.3 points in favor of whites.

In sum, Negroes are handicapped by having poorer parents, less education, and inferior early career experiences than whites. Yet even if these handicaps are statistically controlled by asking, in effect, what the achievement of nonwhites would be if they had the same origins, the same education, and the same first jobs as whites, their occupational chances are still consistently inferior to those of whites. Thus being a Negro in the United States has independent disadvantageous consequences for several of the factors that directly affect occupational success. The cumulation of these distinct, though not unrelated, disadvantages creates profound inequalities of occupational opportunities for the Negro American.

The data on social mobility, just as those on occupational achievement, reveal the disadvantaged position of the Negro. This is by no means self-evident. Quite the contrary, we had expected that Negroes, given their much lower socioeconomic origins, would be less likely to be downwardly and more likely to be upwardly mobile than whites. The findings, however, contradict this expectation; nonwhites are more likely to be downwardly and less likely to be upwardly mobile than whites, as illustrated by the data on long-distance upward mo-

TABLE 6.2.   MOBILITY DISADVANTAGE OF NONWHITES

| Education | Per Cent Very Upwardly Mobile[a] | | Difference |
	Native Whites	Nonwhites	
0 to 8 years	13	5	8
High school, 1 to 3 years	19	8	10
High school, 4 years	27	15	12
College, 1 or more years	38	35	3

[a]More than 25 points from occupation of father.

bility in Table 6.2. The initial expectation rested on the assumption that the serious economic discrimination against Negroes in the parental generation, which is manifest in lower origins, has become attenuated in recent decades. The finding that Negroes, despite their lower points of origin, do not achieve as much upward mobility as whites raises the question of whether the gap between whites and Negroes continues to be widening; we shall come back to this issue later in this chapter.

The likelihood of moving up from social origins a considerable distance increases with increasing education for both whites and non-whites, as Table 6.2 shows. For nonwhites, however, the increment in upward mobility effected by higher education is relatively small except for the college-educated. The result is that the difference between the mobility chances of whites and of nonwhites becomes larger with increasing education until after high school. Education, a path to upward mobility for all, is not as effective a route up for nonwhites as it is for whites. This pattern exists notwithstanding the lower social origins of nonwhites, which should make it easier for them than for whites, if other things were equal, to attain upward mobility.

Education does not produce the same benefits for Negroes as for whites, whether benefits are reckoned in terms of occupational achievement or mobility. The difference between mean occupational status of whites and of nonwhites increases with higher educational levels. Among the least educated, the socioeconomic status of native whites is 6.8 points above that of nonwhites (Table 6.1, column 5); for men with some high school, the difference is 11.1; for high-school graduates, it is 15.0; and for the most educated men, it is 15.7. Although educated Negroes achieve occupations superior to those of the less educated, the more education a nonwhite man acquires the further does his occupational status fall behind that of whites with comparable education. Differences for the nonfarm population are similar except that they show the college-educated Negro to be slightly less disadvantaged than the one who discontinued his education at high-school graduation. For the least educated among these nonfarm men the occupational status of nonwhites is 9.3 points below that of whites; for men with some high school the difference is 11.7; for high-school graduates it is 17.8; and for college men it is not quite so large, being 15.4.

College-educated Negroes are a highly select group. Coming, unlike college-educated whites, from depressed origins,[2] college-educated Negroes have had to overcome more serious obstacles. The fact that they have surmounted these obstacles educationally suggests that they are more highly motivated (or more able) than their white counterparts. Yet despite this greater selectivity of nonwhites with college experience, they do not manage to achieve an occupational level comparable to that of whites and even fail to rise as far above their lower social origins as college-educated whites rise above their higher ones. Whereas the lower occupational status of Negroes may be in part attributable to their more disadvantageous parental background,[3] the latter cannot account for their lesser chances of achieving upward mobility compared to whites, because it provides *more* room above their origins into which to move than is the case for whites. It is very probable that discrimination plays an important role here.

This interaction effect of color and education means that the highly educated Negro suffers more from occupational discrimination than the less educated Negro. At the same time there is reason to believe that the college-educated Negro's greater knowledge and stronger achievement motivation, without which he could hardly have overcome the serious obstacles to going to college he typically encounters, make him particularly sensitive to discrimination in employment and advancement. The implication is that the most educated Negroes, who tend to be most sensitized to and aware of discrimination, are also the ones most likely to experience relative deprivation as the result of occupational discrimination. One would therefore expect

[2] Mean socioeconomic status of fathers is 43.9 for college-educated whites but 26.3 for college-educated nonwhites.

[3] But not for the most part, since social origins exert only a limited influence on occupational status, as the section on path coefficients in Chapter 5 showed.

the educated Negro to be more militant in the struggle for equal opportunities than the uneducated one, and impressionistic observation suggests that this is indeed the case.

Another implication of these findings is that Negroes have less incentive than whites to acquire an education and to make the serious sacrifices that doing so entails for persons from underprivileged socioeconomic classes. The data show that approximately the same amount of educational investment yields considerably less return in the form of superior occupational status or mobility to nonwhites than to whites. Another study[4] found that white–nonwhite income differentials also increase with increasing education. The largest income difference between whites and nonwhites was observed for men with some college. The differential was smaller for men with less education and also for college graduates, indicating that there is a point beyond which educational investment does begin to pay on for nonwhites. The fact that Negroes obtain fewer rewards than the majority group for their educational investments, robbing them of important incentives to incur these costs, may help explain why many Negroes exhibit little interest or motivation in pursuing their education.[5] The school dropouts resulting from this lack of motivation worsen the position of Negroes in the labor market, and the inferior education of most Negroes serves to justify on actuarial grounds occupational discrimination against Negroes in general, thus further lessening the returns Negroes get for the educational investment that they *have* made and their incentives to make more such investments. It takes a strong belief in the value of education for Negroes to stay in school and improve their education, as they have actually done.[6]

Differentials in occupational opportunities are not the ultimate

[4] Paul Siegel, "On the Cost of Being a Negro," *Sociological Inquiry* 35(1965), 44.

[5] Although the data refer to all nonwhites, the findings and conclusions are particularly applicable to Negroes, and the tendencies observed would undoubtly be accentuated if the 6 per cent of the nonwhites who are not Negroes were eliminated from the analysis. Some findings may well not be applicable at all to other nonwhite groups.

[6] The multiple classification procedure used in this section (Table 6.1, columns 6 and 7) makes the assumption that there is no interaction between the control and other variables. Regression analysis supports this assumption fairly well, inasmuch as it shows that the regression slopes and the correlations of father's status are low and vary little with education and race, most being around .20. Although there is not much variation, the relationships are slightly higher for whites than for nonwhites. This suggests that the dominant whites are better equipped than are nonwhites to pass on to their sons status advantages. A likely reason for this difference is that a disproportionate number of Negroes are not raised in the same household with their fathers, and Negro women cannot as easily pass on their occupational status to their sons as Negro men could and as white men can.

economic disadvantage of nonwhite Americans. Nonwhites also tend to receive less income than whites in comparable occupational positions.[7] Schmid and Nobbe's recent analysis of the differences in education, occupation, and income between whites and several nonwhite ethnic groups indicates that the occupational status of both the Japanese and the Chinese is higher than that of the whites, but the income level of whites is nevertheless the highest of all groups.[8] Background and educational handicaps create occupational disadvantages for most nonwhite groups, but there are additional career and income disadvantages that must be attributed to ethnic status itself and probably to the discrimination it evokes.

SOUTHERNERS AND NORTHERNERS

The average socioeconomic status of Southerners is lower than that of Northerners. Although this is by no means unexpected, the data make it possible to ask what about being a Southerner produces occupational disadvantages. Is it the lack of industrialization or the predominance of Negroes in the South, the poor qualification of the Southerner or discrimination against him in the labor market? Men born in the South are compared in this section with men born in the North (any of the other three regions—Northeast, North Central, and West), and further contrasts are drawn between those who have remained in their region of birth and those living elsewhere in 1962. It should be noted that the comparison of Southerners and Northerners who do not live in their region of birth refers to men most of whom live in the North; all Southerners who do not live in their region of birth live, by definition, in the North, whereas most Northerners who do not live in their region of birth do not live in the South, but in the North, having migrated from one to another of the three northern regions. As the North and the South differ greatly in the proportion of their total population that is white, and color has already been shown to exert an independent influence on occupational achievement, northern and southern whites and nonwhites are compared separately.[9]

Southerers are disadvantaged in the struggle for occupational success, not only because economic opportunities in the South are inferior

[7] See Herman P. Miller, *Rich Man, Poor Man*, New York: Crowell, 1964, pp. 85-96.

[8] Calvin F. Schmid and Charles E. Nobbe, "Socioeconomic Differentials Among Nonwhite Races," *American Sociological Review*, 30(1965), 909-922.

[9] In this comparison southern nonwhite is virtually synonomous with southern Negro, whereas northern nonwhite includes a minority mixture of other racial groups.

to those in the North, but also because being raised in the South equips a man poorly for occupational achievement. Table 6.3 shows that the occupational achievement of men born in the South, both white and nonwhite, is inferior to that of Northerners.[10] This inferiority is much greater for southern nonwhites. The socioeconomic status of nonwhites born and living in the South falls 12.7 points behind that of northern nonwhites living in their region of birth, whereas the comparable figure for whites is 2.9. Color does not affect the differences between northern and southern migrants so much (using the term "migrant" here for men not living in their region of birth). The socioeconomic status of northern *white* migrants exceeds that of southern whites who live in the North by 9.4, and the socioeconomic status of northern *nonwhite* migrants exceeds that of southern nonwhites living in the North by 13.0. In general having moved out of the region of birth is associated with higher occupational status. However, this effect is not great enough to offset the inferiority implicit in southern birth: whether white or Negro, Southerners living in the North are inferior not only to northern migrants but also to Northerners who live in their region of birth. These differences persist when social origins, which also are inferior in the South, are controlled. Even after the effect of father's status has been statistically removed, both white and nonwhite Southerners achieve lower occupational status than comparable Northerners, whether the southern-born remain in the South or move north (Table 6.3, column 6). Parallel differences are observed in the first jobs held by Southerners and Northerners (column 3). Men born in the South, whether they remained or left there, and whether white or nonwhite, have first jobs inferior to those of their northern counterparts.

Northerners achieve higher first and higher ultimate occupations than Southerners; for whites there is no difference in the extent of upward movement between the two, though for Negroes there is. Column 4 of Table 6.3 presents the mean distance moved between first job and 1962 occupation by the four categories—white and nonwhite Northerners and Southerners. Northern whites experience hardly more intragenerational mobility than southern whites, the difference being a mere 0.4, whether men who remained in the region of their birth or migrants are considered. Among Negroes, however, southern birth reduces career mobility considerably. Southern nonwhites have moved up much less during their careers than northern ones, whether they

---

[10] Table J6.2 in the Appendix presents the complete data on the gross and net effects of the ethnic-migration classification on occupational status in 1962, status of first job, and educational attainment, by farm background.

TABLE 6.3. EFFECTS OF REGION OF BIRTH AND COLOR, FOR NATIVE MEN OF NATIVE PARENTAGE

Color and Region	Population (in Thousands) (1)	1962 Occ. (Y) Deviations from Mean (2)	First Job (W) Deviations from Mean (3)	Mean Intragenerational Mobility (Y - W) (4)	Education Deviations from Mean (5)	1962 Occ. (Y) Deviations from Mean Controlling for		
						X^a (6)	U^a (7)	X, U, W^a (8)
WHITES[b]								
Born in North								
Living in region of birth	16,513	1.5	.8	11.5	.29	.4	.0	-0.1
Living elsewhere	3,759	8.9	6.2	13.5	.84	5.5	2.9	2.1
Born in South								
Living in region of birth	7,831	-1.4	-1.7	11.1	-.37	-.1	.8	1.1
Living elsewhere	2,101	-.5	-2.8	13.1	-.10	1.1	.5	1.3
NONWHITES								
Born in North								
Living in region of birth	665	-6.3	-4.3	8.8	.14	-4.6	-6.2	-4.4
Living elsewhere	87	-2.3	2.5	6.0	.34	-1.6	-4.5	-8.8
Born in South								
Living in region of birth	2,155	-19.0	-11.6	3.4	-1.69	-13.6	-10.8	-8.6
Living elsewhere	1,672	-15.3	-7.4	2.9	-.92	-11.6	-8.4	-6.9
MEAN[c]	...	36.3	25.5	10.8	4.43	36.3	36.3	36.3

[a] X = Occ. of father.
U = Education.
W = First job.

[b] Native whites of native parentage.

[c] Mean of the total sample, rather than only that portion treated in this table (which excludes men of foreign parentage or birth).

215

remain in the South (5.4 below comparable Northerners) or move to the North (7.1).

One might be tempted to attribute the disadvantaged occupational situation in which the Southerner finds himself to the more restricted opportunities offered by the southern labor market, and this may well be true for the southern Negro, but the most serious handicap of the southern white appears to be the inferior preparation for occupational success men reared in the South receive rather than the lack of good opportunities in the southern labor market. Among whites, the difference between Northerners and Southerners in occupational status is far less for men who have remained in the region of their birth (2.9) than for those who have left it (9.4). In other words, in the case of nonmigrants, when Southerners and Northerners work in different labor markets, Southerners are less inferior in occupational achievement to Northerners than in the case of migrants, which involves Southerners and Northerners both of whom now work in the North.[11] This difference cannot be due to variations in labor-market conditions but must reflect disadvantageous consequences of having been born and raised in the South, undoubtedly because southern training does not prepare a man well for occupational attainment.

The interpretation implies that the occupational handicap of Southerners is due to the inferiority of southern education. To be sure, this study has no information on the comparable quality of northern and southern education, though it is probable that southern schools (both Negro and white) are inferior to northern schools. The present data make it possible, however, to determine to what extent Northerners and Southerners avail themselves of the educational opportunities that do exist by ascertaining the differences in educational attainment between the two. In other words, quite aside from any differences in quality, what are the differences in amount of schooling received by Southerners and Northerners? The answer is unequivocal; Southerners are less educated than Northerners. The average educational score of southern whites who have remained there falls .66 points short (on a scale ranging from 0 to 8) of that of Northerners living in their region of birth, which corresponds to more than a year of schooling. The education of southern whites who have moved North lags .94

[11] These differences are not due to the more rural population of the South. When the farm population is eliminated from the analysis, the differences persist: white Northerners who live in the region of their birth enjoy a status advantage of 2.4 over comparable white Southerners; the occupational status of regionally mobile Northerners is 9.2 above that of Southerners who have moved to the North. The comparable figures for nonwhites are 16.2 for the stayers and 15.9 for the regional migrants.

points—nearly two years—behind that of northern migrants. The comparable figures for nonwhites are even larger, 1.83 and 1.26, respectively. Although southern birth creates an educational disadvantage for whites as well as Negroes, it constitutes a greater handicap for Negroes.

As a matter of fact, Southerners are less likely than Northerners to continue their schooling at every step of the educational ladder. Among whites living in their region of birth, for example, 92 per cent of the Northerners and 75 per cent of the Southerners finish eighth grade; for the corresponding nonwhites the figures are 91 per cent and 49 per cent. Of these nonwhites who have completed elementary school, 91 per cent in the North and 79 per cent in the South go on to high school. Similarly, the proportion of high-school entrants who graduate; the proportion of these who go on to college; the proportion of college students who graduate; and the proportion of these who go on to graduate work—all are higher in the North than in the South, whether whites or nonwhites, men who stay in or those who leave their region of birth are examined.[12]

The finding that Southerners discontinue their education considerably earlier than do Northerners does not demonstrate that the lower occupational achievements of Southerners are the result of their lower educational attainments. The question is whether the differences in education between North and South suffice to account for the differences in occupational status. The answer to this question is presented in column 7 of Table 6.3, which shows the effects net of education for the four categories of Northerners and Southerners. Controlling for education reduces the differences between Northerners and Southerners considerably, but it does not eliminate all of them. The residual differences between Northerners and Southerners are only 2.4 for whites who left and a negative —.8 for whites who remained in the region of their birth, and the corresponding differences for nonwhites are 3.9 and 4.6. It is interesting that, among whites, the Southerner who stays in the South enjoys not lower but slightly higher occupational status than the Northerner who remains in his region of birth. Rather than suffering from a labor market of limited and depressed opportunities, apparently, the southern white benefits from a labor market that is adapted to the educational preparation of the labor force that serves it, allowing him to obtain jobs from which he

---

12 There are exceptions to this among nonwhites at college-graduation and graduate-school levels. These exceptions to the dominant trend, involving very few persons, are most likely simply due to sampling error. See Table J6.3 in the Appendix.

might well be barred in the North as a result of his educational short-comings. The inferior occupational chances of southern whites who have stayed in the South are completely accounted for by their lower education; indeed, given their limited education, southern whites enjoy a competitive advantage by remaining in the South.

Neither the inferior occupational chances of white Southerners who move North nor those of southern Negroes are fully accounted for by differences in education. The remaining handicaps of these groups may be due to the inferior quality of southern school systems, which implies that Southerners learn less in the same number of years of schooling than do Northerners. Such a difference would not be a disadvantage to Southerners who remain in the South, since they compete occupationally primarily with other Southerners. This explanation, though plausible, cannot be tested with the data in our study. Another hypothesis to explain the residual disadvantage of three of the four categories of Southerners is that it is due to discrimination. All Southerners, whether white or Negro, may suffer from discrimination in employment in Northern labor markets, and Negroes may be discriminated against in the South more than in the North.

If this hypothesized explanation is correct and the remaining differences are the result of discrimination, these differences should continue to be in evidence when other background factors are controlled. If, on the other hand, the net effects of region of birth and residence disappear after the influences of social origins, education, and career beginnings have been controlled, it would indicate that the observed differences were not due to discrimination.[13] The results of using this procedure to test the hypothesis are presented in column 8 of Table 6.3.[14] Both the net effects of the classificatory variable and the differences between Northerners and Southerners diminish. Indeed, the residual difference in occupational status between Northerners and Southerners is close to zero or negative in three of the four cases, being .8 for white migrants, —1.2 for white nonmigrants, and

[13] If the discrimination hypothesis is correct the differences must persist, but the persistence of the differences does not necessarily prove the correctness of this hypothesis, since factors other than discrimination might account for such persistence, such as lower achievement motivation of Southerners or inferior quality of southern education. In short, negative evidence for the hypothesis—the disappearance of the differences under statistical controls—demonstrates that discrimination in employment is not responsible for the original difference, but positive evidence permits only an inference that discrimination may be responsible, and the plausibility of this inference compared to possible alternatives must be established on other grounds.

[14] It should be noted that the assumption of no statistical interaction made in this analysis is not completely met here.

—1.9 for nonwhite migrants, whereas it remains 4.2 for nonwhite non-migrants.

Thus, given the inferior background of Southerners—their lower social origins, education, and early occupational experience—the occupational positions of the whites among them are no worse than those of northern whites, and the same is true for the Negroes who have left their region of birth and moved north. Only the occupational chances of Negroes who have remained in the South continue to be inferior to those of their northern counterparts. These results imply that there is little discrimination against Southerners *qua* Southerners in the northern labor market. They also indicate that it is not primarily any motivational handicap associated with southern birth that is responsible for the lower occupational status of Southerners. The lesser occupational chances of southern whites and of southern Negroes who move north are entirely due to their inferior preparation and background, but this is not true for Negroes who remain in the South. The data imply that there is more discrimination against Negroes in the South than in the North, and although this is not the only interpretation the findings permit, it is a highly plausible one.

Regional migration has different implications for the ultimate achievement of southern whites and Negroes. The white profits by remaining in the South, where he need not compete with the superior background, education, and experience of Northerners, and where stronger discrimination in employment against Negroes favors him. The southern Negro, on the other hand, profits by moving north, accepting the handicap of inferior education in exchange for escaping from the more rigorous racial discrimination in the South.

Although it has been shown above that the differences in occupational status between Northerners and Southerners can be accounted for by prior status differences between the two groups (except in the case of southern Negroes who remain in the South), the essential handicap of southern birth remains. It is manifest in the lower educational attainment and more humble first jobs of Southerners, and through them it is transmitted to ultimate occupational status. Their disadvantageous background is what handicaps Southerners in the struggle for occupational success.

THE NEGRO IN THE SOUTH AND IN THE NORTH

The handicap of southern birth is more pronounced for Negroes than for whites. Among men living in their region of birth, who constitute the large majority, southern whites achieve an occupational status that is on the average 2.9 points lower than that of northern whites, whereas southern nonwhites are 12.7 points below northern nonwhites (see column 2, Table 6.3). In other words, the southern Negro is most handicapped, which is also evident when the data are examined from a different perspective, looking at the status difference between whites and nonwhites in both South and North. The status disadvantage of nonwhites is 17.6 for Southerners but only 7.8 for Northerners among men who have remained in their region of birth. This constitutes impressive evidence of the far more serious deprivations Negroes suffer in the South.

Intragenerational mobility from career beginnings to 1962 occupational status manifests a similar pattern of interaction between color and region. Among Southerners who continue to live in the South, whites enjoy a 7.7-point advantage over nonwhites in respect to the distance moved between first job and 1962 occupation, and among Southerners who migrated north whites have an advantage of 10.2 points. Among Northerners, by contrast, the net mobility of whites exceeds that of nonwhites by only 2.7 points for regionally stable men and 7.5 for migrants. In short, the more pronounced discrimination against Negroes in the South finds expression not only in lower ultimate achievement but also in less upward mobility, and the early handicaps of the southern Negro continue to impede him even after he has moved to the less restrictive North.

It has been shown that the disadvantages of southern Negroes in the struggle for occupational success, as distinguished from those of southern whites, are not entirely due to their lower educational achievement. Although education alone does not account for the occupational inferiority of southern nonwhites, it does serve as one means of assuring and perpetuating this inferiority in the South. Whereas the mean educational attainment of northern nonwhites is only .15 points (less than half a year) below that of northern whites, the education of southern nonwhites lags 1.32 points (nearly three years) behind that of southern whites.[15] Not only is the educational disadvantage of Negroes greater in the South than in the North, but educational attainment is a more important determinant of occupational status for southern than for northern Negroes. A comparison of columns 2 and 6 of Table 6.3 reveals that the pronounced inferiority in occupational status of southern Negroes is much reduced when education is controlled statistically, whereas the lesser status inferiority of northern Negroes is not at all reduced by controlling education. This finding indicates that the racial status differential in the South,

[15] For men who live in the region of their birth; for migrants the difference is less; see column 5, Table 6.3.

though not that in the North, rests partly on the Negro's inferior education. Southern Negroes, in addition to being more deprived of the benefits of education than northern ones, are more dependent in their careers on their education and thus more hurt economically by their educational handicaps. In the South, but not in the North, the schools and the educational handicaps they produce for Negroes constitute major means for maintaining Negroes in their subordinate economic positions.

When the three major background variables—social origins, education, and career beginnings—are controlled, however, the remaining disadvantages of skin color are more serious in the South than in the North. The residual difference between whites and nonwhites, for men living in the region of their birth, is only 4.3 points in the North but 10.7 in the South. Undoubtedly these residual handicaps are in large part due to discrimination, and the much greater figure in the South probably reflects that much more discrimination there.

Has this racial discrimination increased or decreased in the past few decades? Is the relative occupational position of the Negro better or worse today than it was 20 to 40 years ago? It is impossible to answer this question conclusively without data for at least two different time periods. However, some inference about time trends can be derived from the examination of the differences between whites and nonwhites of different ages, asking how the relative status of young Negroes compares to that of older ones. To be sure, two patterns are confounded in this comparison, historical trends—changes in the relative position of Negroes since the beginning of this century—and age trends— differences in the career advancements experienced by whites and Negroes as they grow older. Thus the data show that the status difference between whites and nonwhites in the North is least for the youngest cohort and increases rather steadily for progressively older ones (Table 6.4, column 1). This pattern may indicate either that discrimination against nonwhites in Northern hiring practices has decreased in recent decades, or that older nonwhites suffer more serious handicaps in the labor market than younger ones. It is impossible to choose between these two alternative interpretations without further information. In the absence of data collected at different time periods, recall data that refer to different periods can provide such information.

The comparison of the education and of the first jobs of different age cohorts reveals historical trends, whereas these trends are confounded by the influence of career advancements in the comparison of 1962 occupations. For differences in education between age cohorts cannot reflect the influence of growing older, inasmuch as virtually

TABLE 6.4. DIFFERENCE BETWEEN NATIVE WHITES AND NONWHITES FOR SELECTED
FACTORS BY AGE AND REGION, FOR NONFARM MEN LIVING IN REGION OF BIRTH

Age	North			South		
	1962 Occ. (1)	Education (2)	First Job (3)	1962 Occ. (4)	Education (5)	First Job (6)
25 to 34	7.46	.30	5.46	23.37	1.05	14.54
35 to 44	9.31	.36	10.64	18.15	1.45	7.57
45 to 54	7.40	.19	6.40	20.41	1.09	10.45
55 to 64	15.93	1.88	9.91	17.94	1.56	11.28

everybody completes his education by age 25, and they therefore must
reflect historical changes that have occurred in the United States in
this century. The same is true for age differences in first job, since
these too do not distinguish the status achieved by older from that
achieved by younger men but refer rather to the mean occupational
status that men born in different decades had achieved when they
entered the labor market. Since some men quit school and start
to work much earlier than others, however, another problem arises,
though one less serious than the confusion of the influences of career
advancements and historical trends. All members of an age cohort
did not complete their education or hold their first jobs at the same
time, and the periods involved for the different cohorts are overlapping, with each spanning about 20 years instead of 10. Overlapping
though these cohort data are, which makes them less reliable for the
analysis of historical periods than we would wish, they do pertain to
successive historical periods, the beginnings and the ends of which
are roughly 10 years apart.

Table 6.4 shows that the difference between white and nonwhite
Northerners in education and in status of first job is less for younger
than for older men, just as the difference in 1962 status is. The fact
that the three trends are roughly parallel suggests that discrimination
against Negroes in the North has indeed become less severe in recent
decades. The jobs as well as the education of nonwhites who started
to work around the time of World War I were considerably inferior
to those of whites, more than was the case for nonwhites starting their
careers after World War II. The more serious handicaps of the earlier
generation of Negroes seem to have persisted and even become intensi-
fied as they grew older. The trend toward equality is most pronounced
for education, which may indicate that greater educational opportunities constitute the first step on the path toward achieving equal
opportunity in general.[16] No such trend is evident in the South,

[16] The dip in the trends for men aged 45 to 54 in 1962 may be due to the market

however. The difference in either first or ultimate occupational status between nonwhites and whites in the South is *not* smaller for the most recent than for earlier cohorts, and though the educational handicap of southern Negroes is smallest for the youngest cohort, there is no consistent trend.

It must be emphasized that these conclusions are only inferential. First job is not as reliable an indicator as it might otherwise be because, as noted in the first chapter, a substantial number of respondents reported (contrary to instructions) a first job that was begun before schooling was completed. Moreover, though there may be less discrimination against nonwhites in education and in the hiring of youngsters, discrimination in advancement and promotion to more responsible positions may continue unabated. Indeed, this possibility is not at all unlikely. Note that the trend data imply that the gap between Negroes and whites has been closing, at least in the North, whereas the finding reported earlier that nonwhites, despite their lower origins, experience less upward mobility than whites, implies that this gap has been widening. A possible explanation that reconciles the apparent contradiction is that the Negro–white status difference has so far narrowed only at the point of entry into the labor market, in accordance with the narrowing educational gap, but that it is still widening in the course of subsequent career advancement.

A more refined analysis of educational trends than the OCG data permit can be carried out on the basis of data from the U. S. Census of Population. The large number of cases in the 5 per cent census sample makes it possible to derive reliable estimates, based on comparisons of eight birth cohorts, of the trends not only in the proportion completing a minimum amount of schooling but also in the proportions continuing from one level to the next. These data, therefore, can answer some questions left unanswered by the more limited OCG data, such as whether the relative educational position of Negroes in the South as well as in the North has improved, and whether such improvements are confined to a minimum level of education or include also continuation on higher educational levels.

In the South as well as in the North the median education of Negroes has been slowly but steadily converging with the median for whites during the past half a century.[17] In other words, the Census data on median years of schooling confirm the conclusion that the

crash in 1929, when these men were 12 to 21 years old, on the assumption that this stock market debacle had the most adverse effect on potential college students in the middle class, disproportionate numbers of whom are white.

[17] See Table 173, 1960 Census of Population, Volume I, part 1, U. S. Summary.

difference between whites and nonwhites has been narrowing, which was earlier derived from the OCG data on mean years of schooling (Table 6.4). The same basic trend is evident when the proportion who completed at least eight years of school is considered. The difference between whites and nonwhites in this proportion is less for young men today than for those who went to school at the beginning of this century, as columns 3 and 6 in the first panel of Table 6.5 show. (The data are confined to men living in their region of birth in order not to complicate the analysis by the factor of migration.) Graduation from grammar school may be considered the minimum education attained by boys who fulfill the legal requirements and who are not mentally retarded. It is barely a minimum in a society where reading and driving a car are practically essential for working and living. The other four columns in the table show that the proportion who attain this minimum has increased steadily in the last half-century for both whites and nonwhites in both the North and the South. But the rate of increase has been greater for nonwhites, who started much lower, than for whites in the North, thereby narrowing the gap. The trend in the South was similar in broad outline, but it differed in specific detail.

The comparative educational disadvantage of the Negro in the South *increased* during the first decades of this century and started to *decrease* only after the depression of the thirties. The difference between southern whites and nonwhites in the proportion who completed grammar school rises from 27 per cent for the oldest cohort to 36 per cent for men between 45 and 64 years old in 1960, but it subsequently drops to a low of 18 per cent for the youngest cohort. This U-shaped curve, which contrasts with the linear decrease in the corresponding difference in the North, is the result of the fact that the rate of increase in the proportion completing grammar school in the South was greater for whites than for Negroes in the early part of the century and that Negroes began to catch up only in the last two decades or so. It is noteworthy that the gap between white and Negro grammar-school graduates in the South started to narrow only after more than 60 per cent of the whites had reached this educational level (column 4), and that at the earliest time for which data on the closing gap in the North are available, also more than 60 per cent of the whites there had reached this minimum level (column 1). We might speculate whether the dominant white group relaxes discriminatory practices and permits Negroes in growing numbers to attain a certain level of education only after a clear majority of its own members have already attained this level. Though this is mere speculation, the fact is that

TABLE 6.5.   PER CENT CONTINUING THEIR EDUCATION FROM ONE LEVEL TO THE NEXT,
BY REGION, COLOR, AND AGE, FOR MEN LIVING IN THEIR REGION OF BIRTH, 1960[a]

Per cent completing eighth grade

Age	North[b]			South		
	White[c]	Nonwhite	Δ	White[c]	Nonwhite	Δ
22 to 24	96.1	89.9	6.2	86.0	67.9	18.1
25 to 29	95.6	90.4	5.2	82.8	61.0	21.8
30 to 34	94.4	89.3	5.1	79.0	52.2	26.8
35 to 44	93.2	85.8	7.4	73.7	41.9	31.8
45 to 54	86.8	71.4	15.4	64.4	28.5	35.9
55 to 64	77.4	55.8	21.6	55.3	19.4	35.9
65 to 74	67.9	45.0	22.9	45.9	14.1	31.8
75+	61.8	36.3	25.5	39.0	11.7	27.3

Per cent continuing from some high school to high-school graduation

Age	North[b]			South		
	White[c]	Nonwhite	Δ	White[c]	Nonwhite	Δ
22 to 24	77.8	61.0	16.8	72.3	51.2	21.1
25 to 29	77.5	62.7	14.8	72.4	50.9	21.5
30 to 34	72.1	60.3	11.8	68.5	47.6	20.9
35 to 44	71.9	62.5	9.4	67.0	48.0	19.0
45 to 54	64.9	56.7	8.2	59.8	49.2	10.6
55 to 64	60.4	53.4	7.0	56.8	48.6	8.2
65 to 74	59.5	53.2	6.3	60.0	55.1	4.9
75+	62.0	54.7	7.3	65.5	55.1	10.4

Per cent continuing from some college to college graduation

Age	North[b]			South		
	White[c]	Nonwhite	Δ	White[c]	Nonwhite	Δ
22 to 24	39.0	22.4	16.6	34.4	25.8	8.6
25 to 29	53.3	37.0	16.3	51.1	38.5	12.6
30 to 34	59.0	43.6	16.4	54.9	46.8	8.1
35 to 44	54.8	44.1	10.7	52.5	51.1	1.4
45 to 54	51.9	43.5	8.4	46.7	53.2	-6.5
55 to 64	50.0	44.3	5.7	45.0	49.5	-4.5
65 to 74	46.7	54.1	-7.4	40.8	47.1	-6.3
75+	46.2	38.9	7.3	44.1	44.8	-.7

[a]Source: United States Census of Population: 1960.   Subject Report PC(2) 5B,
"Educational Attainment," Table 3 (5 per cent sample).
[b]All non-South.
[c]Native whites.

discrimination against Negroes on higher educational levels has not
declined.

The gap between whites and Negroes in respect to high-school graduation, in contrast to that in respect to grammar-school graduation, has
increased in the last 50 years. The second panel in Table 6.5 presents

the proportion of boys entering high school who graduate. In the North students were more likely to remain in high school until graduation in recent decades than formerly. In the South the trend is not consistent, particularly among nonwhites. The differences between whites and nonwhites in the proportion of entering high-school students who graduate, however, reveal a rather consistent trend in the South as well as in the North. The gap has been widening in both parts of the country, which means that the competitive disadvantage of the Negro in the urban labor market has been increasing.[18] To be sure, these data cannot yet reflect the results of the desegregation decision of the U. S. Supreme Court of 1954. Nevertheless, it is surprising that the apparent progress Negroes have made since World War II is not at all reflected in their chance to graduate from high school. On the contrary, relative to the chances of white students in high school, those of Negroes have worsened.

Discrimination in education against Negroes has not really declined in the United States; it has merely moved to a more advanced level. As eight years of schooling have become a bare minimum necessary for the most menial jobs, restrictions against Negroes on this level have subsided. Simultaneously, however, the handicaps Negroes suffer when continuing their education on higher levels have become more severe. This conclusion, based on the data on students in high school, is confirmed by the data on college students presented in the third panel of Table 6.5. The proportion of college entrants who receive a degree has increased for whites (ignoring the youngest cohorts) but not for Negroes in both North and South, with the result that the difference between whites and Negroes has increased. To be sure, these data undoubtedly do *not* simply reflect an increase in outright discrimination. Thus the finding that Negro college students in the South were more likely than white ones to graduate in the early part of this century clearly calls attention to other factors than discrimination that influence the results, such as the more highly selected group of Negroes who entered college, the inferiority of Negro colleges in the South, and the lesser academic demands segregated Negro colleges in the South made on their students. A full treatment of the problem, which would require detailed analysis of enrollment data, is beyond the scope of this study. But the fact remains that the chances of Negroes who go beyond grammar school to continue their education on more advanced levels have become worse in recent decades compared to those of

[18] The income gap between whites and Negroes has not narrowed in recent decades either; see Miller, *op. cit.*, pp. 40-43.

whites, in the North as well as in the South. This surely poses a serious challenge to the complacent belief that the position of the Negro is gradually improving, particularly in a democratic society that prides itself on the educational opportunities it offers to all its citizens.

IMMIGRATION

The United States has long been known as the land of golden opportunity that welcomed "the wretched refuse of [the] teeming shore" of other countries and gave these immigrants and their children opportunities to get ahead and achieve economic success. Without accepting the legendary rise of a Horatio Alger at face value, the assumption has been that immigrants, although typically having to enter the occupational structure near the bottom, can move up to better positions in the course of their lives and, in particular, provide their sons, the second generation, with much better opportunities for upward mobility. How well does this image, derived from the experience of an expanding continent in the nineteenth century, fit present-day reality?

The twentieth century has witnessed radical changes in the volume and pattern of immigration to the United States. During the decade just preceding World War I this country received about one million immigrants per year. Over the decade of the 1950's, by contrast, the number was just one-quarter as large, and the size of the receiving population had very nearly doubled in the meantime. The gross impact of current immigration on the economy and society is certainly much less now than it was 50 years ago.

There have been changes in the selectivity of immigration as well. Of the immigrants stating an occupation on arrival, no less than three out of five were laborers (farm or nonfarm) during 1905 to 1914. This proportion had dropped to one in seven by 1950 to 1959. The decline in numbers of immigrants was primarily a decline in the number of unskilled persons entering the country. In recent years, indeed, the absolute number of professional and technical workers arriving has been greater than at the turn of the century.

Taking the occupation stated on arrival as an indication of occupational skill or experience, we can calculate crude immigration rates by occupational level (Table 6.6). The figures, unfortunately, are not available by sex. Moreover, they refer exclusively to persons arriving and leave out of account those returning to their home countries and other departures. Only gross contrasts are, therefore, meaningful; but the differences in immigration rates between occupations in the earlier period and the changes over time are, in fact, quite pronounced.

TABLE 6.6. IMMIGRANTS STATING AN OCC. PER 100 OF THE MID-DECADE ECONOMICALLY ACTIVE RESIDENT POPULATION, BY MAJOR OCC. GROUP, FOR THE UNITED STATES, OVERLAPPING DECADES, 1900 TO 1959

Major Occ. Group	Decade										
	1900–1909	1905–1914	1910–1919	1915–1924	1920–1929	1925–1934	1930–1939	1935–1944	1940–1949	1945–1954	1950–1959
Professional, technical, and kindred workers	5.5	6.5	4.7	4.6	4.1	2.0	1.1	1.1	1.5	2.5	2.9
Managers, officials, and proprietors, except farm	8.0	7.5	4.6	3.6	2.9	1.0	.8	1.0	.9	1.0	.9
Clerical, sales, and kindred workers	2.9	3.5	2.5	2.4	2.7	1.4	.4	.3	.7	1.2	1.4
Craftsmen, foremen, operatives, and kindred workers	13.3	13.5	7.4	4.8	4.7	1.8	.5	.2	.6	1.3	1.8
Laborers, except farm and mine	55.4	47.0	24.7	13.7	13.3	4.3	.7	.3	.5	1.3	3.1
Private household workers	50.6	60.6	44.1	28.6	25.7	9.6	2.7	1.0	1.5	4.1	4.9
Other service workers	5.8	6.8	6.8	8.4	6.9	2.5	.6	.3	.5	.9	1.2
Farmers and farm managers	1.6	2.0	1.3	1.6	2.0	1.0	.3	.1	.4	1.5	1.8
Farm laborers and foremen	25.6	42.3	26.0	3.9	4.6	2.8	.5	.1	.1	.8	1.6

SOURCE: (a) Immigration: decade summations of annual figures in U.S. Bureau of the Census, Historical Statistics of the United States, Colonial Times to 1957 (Washington: Government Printing Office, 1960), series C 116–132; U.S. Bureau of the Census, Statistical Abstract of the United States: 1962 (Washington: Government Printing Office, 1962), Table 122. (b) Economically active population: For years ending in 5, average of adjacent years ending in 0; for the latter, Historical Statistics, op. cit., series D 73–88, and U.S. Bureau of Labor Statistics, Special Labor Force Report, No. 14 (April, 1961), Tables C–6 and G–2.

NOTE: both sets of data include both males and females, but exclude persons not economically active (such as housewives, retired persons, and children under 14 years old). Persons failing to report occupation are excluded from immigration series but are distributed in the population series.

At the turn of the century the number of nonfarm laborers arriving amounted to 55 per 100 of the resident working force in this occupation group. The corresponding figure for the professional and technical occupations was one-tenth as great, or 5.5 per 100. Very high rates were also observed for farm laborers—though not for farmers—and for private household (or domestic service) workers. During the 1920's the immigration rate for nonfarm laborers was about three times as high as for professional and technical workers, whereas the 1930's and 1940's actually saw a lower arrival rate for laborers than for professionals. In the most recent decade, 1950 to 1959, the two were about equal.

The occupations stated by immigrants upon arrival were not necessarily those they took up in this country. For an indication of how immigrants were absorbed into the occupation structure we must turn to statistics on the resident population of foreign provenance (Table 6.7). In 1910 not quite half of the white male working force classified

TABLE 6.7. PER CENT OF WHITE MALE WORKING FORCE FOREIGN BORN, BY MAJOR OCC. GROUP, FOR THE UNITED STATES, 1910 TO 1960

Major Occ. Group	1910	1920	1950	1960
All occupations[a]	24.7	22.4	9.9	6.9
Professional, technical, and kindred workers	15.6	14.3	7.5	6.1
Managers, officials, and proprietors, except farm	26.4	25.6	13.0	7.5
Sales workers	18.0	16.1	7.0	5.8
Clerical and kindred workers	10.9	9.9	5.5	4.8
Craftsmen, foremen, and kindred workers	29.6	26.4	11.3	7.7
Operatives and kindred workers	38.0	31.8	10.1	6.7
Laborers, except farm and mine	45.0	37.4	13.1	7.9
Service workers, including private household	36.8	36.3	18.7	13.0
Farmers and farm managers	12.8	11.0	4.5	3.0
Farm laborers and foremen	8.4	8.3	7.4	9.5

[a]Gainful workers 10 years of age and over for 1910 and 1920; experienced civilian labor force 14 years of age and over for 1950 and 1960; includes occupation not reported.

SOURCE: 1910 to 1950, E. P. Hutchinson, Immigrants and Their Children, 1850–1950 (New York: Wiley, 1956), Table 38, p. 202 (indices given by Hutchinson were converted back into percentages; the latter are, therefore, subject to rounding errors). 1960, U.S. Bureau of the Census, "Occupational Characteristics," Subject Report PC(2), 7A, 1960 Census of Population (Washington: Government Printing Office, 1963), Tables 3 and 8.

as nonfarm laborers were foreign-born, in conformity with the high immigration rate for this occupation. In sharp contrast, the proportion foreign-born among farm laborers was only one-third as great as in the entire working force, despite the high immigration rate. Clearly, many of the immigrants arriving as farm laborers found other pursuits in this country. No doubt appreciable numbers of them became farmers. In any event the proportion foreign-born among farmers in 1910 was much larger than the immigration rate for this occupation at the time. On the same reasoning, we infer that white-collar occupations as well as skilled and semiskilled manual pursuits offered opening for immigrants.

Thus the "land of opportunity" served as destination for rural-urban migrants originating abroad and provided channels of upward mobility for large numbers of them as they were absorbed into the working force. At the same time, as has frequently been noted, the entry of disproportionate numbers of immigrants into occupations of low status may have induced upward movement on the part of native workers.[19] To estimate the actual magnitudes of the streams of vertical circulation within the native and foreign-born segments would require a much more detailed study—and, no doubt, a certain boldness in contriving estimates—than anyone has been willing to make. The point is merely that patterns of occupational mobility up to, say, World War I were very much affected by the volume and selectivity of immigration. This catalyst of upward mobility has greatly diminished in force with the decline in the volume and the change in the composition of immigrants.

The data for 1950 and 1960 reveal the net result of a drastic decline in immigration and of substantial occupational mobility on the part of the foreign-born, many of whom had lived in the United States for long periods of time. Although some concentration of foreign-born by occupation remains, it has decreased markedly. The proportion of laborers who were foreign-born as of 1960 was only 7.9 per cent, appreciably but not greatly higher than the figure of 6.9 per cent for the entire white male working force. The only group to show an increase in proportion of foreign-born for 1960 over an earlier year was farm laborer. If, hypothetically, there had been an enforced redistribution of jobs in 1960 so as to equalize the foreign-born proportions over occupations, the number of native workers displaced would have been trivial.

In the future, as in the recent past, we shall experience annual fluctuations in the volume and composition of immigration, and the absorption of immigrants may induce interoccupational movements on the part of native workers. In some localities or for brief periods such induced effects may be noticeable. In the foreseeable future, how-

[19] See Elbridge Sibley, "Some Demographic Clues to Stratification," *American Sociological Review*, 8(1942), 322-330.

ever, these effects will be minor on the whole in comparison with the manifestations of other factors producing horizontal and vertical mobility.[20]

These considerations raise some questions concerning the life chances of immigrants and their children in the middle of the twentieth century. Only the very oldest men in 1962, when our data were collected, had entered the labor market at a time when very large numbers of immigrants were still arriving each year. Most of the foreign-born in the sample had come to this country after the main stream of immigration had subsided, though many of the second-generation sons in the 1960's had parents who had arrived at the height of immigration. Has the United States actually been the promised land of opportunity for these more recent immigrants as well as for the sons of the earlier immigrants? How do the occupational chances of the foreign-born and of the second generation today compare to those of white Americans of native parentage? Furthermore, do differences in ethnic background affect the occupational chances of sons of immigrants?

NATIONAL ORIGINS

To answer these questions, three major white ethnic groups are distinguished from the majority group of native parentage—the foreign-born, the second generation whose parents were born in northern or western Europe or in Canada, and the second generation whose parents were born elsewhere. (If one parent is foreign-born a man is classified as second generation.) These three groups are compared to northern whites with native parents, since most children of immigrants do not live in the South. The foreign-born, who, of course, do not live where they were born, are compared to native northern whites who also have left their region of birth.

Table 6.8 (column 2) shows that the mean occupational status of the foreign-born is inferior to that of native white Northerners, but that of the second generation is not, with the status of men of northern-European or western-European descent being somewhat higher than that of men descended from less prestigeful immigrant groups. Among men who live in the region of their birth, the occupational status of the second generation is higher than or as high as that of white natives, depending on whether they have more (2.4) or less (.1) prestigeful national origins. Among men who have left their region of birth, however, the status of the second generation falls short of that of

---

[20] For example, internal migration from rural to urban areas; see the discussion in Chapter 7.

TABLE 6.8. EFFECTS OF ETHNIC BACKGROUND ON OCC. STATUS AND EDUCATION (DEVIATIONS FROM THE GRAND MEAN)

Ethnic–Migration Class	Population (in Thousands) (1)	1962 Occ. Status		Education		Intergenerational Upward Mobility: Per Cent Moving Up 26 or More Points From their Origins (6)
		No Controls (2)	Controlling for X, U, W[a] (3)	No Controls (4)	Controlling for X, V[a] (5)	
Northern-born whites of native parentage, living						
In region of birth	16,513	1.5	– .1	.29	.08	24%
Elsewhere	3,759	8.9	2.1	.84	.38	28
Second generation North and West European parentage, living						
In region of birth	2,419	3.9	3.2	.04	.01	31
Elsewhere	574	7.2	4.9	.28	.14	33
Other parentage, living						
In region of birth	3,797	1.6	1.3	.05	.41	32
Elsewhere	895	4.7	.6	.49	.67	28
Foreign-born white	2,515	.3	.1	– .27	– .24	23
Mean[b]		36.3	36.3	4.43	4.43	25

[a] X = Occ. of father
U = Education
W = First job
V = Education of father
[b] Mean of the total sample, rather than only that portion treated in this table (which excludes white Southerners and all nonwhites).

the natives (—1.7 for the more and —4.2 for the less prestigeful nationalities).[21]

In sharp contrast to the inferior opportunities of Negroes, therefore, the occupational opportunities of white ethnic minorities, on the whole, differ little from those of whites of native parentage. (Indeed, they are considerably superior to those of southern whites.) Even the inferior position of the foreign-born is largely due to their lesser educational attainment. When the three major background variables —social origin, education, and first job—are controlled (Table 6.8, column 3), the socioeconomic status of the foreign-born is only slightly lower than that of native white migrants and not at all inferior to that of native whites who have remained in the region of their birth.

These controls, however, only accentuate the pattern already observed in attenuated form among the second generation. Standardizing for their less advantageous background, sons of immigrants who live in the region of their birth tend to achieve an occupational status that is superior to that of comparable natives, not only if they descend from more prestigeful (3.3) but also if they descend from less prestigeful nationalities (1.4). Among migrants, on the other hand, only second-generation men whose origins are northern or western European achieve a higher status, when background factors are controlled, than the white natives (2.8), whereas those of less prestigeful origins do not (—1.5). One factor underlying this pattern is that northern European and western European descent gives a man of the second generation an advantage in the struggle for occupational success, perhaps indicating some discrimination against white ethnic minorities of the more recent and less prestigeful immigrant groups. A second underlying factor is of special interest.

The conclusion that emerges is that the occupational achievements of the second generation are superior to those of native whites among men who stayed close to their birth place but not—at least, not consistently—among migrants. This can be explained by the hypothesis that varied experience in different social environments promotes occupational success. Men raised in the American culture and in American schools, but within a family from a different cultural tradition,

---

21 In the nonfarm data (that is, after the elimination of the farm-reared population) the import of national origins is seen to be somewhat more decisive. Men of more prestigeful national origins, regardless of their migration status, hold occupations superior to those of native whites, with a difference favoring second-generation men living in their region of birth by 2.7 points and those living elsewhere by .7 points. On the other hand, the second generation from less prestigeful origins achieves status inferior to that of native whites, whether remaining in their region of birth (—1.7) or moving elsewhere (—4.7).

have such varied experience. This gives them an advantage over men of native parentage who never left the region in which they were born but provides no advantage over natives who have moved to a different region, because such a move to another part of the country also furnishes varied experience.

An alternative explanation of the observed pattern is that both immigrants and migrants are select groups with higher ability and motivation to achieve than men who never took the initiative required to migrate to greener pastures. The intensity of achievement motives might be expected to vary with the difficulty of the move they prompt, which would imply that immigrants have strong achievement motives that they are likely to pass on to their children, the second generation.[22] It is impossible to choose between these explanations on the basis of the present data; indeed, both processes probably contribute to the general finding that men who are geographically mobile over long distances, or whose parents were, are more likely than others to be occupationally mobile; so undoubtedly do other factors, such as the tendency of migrants to move to urbanized areas with superior occupational opportunities. A further analysis of the factors that contribute to the association between geographic and social mobility is reserved for Chapter 7.

The education of the foreign-born is far inferior to that of native whites, and that of the second generation is also, though less, inferior, as indicated by the deviations from the mean educational score presented in column 4 of Table 6.8. Because there is a positive relationship between the education of fathers and that of sons, the low educational as well as occupational attainments of the foreign-born constitute handicaps for the second generation.[23] When these background handicaps are taken into account and educational attainments are examined after standardizing for father's education and occupation, the education of the second generation is no longer inferior to that of native northern whites. Indeed, with these controls, the educa-

[22] For support of this interpretation, see William Caudill and George Decos, "Achievement, Culture and Personality," *American Anthropologist*, **58**(1956), 1102–1126. Need achievement scores for first-generation Japanese were found to be higher than for the second generation who, in turn, revealed higher need achievement than middle-class whites. Actual occupational achievement, on the other hand, favored the second generation and was lowest for the first generation, with whites falling intermediate.

[23] To be sure, the foreign-born in the table are not the fathers of the second generation there, inasmuch as these fathers belonged to an earlier generation. But the data on the actual fathers of our respondents also show that the fathers of the second generation, who themselves are foreign-born, have lower educational attainment than do the fathers of the native whites of native parentage.

tion of the second generation of less prestigeful national origins is superior to that of all other categories (column 5). One might say that the descendants of immigrants from southern and eastern Europe and non-European countries have benefitted most from the immigration of their parents to the United States, though these benefits have as yet found expression only in educational and not in occupational improvements.

The observation that members of ethnic minorities do not attain educational levels as high as natives must be qualified by further noting that the variance in the education of minority whites is much greater than that of natives. The implications of this difference can be clarified with the aid of the data on the percentage of men on each educational level who continue to the next level (Table 6.9). White ethnic minorities seem to have an educational handicap due to their foreign origins, but once this handicap is overcome they are more likely than comparable men of native parentage to continue their education to advanced levels.

Education is, of course, not simply technical preparation for adulthood but becomes behavior that is culturally prescribed regardless of whether it is needed for the performance of occupational roles. Thus high-school graduation is coming to be a cultural norm to which most members of our society are expected to conform, as illustrated by the recent concern with high-school dropouts. The discussion of the dropout problem seems to imply that more youngsters quit high school early today than did so previously. But in actual fact the reverse is the case, with larger numbers now going to high school and graduating than have ever done so before. Present concern with dropouts reflects a new norm. High-school graduation has come to be expected, making withdrawal after 10 or 11 years, once considered more than adequate schooling for most, now a dropout problem. Education beyond the level prescribed by the culture (a level varying somewhat by social origin) has a different meaning. Further education is an avenue of upward mobility for men who are highly motivated but whose birth does not predispose them toward high status, for example, for sons of immigrants.

Given a cultural norm of high-school graduation, we would expect disproportionate numbers of the native white majority to finish high school, whereas fewer of the second generation should reach this level because their background is a handicap and because their immigrant parents may not have assimilated this American norm. But if the second generation or a considerable segment of it has acquired strong achievement motives from immigrant parents, its members would be

TABLE 6.9. PER CENT OF WHITE ETHNIC GROUPS CONTINUING THEIR EDUCATION FROM ONE LEVEL TO THE NEXT

Nativity, Parentage, and Residence	Through Eighth Grade	Eighth Grade to Some High School	Some High School to High-School Graduation	High School Graduation to Some College	Some College to College Graduation	College Graduation to Graduate School
Northern-born whites of native parentage						
Living in region of birth	91.5	85.3	76.7	44.5	51.2	38.8
Living elsewhere	96.3	91.8	79.3	59.0	55.1	42.9
Second generation, north and west European parentage						
Living in region of birth	90.5	76.0	74.5	42.6	54.3	40.9
Living elsewhere	89.6	84.9	75.3	45.0	58.1	64.0[a]
Other parentage						
Living in region of birth	88.9	83.0	69.0	43.6	53.0	42.7
Living elsewhere	91.2	85.0	79.4	54.3	57.2	61.4
Foreign-born white	79.2	72.8	77.7	53.9	58.7	52.7

[a]Based on 86,000 population; the base population in all other cells is more than 100,000.

expected (as would the foreign-born) to be particularly likely to go to college and graduate and even advance beyond, as a means of achieving upward mobility, once they have overcome the difficulties getting through high school entails for the underprivileged.

The data in Table 6.9 support these expectations. (Compare row 1 with rows 3 and 5, and row 2 with rows 4, 6 and 7.) Men of native parentage are most likely to complete eight years of education; to continue to high school if they have completed eighth grade; and, once in high school, to graduate. The migrants among these natives are also more likely than any other high-school graduates to go on to college. Among men who do reach college, however, the second generation and the foreign-born[24] are more likely to graduate than are native whites. Similarly, of all college graduates, the second generation and the foreign-born are more likely to continue on to professional or graduate school. In sum, the educationally handicapped men of foreign descent are less likely than the majority group to attain the cultural norm of high-school graduation. But those who do attain it have a higher probability of going on to graduate from college, and are more likely to pursue graduate training. High levels of education are an avenue of upward mobility well suited for the somewhat disadvantaged—the white ethnic minority—but not equally so for the most seriously disadvantaged—the American Negro.

Since men of the second generation start at somewhat lower social origins than the majority natives and end up very nearly their equals, we would expect their proportions of upwardly mobile to be particularly high.[25] The last column of Table 6.8 shows that this is indeed the case. This column presents the percentage of men in each category whose own 1962 occupation is more than 25 points above that of their father's occupation. One-quarter of the total population achieves such upward mobility, another quarter moves up the shorter distance between 6 and 25 points, slightly more (28 per cent) are occupationally immobile, and a few less (22 per cent) experience downward mobility.

The majority group achieves long-distance upward mobility at the average rate for the total population, though the interregional migrants among them do so in somewhat higher proportions. The foreign-born have somewhat less chance of long-distance upward mobility

24 We must remember that the relatively small numbers of recent immigrants come from much higher educational backgrounds than did the large waves of earlier immigrants. (Some foreign-born have and some have not completed their education before arriving here.)

25 This is not a logical necessity, as the same result could be produced by particularly low proportions of downward mobility.

than the average, and the nonwhites (not shown) have much less chance. On the other hand, all four categories of second-generation men exhibit the highest proportions of the upwardly mobile. Close to one-third have risen 26 points or more from their occupational origins, nearly the distance between semiskilled operatives and clerks or that between clerks and professionals. The strong drive toward success of the second generation combines with relatively low barriers to this success to result in disproportionately high upward mobility, enabling the second generation to surpass the socioeconomic status of the white majority living in the region of birth and nearly to reach the highest level occupied by migrant northern whites (Table 6.8, column 2). The very fact that a man lives far from his own place of birth or that of his parents spells economic success, either because it is indicative of achievement motivation and initiative, which may be passed on to children, or because experience with diverse cultural environments promotes achievement. The migrants among the majority group as well as the second generation share this advantage with the foreign-born without being subject to the same handicaps, with the result that their rates of upward mobility and economic achievement are outstandingly high.

CONCLUSIONS

It is hardly surprising that Negroes in the United States do not have the same occupational opportunities as whites. The lower occupational status of Negroes cannot be fully accounted for by their lower educational attainment, since their chances of success are inferior on every educational level. Neither is it attributable to the fact that the majority of Negroes were born in the South and the staus of Southerners is inferior to that of Northerners, since the occupational status of Negroes remains inferior when region of birth is controlled. Negroes do have less advantageous social origins than whites; their education is indeed poorer than that of whites; disproportionate numbers of them are actually from the South where opportunities are inferior; and they start their careers on lower levels. Yet even when these differences are statistically standardized and we examine how Negroes would fare if they did not differ from whites in these respects, their occupational chances are still inferior to those of whites. It is the cumulative effect of the handicaps Negroes encounter at every step in their lives that produces the serious inequalities of opportunities under which they suffer.

A finding that may be surprising is that the difference between Negroes and whites in occupational status as well as income is even greater among the better educated than among the less educated, with the partial exception of the minority who complete a college education.[26] In short, better educated Negroes fare even worse relative to whites than uneducated Negroes. To be sure, the same number of years of schooling may not provide the same degree of training and knowledge for Negroes as for whites, because the educational facilities that the white majority supplies for Negroes are usually inferior. But whether the discrimination against Negroes actually occurs in the educational system or subsequently in the occupational system —and it undoubtedly occurs to some extent in both—the fact remains that the results of this discrimination are more pronounced for the better than for the less educated Negro. This fact has some important implications.

Since Negroes receive less return in the form of superior occupational prestige and income for their educational investments than whites, they have less incentive to make such investments, that is, to make the sacrifices that staying in school to acquire more education entails, particularly for underprivileged youngsters. Acquiring an education is simply not very profitable for Negroes, which may explain why some Negroes exhibit little motivation to pursue their schooling. Negroes must be strongly imbued with the basic value of education for them to have improved their educational attainments in recent years despite the comparatively low rewards education brings them.[27] Moreover, whereas educated persons are generally considered to be more enlightened and, specifically, to be less prejudiced against Negroes and other minorities than less educated ones,[28] the data show that in actuality there is more discrimination against Negroes in highly than in less educated groups. It can hardly be a pattern of prejudice unique to the uneducated laborers and operatives that forces enlightened employers to discriminate against hiring Negroes on these levels, as is sometimes alleged, for there is even more discrimination on higher

[26] It should be noted that there may be a "floor effect." Since the less-educated whites achieve only relatively low occupational status, the less-educated Negroes cannot be very far below them in status.

[27] Alternatively, we could argue that, given the lower level of rewards for Negroes, less increment in rewards is needed for Negroes than for whites to produce the same marginal utility and hence the same incentive power to acquire more advanced education. In other words, the argument would be that the higher occupational returns whites obtain for the same educational investments compared to Negroes are necessary to produce the same marginal utility and incentive value, precisely because the level of rewards is higher for whites than for Negroes.

[28] Samuel A. Stouffer, *Communism, Conformity, and Civil Liberties*, Garden City: Doubleday, 1955, p. 90; and Robin M. Williams, Jr., *Strangers Next Door*, Englewood Cliffs: Prentice-Hall, 1964, p. 55.

levels. Another anomaly implicit in these findings is that although it is the uneducated Negro who is the main object of the prejudiced stereotype, the educated one being often explicitly exempt from it, it is the better educated Negro who in practice suffers most from discrimination.

Men born in the South, white as well as Negro, have inferior occupational chances, whether they remain there or migrate north. The occupational handicaps of southern whites and of southern-born Negroes living in the North are due to their inferior preparation, as indicated by the finding that the differences between them and their northern counterparts disappear when education and other background factors are statistically controlled. The persisting residual difference for Negroes who have remained in the South is in all likelihood the result of discrimination in employment. There is some evidence that the discrimination against Negroes has declined in recent decades, but progress has been very slow. The improvements in the relative position of the Negro have been largely confined to minimum education and less discrimination in hiring at the point of entry into the labor market. In respect to higher education, necessary for advancement to more responsible positions, the gap between whites and Negroes not only has failed to narrow but actually has continued to widen in the last half-century.

Members of white ethnic minorities, in contrast to Negroes, fare as well as if not better than the dominant majority. This does not mean that there is no discrimination against any white ethnic minorities; as a matter of fact, the occupational differences between the second generation of northern European or western European descent and that of other origins suggests that there is some discrimination against descendants of the less prestigeful immigrant groups, such as Italians and Poles. Whatever discrimination against selected white minorities exists, however, is not so pronounced as to suppress the strong achievement motivation characteristic of many sons of immigrants, and their drive to succeed has apparently overcome their background handicap as well as such discrimination, as manifest in their high occupational achievements and rates of mobility. The finding that these sons of immigrants are more successful in their careers than the sons of the native-born majority who have remained near their homes but not than those sons of the majority group who have left their region of birth indicates that something the second generation and migrants have in common promotes occupational achievements. This may be the varied cultural experiences to which both sons of immigrants and men who live in a different part of the country from where they were raised are exposed, or it may be the fact that migration as well as immigration is selective of men with strong achievement motives that are passed on to sons. Further evidence on the selective nature of migration is presented in the next chapter.

The general conclusion to which these findings point is that the American occupational structure is largely governed by universalistic criteria of performance and achievement, with the notable exception of the influence of race. The close relationship between educational attainment and occupational achievement, with education being the most important determinant of occupational status that could be discovered, testifies to this universalism. So does the finding that there is little discrimination against white ethnic groups in occupational life, though discrimination against selected minorities unquestionably exists, concealed in our data due to the superior accomplishments of some members of the second generation. Most of the groups that are economically disadvantaged, such as those born in other countries and those born in the South, have lower educational attainments commensurate with their lower occupational positions. An important exception to this pervasive universalism is the severe discrimination the Negro suffers at every step in the process toward achieving occupational success. Although there is some indication that discrimination against Negroes has declined in this century, and hence that universalism has continued to spread, the trend is not consistent, does not encompass all areas of occupational life, and has only begun to penetrate into the South. But universalism cannot restore equality. Indeed, the data suggest that the relative position of the Negro in regard to higher levels of attainment has become worse in recent decades.

CHAPTER 7

Geographical and Social Mobility

Racial or ethnic background is not the only status ascribed to a man at birth that influences the occupational status he is likely to achieve later in life. The country where he is born also defines an ascribed status that affects his chances of occupational achievement, for economic opportunities vary widely from one country to another. The career opportunities available in highly industrialized societies are not the same as those existing in agricultural ones. The chances of achieving mobility through education depend on whether the society's elite consists primarily of entrepreneurs who own land, factories, and other means of production that can be inherited, or of managers of large organizations they do not own. Within nations, too, there are differences in occupational opportunities between commercial centers, industrial cities, small towns, rural areas, and farms. The division of labor varies from one type of locality to another, and with it the opportunity structure that affects men's careers.

The occupational restrictions imposed by the community into which a man is born, however, are not as inescapable as his race or ethnic status. Although a man cannot change the color of his skin, he can migrate from his birth place to another in which opportunities are better. Migration provides a social mechanism for adjusting the geographical distribution of manpower to the geographical distribution of occupational opportunities. The need for redistribution results from differences in economic and industrial developments among communities and from differential fertility, which may involve higher reproduction rates in places where sufficient jobs are not available. Migration, of course, is not a perfectly functioning redistribution mechanism, if we may judge by the persistence of regional disparities in wages and unemployment rates. Men do not flow from places of poor to places of good opportunity with the ease of water.[1]

Despite its limitations, migration is an essential adjustive mechanism in industrialized societies, if only because the highest fertility is found where the fewest occupational opportunities are, on farms. The core of this chapter deals with this adjustive process and analyzes the bearing of migration between more and less urbanized communities on occupational mobility. Before examining the significance of migration for occupational achievement, however, the existing differences in the occupational structures between various types of communities will be ascertained.

COMMUNITY SIZE AND OCCUPATIONAL CONDITIONS

Men in the sample are identified in Table 7.1 by place of 1962 residence as living in very large urbanized areas with over one million inhabitants, in large cities between 250,000 and one million, in middle-sized urbanized areas between 50,000 and 250,000, in small cities and towns of 2,500 to 50,000, in rural nonfarm areas, or on farms. The men in the three classes of urbanized areas are further subdivided into residents of the central city and those of its suburban ring. This last distinction makes it possible to examine the occupational differences between city dwellers and suburbanites.

In general, the more successful men in metropolitan communities tend to move to the suburbs, leaving a disproportionate number of the less successful to inhabit the large central cities themselves. Columns 1 and 2 of Table 7.1 show that the mean occupational status of suburbanites exceeds that of the central city residents in all three sizes of urbanized areas, with the difference between the suburbs and the central city being greater in the largest cities (8.5 points) than in relatively smaller ones (2.5 and 3.6 points). The implication of these differences is that the movement to the suburbs of the most successful is greatest in the largest metropolitan centers of the United States. When background factors are controlled (in columns 3 and 4 of Table 7.1) the residual difference is reduced to 4.2 points in the largest cities, 1.4 in the second-largest ones, and it is reversed to −1.0 in medium-sized cities. The disappearance of the original difference when controls are introduced in the relatively small but not in the largest cities implies that superior social background distinguishes suburbanites

[1] For unfortunately eloquent testimony to the geographical inertia of workers even in the face of long-term unemployment, see Alan B. Batchelder, "Occupational and Geographic Mobility," *Industrial and Labor Relations Review,* **18**(1965), 570-583.

TABLE 7.1. EFFECTS OF SIZE OF PLACE ON 1962 OCC. STATUS AND FIRST JOB (IN DEVIATIONS FROM THE GRAND MEAN)

| | 1962 Occ. Status | | | | | | First Job | | | |
| | No Controls | | Controlling for Father's Education & Occ., Own Education & First Job | | Controlling for Father's Occ., Ethnicity, Education, & First Job | | No Controls | | Controlling for Father's Education & Occ. & Own Education | |
Place of 1962 Residence	Central City (1)	Suburbs (2)	Central City (3)	Suburbs (4)	Central City (5)	Suburbs (6)	Central City (7)	Suburbs (8)	Central City (9)	Suburbs (10)
Very large city (1,000,000 +)	-.6	7.9	-1.0	3.2	.1	2.8	2.0	5.1	1.7	1.4
Large city (250,000–1,000,000)	3.9	6.3	2.0	3.4	2.5	3.0	2.0	3.6	.2	1.4
Middle-sized city (50,000–250,000)	.9	4.5	.9	-.1	.8	-.2	-.4	4.9	-.4	1.3
Small cities (2,500–50,000)	.7		.6		.6		-.2		-.2	
Rural nonfarm	-3.0		-.4		-.7		-3.5		-1.5	
Rural farm	-17.4		-8.9		-9.6		-9.8		-3.2	

from city dwellers particularly in smaller and less so in larger metropolitan areas. The data suggest that, although the suburbs of all metropolitan areas, regardless of size, contain disproportionate numbers of superior status, only the suburbs of the largest metropolitan centers seem to be attractive to successful self-made men from lowly backgrounds, whereas the suburbs in smaller metropolitan areas draw from the central city primarily men whose superior present status is rooted in superior background. This conclusion is supported by the findings, shown in columns 7 and 8 of Table 7.1, that the first job of suburbanites exceeds in status that of central city residents by 5.3 points in the middle-sized cities, but only by 1.6 points in large and by 3.1 points in very large metropolitan centers. Although the difference between suburbs and central city in ultimate occupational achievement is most pronounced in the largest metropolis, that in status of first job is most pronounced in the smallest urbanized area. Of course we cannot assume that the first jobs reported were held in the same communities where men now live, but this does not lessen their significance as an indication of background status.

In the small metropolis men of well-established high status are most prone to live in suburbs, whereas in the larger metropolis occupationally mobile men are more likely to do so. This interpretation implies that the correlation between father's and son's occupational status should be higher among small-city than among large-city suburbanites, and it also implies that intergenerational mobility should be less prevalent among suburbanites in the smaller than among those in the largest urbanized areas. Both of these expectations are confirmed by the data. In medium-sized cities the correlation between father's and son's occupational status is larger in the suburbs (.38) than in the central cities (.34); but in very large cities this correlation is not so large in the suburbs (.33) as in the central cities (.38).[2] Among men in the suburbs of medium-sized cities, moreover, 23 per cent have been upwardly mobile more than 25 points (less than in the central cities), whereas 30 per cent of those in the suburbs of very large cities have been that much upwardly mobile (more than in the central cities).

Why are men who have risen occupationally from lowly backgrounds less likely to move to suburbs in the comparatively small than in the very large metropolitan area? At first one might suspect that the more traditional suburbs of the middle-sized city are less welcoming to and perhaps more discriminating against families whose economic afflu-

---

[2] These data are based on men with nonfarm background only.

ence is of recent standing than are suburbs of a large metropolis. Yet it seems doubtful that the social elite of the largest metropolitan areas discriminates less against the *nouveaux riches* than do the upper strata in smaller urbanized areas. A more plausible reason for the difference is that the largest cities have more suburbs and more diversified ones than medium-sized cities. Chicago not only has its Lake Forest but also Glencoe and Park Forest and many newer suburban developments, which provide upwardly mobile men with opportunities to move to suburbs without invading the exclusive environs of the social elite. The diversified suburbs of the largest metropolitan areas probably facilitate the move to suburbs of upwardly mobile men.

Before this conclusion inferred from the findings can be accepted as plausible, however, an alternative interpretation must be considered. Disproportionate numbers of urban Negroes and other minorities are concentrated in the central cities of the largest metropolitan areas, and we know that the occupational achievements of these men, particularly the Negroes, are inferior to those of the white majority group. Hence the persistent occupational superiority of suburbanites over city dwellers in the largest cities, and only there, when occupational and educational background are controlled may simply reflect the disproportionate numbers of underprivileged Negroes in the largest central cities. If this is the case this difference should disappear when race and ethnicity as well as other background factors are statistically controlled. The residual values with ethnic classification (including race) being added to the other controls are presented in columns 5 and 6 of Table 7.1.[3] Although the difference in occupational status between suburbanites and city dwellers is further reduced, some difference continues to be evident in the largest cities. The residual differences between suburbs and central cities are 2.7 for the very large, .5 for the large, and −1.0 for the medium-sized metropolitan areas. In the largest cities we can still observe a tendency for the economically successful to live in suburbs regardless of their background, which is not the case in somewhat smaller cities. The preponderance of Negroes and other minorities in the largest central

3 This is not quite the same as simply adding ethnicity (including race) to the controls in columns 3 and 4. Columns 5 and 6 no longer control father's education, whose effect, in any case, is insignificant once the effects of education and first job are accounted for. The three variables controlled here are X, father's occupational status; W, status of first job; and P, the ethnic-education classification used in Chapter 6. This variable, with fewer educational levels being considered, does not control respondent's education as fully as does the variable U, which is controlled in columns 3 and 4.

cities cannot account for this difference. This finding supports the interpretation advanced that economically successful men with low-status background characteristics are more likely to move to suburbs in the largest than in the somewhat smaller metropolitan centers.

We turn now to an examination of occupational differences associated with size of place, reading the data in Table 7.1 vertically. The occupational achievements of urban men, both those living in suburbs and those living in central cities, are higher than those of rural men. Mean occupational status is directly associated with size of place, whether urban places are represented by their central cities or by their suburbs (columns 1 and 2). The only exception to this is the depressed status of the central cities of the largest urban places. The poverty-ridden slums of the great metropolis, from which successful men flee to suburbs, seem to reduce the average occupational status in the metropolis. (The Negro ghettos in the largest cities do not account for these cities' depressed status, as indicated by the persisting low value in column 5.) With this single exception, however, the larger the community is, the better off the men are who live and work there. These differences, although reduced, persist when background factors are controlled, except that suburbanites as well as city dwellers of the largest places are now inferior to residents of cities with 250,000 to one million inhabitants (columns 3 and 4).

Whereas present occupational status is only roughly associated with community size, since the largest central cities have no advantage over smaller ones, status of first job varies consistently with community size, with the largest central cities no longer being inferior to the next-largest ones (columns 7 and 8 in Table 7.1). When background factors are controlled (column 9), men in the largest central cities are revealed as having the highest-status first jobs. (Their superiority in respect to first jobs is further increased if ethnic status and race also are controlled.) As we have said, one must not assume that these first jobs were held in the same community where the men now live, or in a community of the same size. In part the direct relationship between size of place and status of first job is undoubtedly due to a process of selective migration, with promising men who are able to obtain better first jobs moving to more urbanized places. In any case, men now living in the largest central cities had more auspicious career beginnings than men living anywhere else, but their final occupational achievements are not quite so good as those of men in somewhat smaller cities.[4]

---

[4] Part of this difference in final status, but not all of it, may be due to movement to the suburbs of the most successful men.

The implication is that the opportunity to achieve occupational success in the course of one's career is not so good in the very large metropolis as in the city of less than one million inhabitants. The data on intragenerational mobility from first job to 1962 occupation support this inference. (Lest movement to the suburbs of the most successful confound the findings, the data for men living in central cities and their suburbs are combined here.) Men living in the largest metropolitan areas are less likely to have moved up in the course of their careers by more than 25 points (24 per cent have) than men living in cities between 250,000 and one million inhabitants (28 per cent), though their proportion of upwardly mobile is no less than that of the entire population (23 per cent). Moreover, 18 per cent of the men in the largest urbanized areas have experienced downward mobility (of more than 5 points) from first to 1962 occupation, whereas only 15 per cent of those in the second-largest urbanized areas and 16 per cent of the total population did. In short, the chances of intragenerational upward mobility are less and the risks of downward mobility are greater in the largest metropolitan areas than in the somewhat smaller ones, though with this exception the chances of upward mobility are directly related to size of place.

The differences in average occupational status between communities of varying size provide a rough indication of the different occupational opportunities available in more or less urbanized places. If there are few high-status positions in certain localities men there have little chance to achieve high occupational status.[5] Since the men living in the suburbs of a metropolis work within its economic radius, and often actually in the central city, the data pertaining to them and to city dwellers must be combined in defining the opportunity structure. This indicator of the opportunity structure—the weighted mean 1962 status—is presented below for all six categories of size of place:

Very large city (1,000,000 and over)	40.0
Large city (250,000 to 1,000,000)	41.6
Middle-sized city (50,000 to 250,000)	38.9
Small city (2,500 to 50,000)	37.1
Rural nonfarm	32.9
Rural	17.5

[5] The existing occupational structure in a community is treated here as indicative of occupational opportunities and thus presumably of the demand for various occupational services. It must be noted that this is only a very rough indication of opportunities, since the existing structure is not merely a function of demand but also partly the result of the supply of available manpower with appropriate skills. Regardless of demand, positions for which qualified candidates do not exist cannot be filled.

The slightly depressed opportunities of the largest cities are the only exception to the general tendency for opportunities to increase as community size increases. Certainly the occupations available in urban areas are much superior in status to those available in rural areas, particularly on farms.

GEOGRAPHIC MOTILITY

Since occupational opportunities vary greatly among communities of different types, the place in which a man is born affects his future employment chances both directly, by increasing the likelihood that he will live in this place as an adult, and indirectly, by subjecting him to the background and educational limitations or advantages of his birth place. A man's economic chances are improved by his *motility,* that is, his not being rooted to his place of birth but free to leave it for better opportunities elsewhere. Psychological attachments and economic limitations restrict motility, which refers to the capacity to move, and of which actual migration is simply an operational measure. Geographic movement is associated with superior occupational achievement, regardless of place of birth or destination. The significance of motility is indicated by the data on nativity and ethnic background discussed in Chapter 6. As we have seen, there are differences in the chances of occupational success between men born in the North and those born in the South as well as between Negroes and whites, and there are somewhat lesser differences between men of different national origins. Regardless of these ascriptive factors, however, men who live outside the region of their birth tend to achieve higher occupational status than those who have remained in it.

Evidence for this generalization is presented in Table 7.2. Here six independent comparisons between the occupational status of men

TABLE 7.2.   MEAN DIFFERENCE IN OCC. STATUS AND IN INTRAGENERATIONAL MOBILITY BETWEEN MEN LIVING OUTSIDE AND MEN LIVING IN THEIR REGION OF BIRTH

Ethnicity–Nativity	1962 Occ. Status	First Job	Mean Intragenerational Mobility ($\bar{Y} - \bar{W}$)
Native white, native parentage			
Born in North or West	7.4	5.3	2.1
Born in South	1.0	-1.1	2.1
Second generation			
North and West European parentage	3.3	.9	2.4
Other parentage	3.0	2.6	.4
Nonwhite			
Born in North or West	4.0	6.7	-2.8
Born in South	3.7	3.4	.3

living in their region of birth and that of men living in another region are made. The table shows the differences in scores between "migrants" and "nonmigrants" who are by birth northern whites, southern whites, sons of two groupings of foreign-born, northern nonwhites, and southern nonwhites. It should be noted that the migrants here include men who were taken from their region of birth as children by parents who moved as well as men who moved on their own initiative, and that nonmigrants include an undetermined number of men who have returned to their region of birth after experiencing migration.

The data unequivocally show that migrants have more successful careers than men still living in the region of their birth. All six comparisons reported in column 1 of Table 7.2 indicate the superiority of migrants. Although the occupational significance of migration varies considerably by ethnicity and place of birth, it is consistently positive, with men living outside their region of birth having superior achievements in all six comparisons. The migrants also had better first jobs than others in five of six comparisons, the exception being that southern whites living in the North held lower first jobs than did their compatriots who remained in the South. Despite their generally higher starting points, moreover, migrants experienced greater intragenerational mobility, that is, they moved up further from their career beginnings, again in all but one case, than northern nonwhites (column 3). In brief, men who remain in the region in which they were born start their careers on lower levels and advance less subsequently than those who live outside their region of birth. It appears that something either about migration or about migrants promotes occupational success.

A hypothesis that can explain these findings is that living some distance away from his childhood home frees a man from the restraints and influences his childhood environment imposes on his career. Men who do not live in the region of their birth are, consequently, expected not only to be upwardly mobile in disproportionate numbers, because they are less held back by social obligations and limited opportunities at home, but also to be downwardly mobile in disproportionate numbers, because they receive less support and help from relatives and friends. The basic hypothesis is that physical distance promotes social distance from parental status in both directions. Table 7.3 presents data with which this hypothesis can be tested. Upward mobility is divided into long-distance and short-distance, distinguishing between men moving 26 points or more up from their father's status and those moving up 6 to 25 points. Men moving no more than 5

TABLE 7.3.   INTERGENERATIONAL MOBILITY DISTRIBUTION BY ETHNICITY, NATIVITY, AND
WHETHER LIVING IN REGION OF BIRTH (IN PERCENTAGES)

Region of Birth, Ethnic Classification, and Migration Status	Moving Up 26 to 96 Points	Moving Up 6 to 25 Points	Stable −5 to +5 Points	Moving Down 6 Points or More	Total
Northern white					
Living in region of birth	24.5	23.9	27.6	24.1	100.0
Living elsewhere	27.9	27.7	22.1	22.3	100.0
Southern white					
Living in region of birth	24.6	24.2	30.4	20.8	100.0
Living elsewhere	27.7	28.4	25.6	18.3	100.0
Second generation of north and west European parentage					
Living in region of birth	31.0	22.8	26.2	20.0	100.0
Living elsewhere	33.1	23.6	20.4	22.9	100.0
Other parentage					
Living in region of birth	31.9	28.7	24.8	14.6	100.0
Living elsewhere	28.1	31.6	22.7	17.6	100.0
Northern nonwhite					
Living in region of birth	22.9	24.4	32.7	19.9	100.0
Living elsewhere	8.8	33.3	38.6	19.3	100.0
Southern nonwhite					
Living in region of birth	6.7	13.6	45.6	34.1	100.0
Living elsewhere	10.9	24.9	39.0	25.2	100.0
Total[a]	24.8	24.7	28.1	22.3	100.0

[a]Includes foreign-born white, not shown separately.

points either up or down from their origins are taken to be stable.
Long- and short-distance downward mobility have been combined,
as few move down more than 25 points.

As anticipated, men living outside the region of their birth are
more likely than others to experience upward mobility (either long-
or short-distance). Although neither second-generation men of "other"
descent nor northern nonwhites conform to this pattern, the numbers
of migrants among these are small. The second expectation, that
migrants are also more likely than others to experience downward
mobility, however, is not confirmed by the data. On the contrary,
except for the second generation, migrants are less likely to be
downwardly mobile than men who live in their region of birth. On
the basis of this test the hypothesis must be rejected. But before
risking premature rejection of a correct hypothesis a more refined test
of it should be attempted.

As noted in Chapter 4, it is possible to calculate the mobility distribution comparable to Table 7.3 that would be expected if mobility
were governed exclusively by a model of statistical independence of
father's and son's status within each ethnic-migration category. This
is asking, in effect, how much mobility there would be in each ethnic-

migration category if occupational origins and destinations were independent *within* these categories. The pattern of differences between the observed and the expected mobility distributions can then be examined for evidence of the interaction of migration status with the relationship between social origin and 1962 occupation. By adding these differences to the mobility distribution of the total population, the calculations are converted back to percentage distributions that are standardized for the marginal distributions of occupational statuses. These standardized distributions furnish a more adequate test of the hypothesis.

Does the pattern of standardized mobility confirm the hypothesized association between migration and downward as well as upward mobility? The answer is definitely no. To summarize without presenting the full table here (see Table J7.1 in the Appendix), migrants not only continue to have no greater propensity to be downwardly mobile than nonmigrants, but they now also exhibit slightly less upward mobility than men who have remained in their region of birth. These findings have two implications. First, they require the rejection of the hypothesis that geographical mobility promotes both upward and downward social mobility. Second, they furnish support for the selective migration hypothesis, for they imply that the migrants' greater chances of upward mobility are due to their superior social origins and can no longer be observed once origins have been standardized in terms of a statistical model of independence.

The conclusion, in short, is that migrants enjoy both higher occupational achievements and greater chances for upward mobility than nonmigrants, but their superior chances of success seem to be not so much produced by migration as by initial advantages migrants have. The analysis on which this conclusion is based, however, raises a number of problems that must be clarified by more detailed investigation.

The first and most basic of these problems is posed by the definition of migrant. Men who do not live in the region of their birth include not only those who have migrated on their own initiative but also an unknown number of others who were taken as children by their migrating parents to other regions. To study the significance of migration for occupational life, the first of these two groups must be isolated, men who themselves left their home community. To do so, we shall distinguish men who did not live in 1962 in the same community in which they grew up—specifically, in which they lived at age 16—from those who continued to live where they had been raised.

The conclusion that migrants are more successful in their careers than other men is confirmed when this new indicator of migration is used, as will be seen. However, the basic question regarding the causal nexus underlying this correlation remains. Does migration itself produce greater occupational success, and, if so, for what reason? Or, to the contrary, does the pursuit of successful careers constrain men to migrate, for example because a corporation assigns its best managers to more responsible positions in other communities? Or is the correlation perhaps the result of a third factor, such as individual initiative, that promotes both migration and occupational achievement? Do migrants have superior achievements regardless of the locations from and to which they move, or is their superiority rather attained merely because they move from areas of poorer to those with better opportunities? The analysis, though not furnishing definitive answers to these questions, will permit some plausible inferences.

Finally, some broader questions can be raised concerning the significance of migration for occupational mobility in general, not just for that of the migrants themselves. For example, Lipset and Bendix have suggested that today "migration from rural areas and smaller communities to metropolitan centers influences the placement of people in the occupational structure in the same way that large scale immigration once did."[6] To wit, they propose that rural migrants occupy the lower occupational strata in urbanized areas, just as immigrants to the United States did in the past, and this increases the opportunities for upward mobility of the native urban population. The assumption is that migrants to large cities furnish the impetus for occupational mobility on a wider scale in the urban structure. Do our national data support such a hypothesis?

These problems will be investigated with the aid of a variable that derives migration status from the answer to the question, "Where were you living when you were 16 years old?" Men reporting that they had lived in the same community as in 1962 are identified as nonmigrants. The rest, the migrants, were asked whether they had lived in a large city of 100,000 or more inhabitants or its suburbs, a smaller city, or a rural area. The last category was subdivided by father's occupation into rural nonfarm and farm. Four roughly comparable categories of the Bureau of the Census (rather than self-identification) were used to classify men by present residence. Hence we can not only compare migrants and nonmigrants but also examine separately the influence on occupational life of being raised and of living as adults in large cities, in small cities, in rural nonfarm areas, and on farms. (A more

[6] Seymour M. Lipset and Reinhard Bendix, *Social Mobility in Industrial Society*, Berkeley and Los Angeles: Univer. of California Press, 1963, p. 204.

detailed description of the classification procedure is provided in Appendix I.)

It is of interest to estimate when men classified as migrants actually left the community in which they were reared. For men in this sample, 38.5 per cent of the 20- to 24-year-olds have moved from their place of residence at age 16, and about another 17 per cent seem to have moved between 25 and 34, since a total of 55.9 per cent of the 25- to 34-year-old cohort live elsewhere than their community at 16 years of age. Beyond this point, however, increasing age does little to increase the proportion of migrants. An additional 4 per cent of men seem to have moved between 35 and 44 years, and another 3 per cent between 55 and 64 years, yielding a final total of migrants in the oldest cohort of 63 per cent. Although these round calculations inferred from cohort comparisons cannot resolve all problems of the timing of migration, they suggest that about three-fifths of all men leave their home community after age 16, and that the large majority of these do so in late adolescence or early adulthood, before they reach the middle thirties.

THE SIGNIFICANCE OF MIGRATION

With about three-fifths of adult men living outside the community in which they were raised, migration is clearly the prevailing pattern in our industrial society. The majority of men at all ages over 25 are migrants, leaving only 43 per cent of the total sample identified as nonmigrants. These figures can only underestimate the true proportion of the population that has experienced migration at one point or another in adult life, as some unknown number of men return to the community in which they were raised after having migrated elsewhere and hence escape our count. In addition to the primary distinction between migrants and nonmigrants, two broad categories of migrants are identified, those who live in the same type of community, in terms of degree of urbanization, as that in which they were raised, and those who live in a different type of community. One-fifth of the sample are migrants between communities of the same type, and 37 per cent have moved from one type of community to another.[7]

There are only minor differences among age cohorts in the distribution of men with various migration experiences. (For a full tabular presentation of the cohort distributions, see Table J7.2 in the Appendix.) Let it suffice to note that older men are less likely than younger

[7] If more categories of places were used, the proportion of migrants moving to communities of different types would, of course, be larger.

ones to live where they were reared and more likely to have moved between communities of different types. This is the case for seven of nine comparisons, with the two exceptions being the larger proportions of younger cohorts who have moved from large cities to small ones and from urban to rural areas, that is, counter to the main stream of migration toward more urbanized places.[8] This pattern, including the two exceptions, is largely a function of differences in community origins between younger and older cohorts. The oldest cohort has more diverse origins (for rural areas claimed a larger proportion of the population in 1920 than in 1950) from which they could move to large cities, where most of them are now. Conversely, in 1950 there was a much greater proportion of adolescents in large cities than had been the case 30 years earlier, that is, a greater number of men in large places who could move to smaller ones. Although the pattern is partly a function of the marginal distribution, it does reveal some differences in the migration experience between age cohorts.

Migrants in general have more successful careers than other men, as previously noted. But this should be expected, as the main stream of migrants moves from less to more urbanized places where occupational opportunities for all, migrants and nonmigrants alike, are better. The important question is whether migration as such, as distinguished from the change in the occupational structure in which a man competes resulting from migration, is associated with occupational success. To answer this question, nonmigrants in the four types of communities are compared with those migrants who both live now and were raised in communities of the same type—that is, with migrants who moved from one large city to another, from one to another small city, from one rural nonfarm area to another, or from one farm area to a farm elsewhere. This procedure holds constant the occupational structure associated with communities of a given type.

Table 7.4 presents a series of comparisons between nonmigrants and migrants within the same community type. The top panel of the table shows that migration as such, independent of differences in degree of urbanization, is clearly associated with occupational achievement. The superiority of migrants over nonmigrants is pronounced in urban areas, being 6.7 points in large cities and 9.0 points in small ones; it is a good deal smaller, 2.4 points, in rural nonfarm areas,

---

[8] We must not attach undue significance to the increased volume of urban to rural migration among younger cohorts. Undoubtedly, the great bulk of this migration is to nonfarm areas, frequently in the immediate vicinity of a city though beyond the limits of what is identified as the built-up urbanized area.

TABLE 7.4.   MEAN STATUS CHARACTERISTICS BY COMMUNITY TYPE AND MIGRATION FOR MEN LIVING IN SAME TYPE OF COMMUNITY AS AT AGE 16 (IN DEVIATIONS FROM THE GRAND MEAN)

Characteristic and Migration	Large City	Small City	Rural Nonfarm	Rural Farm
Occupational status				
Nonmigrant	2.7	-3.5	-5.8	-15.3
Migrant within community type	9.3	5.5	-3.4	-19.1
Difference	6.7	9.0	2.4	-3.8
Education				
Nonmigrant	.21	-.14	-.33	-.95
Migrant within community type	.70	.46	-.32	-1.29
Difference	.49	.60	.01	-.34
First job				
Nonmigrant	3.0	-2.4	-4.8	-9.8
Migrant within community type	8.4	5.3	-4.5	-11.7
Difference	5.4	7.7	0.3	-1.9
Father's occ.				
Nonmigrant	4.6	-.5	-.4	-15.0[a]
Migrant within community type	10.5	4.2	-1.2	-14.9[a]
Difference	5.7	4.7	-.8	.1
Occupational status controlling for education & first job				
Nonmigrant	1.2	-1.7	-2.1	-7.4
Migrant within community type	2.9	1.2	-.4	-9.1
Difference	1.7	2.9	1.7	-1.7

[a]Subject to slight downward bias owing to calculation from midpoints of class intervals.

and there is a reversal of the pattern on farms, with the status of non-migrants exceeding that of migrants by 3.8 points.

To be sure, labor-market conditions have not actually been held constant in these comparisons, for these conditions may vary widely among communities of the same size, quite aside from the fact that considerable variations of size exist within our broad category of large cities. Nevertheless, the important variations of occupational opportunities between farm areas, other rural areas, small towns, and large cities have been held constant in our comparisons, which consequently indicate that the superior economic success of migrants is *not* primarily the result of the disproportionate numbers who move from rural areas to urban ones, where occupational opportunities are better.

These findings are consistent with the interpretation that migration is selective of men predisposed to occupational success. However, they are likewise consistent with the alternative hypothesis that migration is an advantageous experience that improves a man's occupational abilities. To try to distinguish between these two interpretations we can examine differences in background characteristics between migrants and nonmigrants. If the economic superiority of migrants is, at least in part, the result of a process of selective migration, it follows that men who later migrate must already be superior to others in some relevant respects before they move.

Education is such an early indicator of superior potential for achievement. The second panel of Table 7.4 shows that urban migrants have, indeed, acquired more education than urban nonmigrants. In contrast to the differences favoring migrants in urban areas, there is no difference in rural nonfarm areas, and on farms nonmigrants have actually some educational superiority over migrants. In addition to their educational advantages, urban migrants had first jobs that were superior to those of nonmigrants, as the third panel shows. The pattern here is the same as that for education, with the superiority of migrants being confined to urban areas. To be sure, not all migrants completed their education and held their first jobs before they left their parental home, though many undoubtedly did. But another background variable, father's occupation when the respondent was 16 years old, precedes migration by definition, since only migration after age 16 is under consideration. Any differences in social origins between migrants and nonmigrants must therefore reflect selective factors. The fourth panel of Table 7.4 shows that urban migrants come from origins superior to those of nonmigrants, whereas there is again no such difference for rural men.

These data regarding differences in social origins, education, and first jobs between same-community-type migrants and nonmigrants reveal superior conditions of migrants that already existed, at least for most of them, at the time of their migration and thus could not have been produced by the experience of migration. Hence the superiority of same-environment urban migrants over nonmigrants in social origins, education, and career beginnings supports the conclusion that urban migration is selective of men with greater potentialities for occupational success, although farm-to-farm migration does not exhibit such a process of selection. However, these findings do not demonstrate that the same urban migrants who enjoy the greatest occupational success are also the ones with the superior background, as implied by the selective-migration hypothesis. The question is whether the differences in occupational achievements between migrants and nonmigrants are accounted for by their differences in early qualifications. The last panel of Table 7.4 helps answer this question by presenting the effects of migration on 1962 occupational status net of education and first job. When these two variables are controlled the original differences in status between migrants and nonmigrants are greatly reduced, but the residuals reveal the same pattern, that is, they show the migrants to be superior except in the farm population.

The inference, therefore, is that urban migration is selective of men with superior qualifications for success, whereas farm migration is not selective of the most able. Urban migrants are men with greater potential for occupational achievement, and they realize this potential in the course of their careers. A possible explanation of the exceptional case of rural farm migrants, whose achievements are inferior to those of farm nonmigrants, is that a significant portion of this group (which is less than 2 per cent of the total sample) are migratory farm laborers. The rewards available in this occupation are manifestly inadequate to attract men of high potential.

Although the data clearly support the hypothesis that migration is selective of men with higher potential for occupational achievement, the residual differences when training and early experience are controlled lend credence to the notion that migration also promotes (or is required for) occupational success. However, the evidence is equivocal on this point. The residual superiority of migrants may be due to some other background factors that are not reflected in education or first job, such as initiative. Alternatively, the residual differences between migrants and nonmigrants may be indicative of the fact that migration increases chances of success simply because it improves the occupational opportunities in a man's environment, inasmuch as only some and by no means all variations in opportunity structure have been controlled in the foregoing analysis. Some evidence can be brought to bear on this last inference by investigating how the changes in economic opportunities resulting from migration influence the occupational achievements of migrants to different types of communities.

OPPORTUNITY STRUCTURE AND MIGRATION PROCESS

Let us turn now to a consideration of the significance of the change in occupational environment produced by migration, the very factor we attempted to control in the preceding analysis of the significance of migration as such. We shall first examine the influence of the degree of urbanization of the community to which migrants come and ask whether natives and migrants from various places are similarly affected by differences in the degree of urbanization of their social environment and the correlated differences in opportunity structure. Then we shall turn attention to the influence of the type of community in which a migrant was raised on his subsequent career elsewhere.

As has been previously mentioned, occupational opportunities are directly related to the degree of urbanization of a community, with opportunities being worst on farms and improving steadily with movement toward nonfarm rural areas, toward small cities, and finally toward large cities.[9] These differences in opportunity structure are clearly evident in the occupational achievements of nonmigrants. The first row of Table 7.5 presents the mean occupational achievement of

TABLE 7.5.   MEAN 1962 OCC. STATUS BY TYPE OF COMMUNITY AT AGE 16 AND IN 1962 AND MIGRATION STATUS (IN DEVIATIONS FROM THE GRAND MEAN)

	1962 Residence			
Residence at Age 16	Large City (50,000+)	Small City (2,500 to 50,000)	Rural Nonfarm	Farm
Same Community	2.7	-3.5	-5.8	-15.3
Different Community				
Large City (100,000+)	9.3	11.7		
Small City (2,500 to 100,000)	5.7	5.5	4.2	
Rural Nonfarm	-2.1	-1.5	-3.4	-18.6
Farm	-4.5	-1.6	-6.6	-19.1

nonmigrants in the four types of communities in terms of deviations from the total population mean.[10] The more urbanized the environment, the higher the mean occupational status of natives. The occupational position of migrants, on the other hand, does not accurately mirror these differences in opportunities, as the other four rows of the table indicate. To be sure, migrants as well as natives have more successful careers in urban than in rural areas. However, whereas the nonmigrant's position is highest in large cities, the migrant's is best in small cities. This is the case not only for migrants from rural areas, who might be expected to do better in small cities, which contrast less with their rural background, but also for those who themselves come from large cities. Surprisingly, migrants who come from small cities are the only ones who do not fare best in small cities; they

[9] The slightly lower opportunities found in very large metropolitan centers of over one million inhabitants do not affect the present analysis in which these largest cities are combined with other large ones into a single category.

[10] Since the opportunity structure is defined by the total distribution of occupations in a community, the relationship between the occupational achievements of a large proportion of this population, such as the nonmigrants, and the occupational structure is largely tautological. However, the differences in achievements between migrants from various places and nonmigrants within the same community can be meaningfully related to the opportunity structure.

do as well in large cities as in small ones. Moving to a similar place appears to have no advantage.

Data on upward mobility from social origins confirm the conclusion that the small city provides exceptional opportunities for the migrant (Table 7.6). The native's chances of experiencing considerable upward

TABLE 7.6.   PER CENT UPWARDLY MOBILE FROM FATHER'S OCC. MORE THAN 25 POINTS, BY TYPE OF COMMUNITY AT AGE 16 AND IN 1962 AND MIGRATION STATUS

| | 1962 Residence | | | |
Residence at Age 16	Large City (50,000+)	Small City (2,500 to 50,000)	Rural Nonfarm	Farm
Same Community	25.4	20.5	15.4[a]	
Different Community				
Large City (100,000+)	29.1	35.3	26.0	
Small City (2,500 to 100,000)	27.1	31.3		
Rural[a]	29.7	37.4	25.3	6.1

[a]The distinction between farm and nonfarm used in Tables 7.5, 7.7, and 7.8 is not available for this tabulation.

mobility (over 25 points) are greater in large cities (25 per cent), than in small ones (20 per cent), where they are still greater than in rural areas (15 per cent). But migrants find their best chances for upward mobility in small cities, regardless of whether they were raised in large cities, small cities, or rural areas. The superior occupational opportunities in large cities notwithstanding, migrants to small cities are the ones most likely to achieve upward mobility and high occupational status. As a result of the apparent advantages migrants enjoy in small cities, those of rural as well as those of urban origins are more successful than natives there (Table 7.5, column 2). In large cities, on the other hand, only urban migrants are superior to natives, and the achievements of migrants from rural areas are inferior to the natives' (column 1). These differences are not entirely due to the superior background qualifications of urban migrants. When the effects of education and first job are controlled (Table 7.7), the same pattern emerges, though the differences are greatly reduced.

Although migrants achieve their greatest success in small cities, it should be noted that urban-raised migrants to large cities are more successful than natives there. In the light of this one can hardly argue that migrants are handicapped in large cities. Yet it is clear that migrants to large cities do not do as well as migrants to small cities, whereas natives are more successful in large than in small cities. This holds whether we examine mean occupational achievement, per cent

TABLE 7.7.   MEAN OCC. STATUS BY TYPE OF COMMUNITY AT AGE 16 AND IN 1962 AND MIGRATION STATUS, CONTROLLING FOR EDUCATION AND FIRST JOB (IN DEVIATIONS FROM THE GRAND MEAN)

Residence at Age 16	1962 Residence			
	Large City (50,000+)	Small City (2,500 to 50,000)	Rural Nonfarm	Farm
Same community	1.2	-1.7	-2.1	-7.4
Different community				
Large city (100,000+)	2.9	4.3	1.3	
Small city (2,500 to 100,000)	1.3	1.2		
Rural nonfarm	.2	2.0	-.4	-9.5
Farm	1.0	2.1	-.5	-9.1

upwardly mobile, or occupational achievement when background factors are controlled—a puzzling finding to be further explored later.

The community in which a boy is raised affects his career as an adult, just as the region where he was born does. The socioeconomic structure of the community where a boy grows up probably serves as an ascriptive determinant of his later behavior in a manner somewhat similar to his family origins. The adolescent doubtlessly is more aware of career lines to which he has been exposed in his home town, more interested in jobs for which role models exist in his experience, and better prepared for occupations to which the local school system is oriented. Thus we would expect the occupational structure of the community in which a man was raised to influence his future career—and occupational structures vary, of course, with degree of urbanization.

The larger the place where a man was reared, the better are his chances of occupational success. This positive association between degree of urbanization of place of origin and occupational achievement can be observed among both migrants and nonmigrants, and it is independent of the size of the community to which a migrant moves and in which he lives and works. The pattern is perfectly consistent. The degree of urbanization of the place where a migrant grew up is directly associated with his later occupational achievement elsewhere, as can be seen by reading down from row 2 in each column of Table 7.5. The same influence of place of origin is revealed by the finding that the occupational status of nonmigrants is directly related to size of nonmigrants the present community is, naturally, identical with the one where they lived at age 16.

The influence on occupational life of the size of the place of origin is both more pronounced and more consistent than the effect of size of present community. This finding contradicts the common-sense expectation that where a man works should affect his career more than where he grew up. As a matter of fact, the less consistent findings on present place might be reinterpreted in terms of the more clear-cut ones on place of origin. Perhaps the association between size of present place and occupation differs for natives and for migrants because the influences of the environment in which a man was reared and of the environment where he presently lives cannot be separated for nonmigrants. The case of migrants, in which these two influences can be separated, shows that having been reared in a large city gives a man the greatest occupational advantage, whereas working in a large city is less advantageous than working in a small one, other conditions being equal. The implication is that the high occupational achievements of natives in large cities are primarily due to their having been raised and trained there rather than merely to their working there.

The importance of the type of community in which a man was brought up for his occupational success can only mean that more urbanized environments prepare youngsters better for high-status occupations. In the absence of more comprehensive measures, education may serve as an indicator of occupational preparation. Indeed, the larger the community in which a man lived as an adolescent, the greater his educational attainment tends to be, regardless of the type of community in which he later works. The data in Table 7.8 show

TABLE 7.8. MEAN EDUCATIONAL ATTAINMENT BY TYPE OF COMMUNITY AT AGE 16 AND IN 1962 AND MIGRATION STATUS (IN DEVIATIONS FROM THE GRAND MEAN)

Residence at Age 16	1962 Residence			
	Large City (50,000+)	Small City (2,500 to 50,000)	Rural Nonfarm	Farm
Same community	.21	-.14	-.33	-.95
Different community				
Large city (100,000+)	.70	.78	.36	
Small city (2,500 to 100,000)	.53	.46		
Rural nonfarm	-.31	-.35	-.32	-1.23
Farm	-.68	-.47	-.73	-1.29

this pattern again to be perfectly consistent for all five comparisons (migrants in four destinations and nonmigrants). Furthermore, the educational differences among migrants raised in various communities (read vertically) are somewhat larger than the differences among non-migrants raised in comparable communities (read first row). This is in accord with the superior achievements of migrants, suggesting that, as potential achievers, they are more likely to take advantage of the better educational facilities of urban places.

Early work experiences also help prepare a man for his later career. The more urbanized a community is, the greater is the variety of promising first jobs that prepare youngsters well for occupational success. The expectation is, therefore, that the quality of first jobs is directly associated with the size of the place in which a man grew up, just as education is, and the data in Table 7.9 confirm this expectation. The mean status of first job exhibits the same pattern as mean educational attainment. It is directly related to the size of the community in which a man was raised, whether he remained there or migrated to another and regardless of the size of the community to which he migrated.

TABLE 7.9. MEAN STATUS OF FIRST JOB BY TYPE OF COMMUNITY AT AGE 16 AND IN 1962 AND MIGRATION STATUS (IN DEVIATIONS FROM THE GRAND MEAN)

Residence at Age 16	1962 Residence			
	Large City (50,000+)	Small City (2,500 to 50,000)	Rural Nonfarm	Farm
Same community	3.0	-2.4	-4.8	-9.8
Different community				
Large City (100,000+)	8.4	7.7	2.9	
Small City (2,500 to 100,000)	4.0	5.3		
Rural nonfarm	-4.0	-5.9	-4.5	-11.1
Farm	-7.3	-5.2	-7.9	-11.7

These observations suggest that the superior education and early work experience of men reared in more urbanized communities account for their more successful subsequent careers. Data to test this expectation are supplied in Table 7.7, in which variation in mean occupational status net of the effects of education and first job is shown. (Differences among nonmigrants are read across row 1; those among migrants, down from row 2 in all columns.) The importance of the community in which a man was raised for his occupational status is greatly reduced by controlling education and first job. For nonmigrants, the residual differences reveal the same general pattern that existed before controls were applied (compare Table 7.7 to Table 7.5). For migrants, on the other hand, the pattern has remained the same only in broad outline, not in specific detail. Migrants raised in large cities continue to enjoy higher status than those raised in small towns or rural areas. However, migrants raised on farms are no longer inferior in status to those raised in other rural areas once the effects of education and first job are eliminated, and men raised in small cities are not consistently superior to those raised in rural nonfarm places.

The residual differences among nonmigrants, moreover, are not only more consonant with the original direct relationship between occupational status and place size but also far more pronounced than those among migrants.

With two notable exceptions, the better education and early work experience of men raised in more urbanized areas largely explain their more successful subsequent careers. The first exception is that the occupational achievements of nonmigrants vary directly with community size even among men with the same education and career beginnings. This undoubtedly reflects the superior occupational opportunities available in the larger communities. Differences in these opportunities benefit, of course, only those men raised in urban places who remain there, not those who have moved elsewhere. Men who moved from their home community to another of the same type, however, also retain the benefits or disadvantages of the opportunity structure of this community type. The interpretation implies, therefore, that differences parallel to those found among nonmigrants should be observed among migrants if only those within the same community type are considered. This is in fact the case, as the values in the diagonal of the migrant portion of Table 7.7 show. For these migrants within community type, controlling for education and first job, mean occupational status declines from 39.2 in large cities to 37.5 in small ones, 35.9 in rural nonfarm areas, and 27.2 on farms.[11] Note that the range for same-environment migrants is greater than that for nonmigrants, for whom the corresponding values, in order, are: 37.5, 34.6, 34.2, and 28.9. The greater range for migrants suggests that these men with high potentials take more advantage than others of existing occupational opportunities, just as they take more advantage of existing educational opportunities.

The second major exception to the generalization that the better preparation of men raised in more urbanized places accounts for their more successful careers is that migrants as well as nonmigrants raised in large cities enjoy career advantages over other men beyond those resulting from their better education and early work experience. The wider scope and better quality of the educational facilities in the metropolis, as exemplified by specialized high schools, may give boys going to school there a competitive advantage. Another relevant factor probably is that the highly diversified labor market in a metropolis provides youngsters growing up there with knowledge and sophis-

[11] These cell means are calculated simply by adding 36.3, the total population mean, to the value in each cell of Table 7.7, which represent the deviations from the grand mean.

tication about possible careers and employment conditions that stand them in good stead later in their careers. Such big-city experiences seem to benefit most those men who later move to small cities, where they can become, so to speak, big fish in small ponds.

Although most aspects of occupational success are directly associated with the size of the place in which a man was raised, the reverse is the case for the social distance that migrants to large cities move up in the course of their careers. Among migrants to large cities, those who came from other large cities move up from their first to their 1962 occupation an average of 11.7 points on the occupational status scale. The smaller the community from which migrants to the large cities have come, the larger is the mean distance moved, being 12.4 points for men from small cities, 12.6 points for those from rural nonfarm areas, and 13.5 points for men raised on farms.[12]

This pattern reflects the superior career beginnings of migrants from more urban communities. The more urban the place in which a migrant to a large city grew up, the better are his chances of achieving high occupational status, but the greater also is the likelihood that he started his career at a relatively high level, and the worse, consequently, are his chances of experiencing upward mobility in the course of his career. No similar pattern, however, is observed among migrants to places other than large cities. Migrants to small cities or rural areas do not move up from their first jobs to higher ones any less (on the average) if they were raised in larger than if they were raised in smaller places, although status of first job is directly associated with size of place of origin for these migrants too (Table 7.9). The implication is that having been reared in a highly urbanized place gives men who work in such a place as adults less of a competitive advantage than it gives men who work in less urban places, and that rural upbringing has, unexpectedly, least disadvantages for career mobility in large cities, whose outstanding opportunities outweigh the educational handicaps of rural migrants.

THE DYNAMICS OF SOCIAL AND SPATIAL MOVEMENTS

The fact dominating the findings of the last section is that urbanization—of place of origin as well as present residence—promotes occupational success. In terms of a man's career the city is a better place than the country, not only as a place to work, but also as a place to grow up. There is, however, an important subsidiary pattern that in

---

[12] These values are the differences between the values in the first columns of Tables 7.5 and 7.9, plus 10.8, which is the difference between the grand means of 1962 and first occupation (36.3 − 25.5).

a sense runs counter to this dominant one. This subsidiary pattern can be observed when the occupational achievements of migrants from smaller to larger communities are compared to those of migrants moving in the opposite direction.

Despite the fact that occupational opportunities are generally better in larger than in smaller communities, migrants who move from a smaller to a larger place consistently fail to achieve as high an occupational status as those moving the other way. Thus the mean status of migrants from small to large cities is 6.0 points lower than that of migrants from large to small ones (Table 7.5). Similarly, the status of migrants from rural to urban areas, the weighted mean of 34.1, 34.8, 31.8, and 34.7, is considerably lower than that of migrants from urban to rural areas, 40.5. The single exception is that the status of men moving from farms to other rural areas is higher than that of those moving from rural nonfarm places to farms. A possible reason for this exception is the probable underevaluation of farm occupations on the status scale, which has been previously noted.

The superiority of men moving from larger to smaller communities over those moving in the other direction is not restricted to ultimate occupational status. The educational attainments of migrants who have moved in opposite directions in terms of community size reveal the same pattern (see Table 7.8), and so do their first jobs (Table 7.9). Indeed, at every educational level, as shown in Table 7.10, the likelihood that a man will continue on to the next is greater if he is a migrant from a large to a small city or from an urban to a rural area than if his migration carried him the other way.

TABLE 7.10. PER CENT CONTINUING THEIR EDUCATION FROM ONE LEVEL TO THE NEXT FOR MIGRANTS MOVING BETWEEN DIFFERENT TYPES OF COMMUNITIES

Type of Migration	Through Eighth Grade	Eighth Grade to Some High School	Some High School to High-School Graduation	High-School Graduation to Some College	Some College to College Graduation	College Graduation to Post-Graduate
Large city to small city	90.5	93.1	83.0	58.6	66.5	48.1[a]
Small city to large city	90.4	88.0	79.9	55.0	60.5	43.3
Urban to rural	88.6	89.6	75.9	50.7	59.7	40.3
Rural to large city	76.1	75.4	70.8	39.3	46.5	35.7
Rural to small city	79.9	73.3	70.1	41.6	53.3	41.0
Total population	84.9	84.0	73.6	45.8	51.2	41.1[a]

[a]Estimated population in less than 100,000.

As the standardized values in Table 7.7 show, these differences in education and first job account only in part for the differences in occupational achievements between men migrating in opposite directions. The residual difference between farm-to-rural-nonfarm migrants and those making the opposite move remains a substantial 9.1 in favor of men moving off the farm. The residuals for the remaining comparisons also reflect the original differences in attenuated form. Among urban migrants the differences are still considerable, with the standardized status of men moving from small to large cities being 3.0 points lower than that of men moving from large to small ones. However, when the effects of education and first job have been eliminated, the status of migrants from rural to urban areas is a mere 0.2 points below that of migrants from urban to rural places.[13]

One reason for the existence of this pattern is the previously noted finding that place of origin influences occupational achievement more than place of present residence. Migrants coming from more to less urban places must be more successful than those going the opposite way if being raised in a more urbanized place furthers occupational success more than working in one does. However, the pattern has further implications for the relationship between migration and mobility.

The dominant stream of migration is from less to more urban areas. More than four million men moved as adolescents from small cities to large cities, whereas only half a million men raised in large moved to small cities. Close to five million men moved from rural to urban areas, in contrast to less than three million who moved from urban to rural ones.[14] It is probable that special incentives are necessary to induce a man to move against this predominant stream. He is unlikely to migrate from a larger to a smaller place unless he has reasonable expectations that doing so will have special advantageous consequences for his career. Thus a process of selection of men with exceptionally good occupational prospects, an extreme case of the general process of selective migration, helps explain the superior occupational status of men who have moved from more to less urban places.[15]

Let us reexamine several findings simultaneously to infer the dynamic processes produced by migration and urbanization in the occupational structure. The superior occupational opportunities in more urban communities attract disproportionate numbers of men from

---

[13] The weighted mean of the four cells of rural to urban migrants is 1.1.

[14] Population estimates are based on our sample; see Table J7.2 in the Appendix. The discrepancies in the percentages are greater than those expected by a model of independence.

[15] Another possible reason why men who moved from larger to smaller places have disproportionately high status is that the most successful men in the metropolis often move to rural areas or small towns beyond the suburban fringe, such as Bucks County and upper Long Island.

smaller places. As a result of the process of selective migration, these migrants to cities tend to achieve higher occupational positions, other things being equal, than the natives there. However, other things are not equal. The inferior training and skills of men raised in rural areas counteract the influence of selective migration, so that the occupational achievements of rural migrants to large cities are inferior to those of the natives. That is, migrants from rural to urban places are more successful than the rural men they leave behind, which reflects both selection and superior opportunities in cities, but less successful than other residents of large cities, an inferiority almost wholly explained by their inferior background and preparation. The greater success of rural migrants to small cities than that enjoyed by natives there implies that their background and qualifications are not so great a handicap in small cities as in large ones.

It bears repeating that rural migrants to large cities are better off than they would be had they remained at home but not so well off as natives or urban migrants there.[16] For this fact underlies the dynamics of the occupational structure in large cities. The superior opportunities available in large cities prompt men of rural origins to move to these cities in large numbers. Eight and a half per cent of the sample has done so, representing three and a half million men. These rural migrants to large cities achieve higher occupational status than their counterparts who remain in rural areas, even though their inferior qualifications force them to accept jobs that rank low in the urban occupational structure. The natives in large cities as well as the migrants from other urban places gain from the influx of rural migrants into the least desirable occupational positions there, for this influx means that fewer natives must occupy the lower positions than would otherwise be necessary. Thus more of them are enabled to take advantage of the superior educational and training facilities in their urban environment and acquire the qualifications needed to move into higher occupational positions. Given the poor occupational opportunities in rural areas, particularly on farms, rural migrants to cities tend to experience upward mobility although they occupy relatively low positions in the urban occupational hierarchy. By preempting these lowest positions they provide a structural impetus to upward mobility for the other men in large cities.

These observations and inferences confirm the previously men-

16 This is the case for 1962 occupation, without and with controlling background, for education, and for first job. Note that in all the tables (7.5, 7.7, 7.8, and 7.9), the figures in the lower left, representing rural migrants to large cities, are higher than those in the lower or upper right, referring to men who remained in or moved to rural areas, and lower than those in the upper left, referring to urban men in large cities.

tioned hypothesis of Lipset and Bendix that rural migrants to cities have taken the place in today's large cities formerly occupied by immigrants.[17] Migration, then, promotes social mobility among nonmigrants as well as among migrants, even though it is not a simple case of migration causing occupational success. Men with ambition and initiative born amidst the poor opportunities of rural areas must move to cities to achieve upward mobility. Such migration tends to accomplish its goal, if only because there are many more high-status jobs in the urban occupational structure than in the rural labor market. Despite the fact that their poor qualifications force rural migrants to the bottom of the occupational hierarchy of the large city, they tend to achieve upward mobility. Simultaneously, the influx of these migrants at the bottom stimulates upward mobility of others. Hence, migration has a structural effect on social mobility in large cities, promoting that of men who never migrated as well as that of the migrants themselves.[18] This effect of migration as a catalyst of social mobility is only indirectly related to its function as a selective mechanism through which occupational demand and population supply in large complex societies are adjusted.

Have there been any changes in the dynamic interplay between migration and social mobility in recent decades? Age cohort comparisons permit some inferences that help answer this question. In general the occupational advantages migrants enjoy over nonmigrants are greater for younger than for older men. Concern here is with age trends in the significance of migration as such, as trends in the occupational structure have been discussed in Chapter 3. For this purpose, nonmigrants are compared with migrants in the same type of community. Table 7.11 presents the differences in occupational status, education, and first job between same-environment migrants and nonmigrants.[19]

The occupational superiority of migrants within community type over nonmigrants is greater for younger than for older men, notably in urban areas, and less consistently in rural ones. These differences might indicate that the economic advantages enjoyed by migrants, who are, as we know, a selected group with high occupational qualifications, are manifest primarily early in their careers and become reduced with increased age and experience. However, the differences

---

[17] Lipset and Bendix, loc. cit.

[18] This is, of course, not the only source of occupational mobility in large cities, which far exceeds the amount that can be reasonably attributed to the influx of rural migrants. On the concept of structural effects, see Peter M. Blau, "Structural Effects," American Sociological Review, 25(1960), 178-193.

[19] These data are restricted to men with nonfarm background.

TABLE 7.11. DIFFERENCES BETWEEN MIGRANTS WITHIN COMMUNITY TYPE AND NONMIGRANTS IN 1962 OCC. STATUS, EDUCATION, AND FIRST JOB, BY AGE, FOR MEN WITH NONFARM BACKGROUND

Characteristic and 1962 Residence	Age (years)			
	25 to 34	35 to 44	45 to 54	55 to 64
1962 occ.				
Large cities	9.0	6.3	5.2	2.8
Small cities	15.1	9.9	6.7	4.1
Rural nonfarm areas	8.5	-2.0	3.9	6.1
Education				
Large cities	.64	.51	.51	.45
Small cities	.90	.86	.54	.31
Rural nonfarm areas	.43	-.12	.16	-.15
First job				
Large cities	7.6	5.3	1.4	5.0
Small cities	14.5	4.9	7.8	3.7
Rural nonfarm areas	1.0	-.1	1.0	-1.6

between urban migrants and nonmigrants in educational attainment and in status of first job also are greater for younger than for older men, and these variations among age cohorts cannot be due to the impact of having grown older, since the educational attainments and career beginnings of the older as well as the younger cohorts refer, of course, to the time when they were younger.

These data suggest, therefore, that migration has become increasingly selective of high potential achievers in recent decades. Urban migrants who started their careers 30 or 40 years ago were better educated and could enter the labor market on a higher level than nonmigrants, but migrants who started their careers in the past decade are still more superior to nonmigrants in these respects. In addition, rural migrants, who were not consistently superior to nonmigrants in the past, are clearly superior among the youngest men. Inasmuch as migration has become increasingly selective of men well prepared for occupational success in recent times, the finding that young migrants exceed the rest of their contemporaries in occupational status more than old migrants exceed theirs probably reflects largely this secular trend in selective migration rather than the waning significance of the migration differential with age. In brief, the probable inference is that migration today is a more effective screening test for potentially high achievers in occupational life than it was some decades ago.

CONCLUSIONS: MIGRATION AND UNIVERSALISM

The basic finding of this chapter is that the careers of migrants are, in almost all comparisons, clearly superior to those of nonmigrants, and the rest of the analysis has been designed to refine and explain this finding. Whether migration between regions or between communities is examined; whether migration since birth or only after adolescence is considered; whether migrants are compared to nonmigrants within ethnic-nativity groupings or without employing these controls; whether education and first job are held constant; and whether migrants are compared to natives in their place of origin or their place of destination—migrants tend to attain higher occupational levels and to experience more upward mobility than nonmigrants, with only a few exceptions.

Men who migrated after age 16 from the community in which they grew up typically achieve higher occupational status than nonmigrants in the community to which they have moved as well as higher status than nonmigrants in the communities they left. Migrants from urban places, though not those from rural areas, enjoy higher status than the natives in the community to which they have come, regardless of its size. When nonmigrants are compared to migrants who have moved between two communities of the same type, the occupational status of migrants is superior in all cases except on farms.

If we turn the first row of Table 7.5 by 90 degrees and place it as a column next to the other four, we can compare the entries for nonmigrants in this new column horizontally with those for migrants in the other four columns, yielding comparisons by place of origin. In 11 of 13 comparisons, the occupational status of migrants, regardless of the type of community to which they have moved, is superior to that of the nonmigrants they have left behind. The two exceptions are the two groups of rural migrants working on farms, whose inferior mean status may be due to the inclusion of transitory farm laborers in these groups.

Occupational opportunities improve as the size of place increases. The achievements of nonmigrants in the various community types parallel the differences in opportunity structure, but the achievements of migrants do not. To be sure, migrants do better in urban areas than in rural areas, but they do less well in large cities than in small ones. Indeed, migrants from a larger to a smaller place tend to be more successful than those migrating in the opposite direction, with the single exception of migrants to farms. The success of urban migrants to large cities is greater than that of the natives there, notwithstanding the fact that the achievements of natives are nowhere better than in large cities, whereas those of migrants are better in small cities.

These findings can largely be explained in terms of selective migration and the conditions associated with the degree of urbanization—differential fertility, variations in opportunities, and differences in preparation. The better opportunities in more urban places, reinforced by population pressures created by differential fertility, attract men from less to more urbanized environments. The initiative required for migration tends to be more characteristic of men with higher potential for success—with superior social origin, education, and work experience—rendering migration a selective process that moves men most likely to succeed anywhere to the places in which the greatest opportunities for success are available to anyone. However, the inferior training youngsters receive in rural areas compared to that of urban youngsters, particularly in large cities, handicaps rural migrants to large cities relative to the natives there. Inasmuch as migration is selective of men with high potential, the achievements of migrants are superior not only to those of the men they left behind but also to those of the men they have joined in their new community, except when background differences are extreme, as in the case of rural migrants to large cities.

Since the general superiority of economic opportunities in more urban places supplies incentive for migration to them, the prevailing stream of migrants moves, in response to these opportunity differentials, from less to more urban places. Particularly good occupational prospects are probably required to induce a man to migrate against this stream to a place less urban than where he was raised. The assumption is that men are likely to migrate to communities in which opportunities are generally worse than elsewhere only if their personal prospects there are quite good, which adds another source of selection. In sum, the interpretation suggested is that migrants from larger to smaller communities achieve higher occupational status than their replacements moving in the opposite direction because the former are a more highly selected group, screened not only in terms of superior qualifications, as migrants generally are, but also on the basis of superior prospects. Another reason for this finding is the greater importance of origin than destination community for chances of career success.

Urbanization has paradoxical consequences for the migration-mobility complex. The better opportunities in cities attract the main stream of migration and improve the opportunities of most migrants, as migration tends to flow in the direction of greater opportunities. But this very process has an adverse effect on the preparation of the majority of migrants, who come from relatively less urban areas in which they received poor training for successful work in highly urbanized labor markets. In short, the fact that migration tends to flow from less to more urbanized places means that migrants have better opportunities but worse qualifications for occupational success than would otherwise be the case. These two opposite influences exert their full force on occupational chances in the polar case of rural migrants to large cities, and they consequently become manifest in the occupational achievements of these migrants, though other factors, such as selective migration, complicate the pattern in the case of other migrants.

The average occupational achievements of rural migrants to large cities are superior to those of rural men who have remained in rural areas, reflecting the better urban opportunities, but inferior to those of urban men in these cities, reflecting the poorer occupational preparation of men raised in rural areas. The influx of rural migrants into the lower ranks of the occupational hierarchy in the large city creates additional opportunities for upward mobility for other city dwellers. The advantage the natives in large cities gain from the upward push produced by the flow of rural migrants into lower occupational positions makes their chances of high achievement better than those of natives in smaller places, though not as good as those of urban migrants to large cities, whom selective migration gives a further competitive advantage. Thus rural migration to large cities promotes social mobility both directly and indirectly, as it increases the chances of occupational success not only of the men involved in this migration but also of the other men in large cities.

Migration can be considered a social mechanism for the distribution of qualified human resources in accordance with the need for occupational services, though it surely is not fully adequate for this purpose. As a mechanism of selection and redistribution of manpower, migration furthers occupational mobility. Indeed, it is essential for occupational mobility on a wide scale in a highly diversified society, because it alone can alter the opportunity structure in which a given man competes. The principle of selective migration is by no means incompatible with the proposition that migration promotes social mobility both directly and indirectly.

It appears that migration has in recent decades become increasingly effective as a selective mechanism by which the more able are channeled to places where their potential can be realized. The only basis for this conclusion in a cross-sectional study such as this is a comparison of differences between migrants and nonmigrants among age cohorts. The superiority of migrants within the same community type over nonmigrants in education and in status of first job as well as in occupational achievement is greater for younger than for older men, which implies that migration has become increasingly selective of men well qualified for occupational success.

The community in which a man is raised, just as the race or ethnic group into which he is born, defines an ascriptive base that limits his adult occupational chances. Migration, however, partly removes these ascribed restrictions on achievement by enabling a man to take advantage of opportunities not available in his original community. To be sure, the ascriptive status of place of birth continues to limit occupational achievement, because not all men migrate, and because it affects the occupational qualifications of those who do. Nevertheless, selective migration strengthens the operation of universalistic criteria of achievement, and the trend toward increasing selectivity in migration manifests an extension of universalism in our occupational structure.

CHAPTER 8

Farm Background and Occupational Achievement

The OCG study describes occupational mobility during a period near the end of a long-term transition to a completely industrialized society. Accompanying the transformation of technology and economic organization involved in this transition there has been, during its final phase, an absolute as well as a relative reduction in the number of persons living on farms, gaining a livelihood in agriculture, and pursuing farm occupations. It is commonly supposed that there are two main reasons for this reduction. First, the demand for agricultural products is relatively inelastic with respect to income. Hence as nonfarm incomes have risen there has not been a proportional rise in agricultural output or in the employment required to produce this output. Second, with mechanization of agriculture, increased capital inputs (use of fertilizer and the like), and improvements in varieties of crops and in techniques of cultivation, the labor productivity of agricultural workers has been greatly enhanced. A reduced number of workers, therefore, can produce the same or a larger volume of products.

Both of these factors operated to reduce the demand for farm employment and thus to engender movement off farms. Another factor augmented this movement—the high levels of natality of farm families, compared to nonfarm families.

This chapter supplements Chapter 7, "Geographical and Social Mobility," by considering in some detail a specific type of migration stream—that off the farm—and the bearing of farm origin on subsequent occupational achievement. We shall examine first the over-all magnitude of this movement and its selectivity. We next report on the uneven distribution in the nonfarm occupational structure of men with farm origins. An analysis of differential achievement of men with farm and nonfarm backgrounds, with a consideration of the sources of this differential, concludes the discussion.

MIGRATION FROM FARMS

The substantial magnitude of this movement is reflected in the OCG data by the contrast between the number of men originating on farms (as indexed by father's occupation) and the number engaged in farm

TABLE 8.1. PER CENT OF MALES WITH FARM BACKGROUND (AS INDICATED BY FATHER'S OCC.) LIVING IN NONFARM RESIDENCES IN MARCH, 1962, BY SELECTED CHARACTERISTICS

Subject	Total (Thousands) with Farm Background	Number (Thousands) with Nonfarm Residence, 1962	Per Cent Leaving Farm
ALL MEN, 20 TO 64 YEARS OLD	12,104	9,290	76.8
AGE (YEARS)			
20 to 24	726	436	60.1
25 to 34	2,176	1,722	79.1
35 to 44	3,130	2,465	78.8
45 to 54	3,225	2,490	77.2
55 to 64	2,847	2,177	76.5
NATIVITY AND COLOR			
Native white, native parentage	8,476	6,357	75.0
Native white, foreign or mixed parentage	1,287	932	72.4
Foreign-born white	565	537	95.0
Nonwhite	1,776	1,465	82.5
REGION OF BIRTH (FOR SPECIFIED GROUPS)			
Native white, native parentage			
Total[a]	8,650	6,481	74.9
Born in North or West[a]	4,664	3,373	72.3
Born in South	3,986	3,108	78.0
Nonwhite			
Total	1,776	1,465	82.5
Born in North or West	167	157	94.0
Born in South	1,609	1,308	81.3
NUMBER OF SIBLINGS AND BIRTH ORDER			
No siblings	356	276	77.5
Oldest child			
1 to 3 younger siblings	1,170	825	70.5
4 or more[b] younger siblings	975	718	73.6
Youngest child			
1 to 3 older siblings	1,043	777	74.5
4 or more[b] older siblings	1,027	790	76.9
Middle child			
2 or 3 siblings			
No older brother	466	391	83.9
At least 1 older brother	627	493	78.6
4 or more[b] siblings			
No older brother	914	726	79.4
At least 1 older brother	4,764	3,712	77.9
10 siblings, or number or order not stated[c]	764	583	76.3

work or living on farms in 1962. Over one-fourth of the men in the OCG population—12 million out of 45 million—had fathers who were farmers, farm managers, farm laborers, or farm foremen (at respondent's age of 16). Three-quarters of these—9.3 million men— had taken up nonfarm residence by 1962. As an estimate of the amount of movement off the farm this particular figure is only approximate, for the basis of classifying origin is occupational whereas the classification of 1962 status is residential. Nevertheless, variation in this quasi-rate of off-farm movement among population subgroups should be indicative of any pronounced pattern of selectivity in this movement.

Table 8.1 shows per cent leaving the farm by selected background characteristics. We shall interpret the differences among subgroups as

Subject	Total (Thousands) with Farm Background	Number (Thousands) with Nonfarm Residence, 1962	Per Cent Leaving Farm
FATHER'S EDUCATION			
Not reported	1,424	1,136	79.8
No school	1,077	846	78.6
Elementary			
1 to 4 years	1,900	1,454	76.5
5 to 7 years	2,675	2,064	77.2
8 years	3,226	2,367	73.4
High School			
1 to 3 years	802	608	75.8
4 years	657	531	80.8
College, 1 or more years	344	285	82.8
RESPONDENT'S EDUCATION			
No school	275	207	75.3
Elementary			
1 to 4 years	1,077	772	71.7
5 to 7 years	1,955	1,510	77.2
8 years	2,654	1,938	73.0
High school			
1 to 3 years	2,114	1,693	80.1
4 years	2,738	2,063	75.3
College			
1 to 3 years	721	587	81.4
4 years	367	324	88.3
5 or more years	204	198	97.1
RESPONDENT'S EDUCATION (FOR SPECIFIED GROUPS)			
Native white, native parentage			
Elementary, 0 to 8 years	3,653	2,616	71.6
High school, 1 to 3 years	1,537	1,210	78.7
4 years	2,212	1,617	73.1
College, 1 or more years	1,074	914	85.1
Nonwhite			
Elementary, 0 to 8 years	1,208	973	80.5
High school, 1 to 3 years	322	278	86.3
4 years	175	151	86.3
College, 1 or more years	71	63	88.7

[a] Includes native white of native parentage with state of birth not reported.
[b] Except 10.
[c] The majority are men with 10 siblings.

differential out-migration rates, recognizing that neither the definition of out-migration nor its time reference is as specific as would be desirable.

Disregarding the men 20 to 24 years old, there is some rise in the proportion leaving farms, from 76.5 per cent of men now 55 to 64 to 79.1 per cent of men aged 25 to 34. As for the men aged 20 to 24, some caution is indicated in interpreting the figure of 60.1 per cent. Some of these men may, of course, leave the farm later on. It should be borne in mind, moreover, that the OCG data do not cover an appreciable number of men of this age who may, for all intents and purposes, be on their way to nonfarm residences—members of the Armed Forces. To make a rough estimate, it was assumed that all Armed Forces personnel not covered by OCG (see Appendix C) are or will become nonfarm residents and that the proportion of them with farm background is the same as among men of the same age covered in OCG. This leads to an estimate of 65 per cent off-farm movement for men 20 to 24 and 80 per cent for men 25 to 34 years old; estimates for the remaining age groups hardly differ from those shown in Table 8.1. We must suspend judgment on the question of whether the reversal at age 20 to 24 portends an alteration of the long-run rate of movement from farms. It is evident, however, that during the greater part of the period covered by OCG experience there was no sustained interruption of the heavy outflow.

Nonwhite men have left farms at a somewhat higher rate than native white men (Table 8.1). Among the latter, the data suggest, off-farm movement has been a little higher for men with native parents than for men with one or both parents foreign-born. By definition, foreign-born white men must have moved from their birthplace to be in this country; the very high rate, 95 per cent, of movement off farms for this group indicates that rural background in the country of birth does not induce the immigrant to take up farm residence in this country. Among native whites, off-farm movement has been more pronounced for those born in the South than for those originating in other regions. The opposite differential appears for nonwhites, but the number of nonwhites born in the North and West and having farm fathers is so small as to make the comparison questionable. (In the West, disproportionate numbers of nonwhites originating on farms may be Orientals or American Indians.)

Discussions of rural-urban migration sometimes refer to the push from the land occasioned by the large size of farm families, which cannot transmit farm holdings to all sons. Vestiges of primogeniture might make this factor somewhat more salient for the later than for the earlier-born sons. The data support some implications of these ideas, though only partially. The oldest among a group of siblings was least likely to leave the farm, and the middle child in a sibship was most likely to leave ("middle" here merely means there is at least one older and one younger sibling). But among middle children from either small or large families, men with no older brother—respondents who were in fact the first-born *sons*—were *more* likely to leave than those with one or more older brothers, contrary to the implications of primogeniture. Curiously, too, the only child was no more likely to stay on the farm than the average man in all other sibling positions. Altogether, the variation by birth order and sibling position is perhaps neither as great as nor assumes the pattern one might expect.

The data on education in Table 8.1 show that respondents whose fathers were high-school graduates moved off the farm at a somewhat higher rate than those with less well educated fathers. Acquisition of college training on the part of the respondent led to higher than average off-farm movement—as well it might, because college attendance itself would probably have initiated such a move. Below the college level, at least for native white men of native parentage, the relationship of the rate of off-farm movement to educational attainment fluctuates erratically. Why the high-school graduate should be less likely to leave the farm than the high-school dropout is not readily apparent. The grammar-school graduate, similarly, is less likely to leave the farm than youngsters with five to seven years of schooling. Migrants off the farm may be a bimodal group, consisting of the unsuccessful school dropouts, on the one hand, and the college men, on the other.

DISTRIBUTION OF MEN WITH FARM BACKGROUND

We now examine the movement off farms in terms of differentials at the point of destination. The proportion of men with farm background in any subgroup of the population living in nonfarm residences is interpreted as a crude rate of in-migration from farms for that subgroup.

It should be observed, first, that the criterion for identifying men with farm background will produce somewhat different results from those obtained on another criterion, such as place of birth or residence history. In the OCG data just over one-fourth (26.9 per cent) of male respondents 20 to 64 years old in March 1962 are classified in the farm-background category. Data on the entire civilian population 18 years old and over in May 1958 indicate that 23.7 per cent were farm-born.[1]

---

[1] Calvin L. Beale, John C. Hudson, and Vera J. Banks, "Characteristics of the U. S. Population by Farm and Nonfarm Origin," *Agricultural Economic Report*, No. 66 (Washington: Economic Research Service, Department of Agriculture, December, 1964). This report includes a useful bibliography.

A 1952 study by the Survey Research Center classified one-third of the adult *nonfarm* population as farm-reared, with positive answers to the question, "Were you brought up mostly on a farm?"[2] For comparison the proportion of farm-born among nonfarm residents in the 1958 data is 17.2 per cent. (An additional 3.4 per cent are shown with some history of farm residence.) The discrepancies doubtlessly reflect actual changes but also variation due to differences in the criteria of farm origin.

In computing in-migration rates it is important to maintain a stratification by size of the destination community. We know that the bulk of migration occurs over short distances. Because small places are more numerous than large, a short-distance move off the farm is more likely to take the migrant to a small than to a large place. This deduction is borne out by one-year off-farm migration rates for the total U. S. population, 1949 to 1950. There is a perfect inverse association with size of place. The number of in-migrants from farms per 1,000 of the resident population varies from 2.5 for urbanized areas of three million or more to 33.1 for rural incorporated places of less than 1,000 inhabitants.[3]

The rates just cited are not directly comparable with OCG rates, since the latter are not time-specific. Nevertheless, the same inverse pattern obtains. In urbanized areas of one million or more 13 per cent of the OCG men have farm background, that is, have moved from farms at some time in the past; in the smallest urban places the rate is 28 per cent; and in the rural nonfarm population it is as high as 36 per cent (Table 8.2, first row).

Specific in-migration rates, within size-of-place categories, are shown for several characteristics in Table 8.2. With this much detail in cross-classifications the figures are subject to rather high sampling error. Accordingly, it seems conservative to emphasize general patterns of differentials rather than specific paired comparisons of rates.

Within subcategories of most characteristics the general inverse relationship of in-migration rates to size of community holds. Perhaps the most interesting departure from this pattern occurs for the non-white population. Nonwhite in-migration rates are measurably higher in urbanized areas of one million or more than in smaller urbanized areas. In the largest urbanized areas of the South no less than two-fifths of the nonwhite men have farm background. This is markedly

[2] Ronald Freedman and Deborah Freedman, "Farm-Reared Elements in the Nonfarm Population," *Rural Sociology*, 21(1956), pp. 50-61.

[3] Otis Dudley Duncan and Albert J. Reiss, Jr., *Social Characteristics of Urban and Rural Communities, 1950*, New York: Wiley, 1956, Table 23 (p. 85).

TABLE 8.2. PER CENT WITH FARM BACKGROUND, BY SELECTED SOCIAL AND ECONOMIC CHARACTERISTICS, BY SIZE OF PLACE OF RESIDENCE.

| | | Residence in March 1962 | | | | | |
| | | Urbanized Areas | | | | Rural | |
Subject	All Places	1,000,000 or More	250,000 to 1,000,000	50,000 to 250,000	Other Urban	Nonfarm	Farm
TOTAL MALES, 20 TO 64 YEARS OLD	26.9	12.8	18.1	19.8	28.3	35.9	77.8
COLOR AND REGION							
White							
Northeast	11.1	6.3	6.0	7.6	12.9	19.5	62.2
North Central	30.9	14.1	14.8	24.0	27.2	38.5	82.1
South	36.4	11.6	21.9	26.8	32.2	42.6	76.8
West	22.4	13.0	17.7	14.7	31.9	30.2	70.5
Nonwhite							
North and West	28.9	27.1	25.7	17.6	37.7	49.1	100.0[b]
South	49.6	39.6	34.5	32.0	40.7	58.1	80.2
NATIVITY AND COLOR							
Native White, Native Parentage							
Born in North or West	23.0	8.3	12.6	17.2	23.5	29.7	77.8
Born in South	40.1	25.8	27.5	30.4	36.2	44.3	77.0
Native White, Foreign or Mixed Parentage							
Parent(s) Born in Northern or Western Europe	21.5	6.4	12.9	10.7	25.8	34.4	81.0
Parent(s) Born Elsewhere	10.0	3.9	8.2	4.8	15.6	23.4	74.5
Foreign-Born White	22.5	20.5	17.5	20.9	28.2	29.5	61.4[a]
Nonwhite							
Born in North or West	22.1	6.8	13.6	11.1	33.7	62.0	100.0[b]
Born in South	42.0	33.6	33.9	29.2	40.9	54.6	80.5
NUMBER OF SIBLINGS							
None	12.2	6.2	7.1	7.1	12.8	18.8	68.4
1 to 3	17.7	7.0	11.1	13.2	20.1	24.7	74.3
4 or More	36.0	19.4	26.1	27.7	36.5	44.7	79.8
INCOME IN 1961							
Under $1,000	39.1	16.8	12.3	17.4	28.3	47.2	81.0
$1,000 to 1,999	36.5	18.9	11.4	20.8	29.6	39.3	84.0
2,000 to 2,999	37.0	14.3	20.9	27.3	30.7	47.8	76.0
3,000 to 3,999	31.1	21.3	12.3	27.3	26.0	40.3	77.7
4,000 to 4,999	27.5	16.9	16.9	22.8	30.9	36.6	76.2
5,000 to 5,999	24.5	13.9	22.2	20.9	35.2	32.2	54.3
6,000 to 6,999	19.9	9.2	20.7	16.2	24.6	30.3	76.1
7,000 to 9,999	18.4	8.3	15.2	17.9	29.9	25.6	69.5
10,000 and Over	11.7	6.3	14.2	5.2	17.2	17.2	64.9
OCCUPATIONAL SOCIOECONOMIC INDEX							
0 to 19	41.0	20.7	26.7	27.8	34.3	46.8	81.6
20 to 39	24.5	13.7	17.4	21.1	32.2	34.7	64.8
40 to 59	19.8	8.6	17.9	17.0	28.3	31.4	60.8
60 to 79	12.9	6.3	10.3	11.3	19.5	19.4	62.7
80 and Over	10.2	3.4	12.2	9.7	15.7	16.5	45.2[a]
Not in Experienced Civilian Labor Force	26.0	15.8	18.2	19.3	23.4	32.9	73.9
EDUCATION BY NATIVITY AND COLOR							
Native White, Native Parentage							
Elementary, 0 to 8 Years	50.2	27.8	32.8	45.0	43.5	52.7	82.4
High School, 1 to 3 Years	28.3	11.5	20.2	19.3	28.4	35.5	70.5
High School, 4 Years or More	20.0	7.5	13.9	16.4	22.5	23.5	74.9
Native White, Foreign or Mixed Parentage							
Elementary, 0 to 8 Years	30.8	11.4	23.3	15.2	31.8	46.6	82.8
High School, 1 to 3 Years	12.6	3.8	8.9	9.2	15.7	29.0	70.3
High School, 4 Years or More	7.6	2.3	5.8	4.2	14.6	18.0	66.3
Foreign-Born White							
Elementary, 0 to 8 Years	36.5	34.8	23.6	33.9	43.3	46.5	67.7[a]
High School, 1 to 3 Years	12.7	11.8	13.3[a]	9.4[a]	4.2[a]	13.8[a]	100.0[b]
High School, 4 Years or More	12.1	10.5	14.7	11.5	15.0	15.6	12.5[b]
Nonwhite							
Elementary, 0 to 8 Years	53.8	49.3	42.9	37.1	51.8	61.4	79.4
High School, 1 to 3 Years	31.3	20.6	13.4	26.9	46.3	58.3	84.6
High School, 4 years or More	19.0	13.0	17.2	7.0	12.5	42.3	88.9[a]

| Subject | All Places | Residence in March 1962 | | | | | |
| | | Urbanized Areas | | | | Rural | |
		1,000,000 or more	250,000 to 1,000,000	50,000 to 250,000	Other Urban	Nonfarm	Farm
EDUCATION BY AGE							
Total, 20 to 64	26.9	12.7	18.1	19.8	28.3	35.9	77.8
Elementary, 0 to 4 Years	54.9	42.8	41.8	39.6	48.1	60.5	80.0
Elementary, 5 to 7 Years	45.3	31.0	30.4	37.1	45.4	50.7	80.1
Elementary, 8 Years	43.3	24.2	30.5	38.1	39.5	50.9	83.8
High School, 1 to 3 Years	24.9	11.0	16.8	17.8	28.6	35.6	71.8
High School, 4 Years	21.4	8.1	14.6	18.0	23.9	26.9	77.1
College, 1 to 3 Years	13.6	6.1	13.1	10.1	15.1	20.3	65.0
College, 4 or More Years	10.3	4.2	8.1	7.4	18.2	16.0	66.7
20 to 24	14.4	2.9	5.5	10.4	11.7	19.8	71.1
Elementary, 0 to 8 Years	28.6	13.3	13.0[a]	27.6	13.7	27.6	70.4
High School, 1 to 3 Years	17.0	4.2	9.1	10.7	18.3	22.2	64.9
High School, 4 Years or More	11.3	1.6	4.1	6.9	9.8	16.5	73.4
25 to 34	20.5	11.0	14.7	14.2	20.9	25.2	73.3
Elementary, 0 to 8 Years	38.8	31.9	28.1	23.4	31.6	39.4	74.4
High School, 1 to 3 Years	22.3	10.7	17.4	12.7	28.5	28.3	72.8
High School, 4 Years or More	15.2	6.9	11.6	13.3	16.1	19.4	72.4
35 to 44	27.0	12.1	20.4	18.5	29.1	36.9	76.5
Elementary, 0 to 8 Years	47.2	30.0	36.3	38.5	43.4	78.3	78.3
High School, 1 to 3 Years	26.0	14.2	20.8	22.6	24.3	34.9	66.3
High School, 4 Years or More	18.4	6.5	13.6	11.9	23.4	26.1	79.3
45 to 54	31.7	14.9	22.3	23.8	35.0	43.2	81.4
Elementary, 0 to 8 Years	49.2	30.3	39.1	43.7	42.8	55.6	86.2
High School, 1 to 3 Years	26.2	10.0	12.3	15.3	38.5	40.9	74.3
High School, 4 Years or More	20.0	7.6	17.4	16.0	28.6	27.0	74.3
55 to 64	37.6	19.1	23.0	31.1	42.8	52.3	81.9
Elementary, 0 to 8 Years	48.7	28.3	27.8	40.0	53.7	60.1	84.9
High School, 1 to 3 Years	30.7	11.6	23.6	25.9	29.4	54.1	81.7
High School, 4 Years or More	22.1	10.8	17.0	23.0	30.2	33.2	62.1

[a]Base population 20,000 or less.
[b]Base population 21,000 to 50,000.

higher than the fraction, just over one-fourth, of nonwhites with farm background in the largest cities of the North and West.

For the white population as well, the rate of in-migration to urban communities from farms is higher in the South than in the other regions, among which the Northeast has notably low rates. Roughly speaking, the Northeast appears to be a generation ahead of the South in regard to the assimilation of farm migrants into urbanized areas.

When men are classified by size of family of orientation, in-migration rates for communities of all sizes are markedly higher for men from large families. This finding may have implications for studies of urban kinship behavior. Among persons in urban areas with large numbers of siblings, disproportionate numbers have farm antecedents. In view of the high rate of off-farm migration and the minor degree of selectivity by birth order and number of siblings we can presume that the majority of the siblings will likewise be found in nonfarm residences. These data do not indicate, however, whether siblings tend to move from the family farm to the same urban areas, although this probably does happen in many cases. If we foresee a time when in-migrants from farms are a negligible fraction of the urban population we may anticipate a weakening of the importance of consanguine ties on the sheer basis of reduction in number of siblings.

Socioeconomic variables—income, occupational status, and education—are covered in considerable detail in Table 8.2. As one might expect, migrants from farms are underrepresented among men with comparatively high incomes. However, the highest in-migration rates to urban areas do not necessarily occur at the very lowest income levels. There is no greater concentration of men with farm background at the poverty level than at the level of modest means. This observation may provide some support for those who have argued that the problem of urban poverty is as much a problem of poor economic performance of the indigenous urban population as it is a problem of the assimilation of impoverished rural migrants.

The inverse relationship of in-migration rate to socioeconomic status is much clearer when measured in occupational terms. Men with farm background are markedly underrepresented in occupations at the high end of the status scale and overrepresented at the low end. Later in this chapter we consider the sources of this differential.

A similarly clear pattern obtains in the case of education. In-migration rates are high for the poorly educated and low for the well educated, both in the aggregate and for age and color-nativity subgroups. The influx of migrants from farms clearly retards the rate of educational upgrading in the urban population. This source of retardation, however, is rapidly diminishing in importance, as the in-migration rates are much lower for the younger cohorts than for their predecessors.

In this section the process of urbanization has been viewed in terms of the impact of off-farm migration on the urban communities of destination. From one point of view we can see that our cities have been confronted with a continuing problem of assimilating newcomers with educational and racial handicaps, although the impact of this movement on poverty as measured in strictly monetary terms may not have been quite so great as might be expected. On the other hand, this movement may be seen as contributing disproportionately to the supply of untrained and less-skilled labor. In the competition for higher status jobs the indigenous nonfarm population has had an advantage relative to the off-farm migrants.

Both the problem and the relative advantage are due to assume a lessening quantitative importance in the years ahead. Already we can

see that in-migration rates to urban areas were only half as large for
the 1927 to 1936 cohorts as for the 1897 to 1906 cohorts. Further reduction will be the consequence of diminution in the proportion of the
American population born and reared on farms. The patterns of social
mobility that will emerge as an adjustment to this major alteration
of a set of historic forces can only be dimly perceived at this time. It
seems likely that in the foreseeable future other factors than farm
background will assume the role of prime generator of migration and
mobility.

FARM BACKGROUND AND THE PROCESS OF STRATIFICATION

Having documented the fact that large numbers of men with farm
background have found their way into nonfarm pursuits and that
they appear to suffer some handicap when placed in competition with
men with nonfarm background, we now re-examine the model of the
process of stratification presented in Chapter 5. The first question at
issue is that of the relative occupational achievement of men with farm
and nonfarm background. Is farm background a handicap to an
extent greater than we would infer from just the socioeconomic level
of origin of the men with farm background? Second, if the stream
of migrants from farms is necessarily destined to continue its shrinkage
in size, then nearly all men in future cohorts will be of nonfarm origin.
Do the OCG data shed any light on what the process of stratification
may look like in such a population? Finally, as a methodological point,
we are not wholly confident of the status score as an index of the socioeconomic position of farm occupations. We know that the prestige
ratings given farming by the general public run higher than would be
expected from the value of the socioeconomic index for this occupation. When the index was constructed the possibility of bias in this
score was noted.[4] We cannot resolve this issue here, but we can treat
the data in such a way that the distortion from this source, if any, is
greatly reduced.

Table 8.3 provides an initial summary of the simple correlations
for the two subpopulations: the men with nonfarm background and
those whose fathers were farmers or farm laborers. The first comparison we wish to suggest is with the correlations for all men given
earlier, in Chapter 5 (Table 5.1). The three correlations among Y, W,
and U hardly differ in the total population from those observed for
men with nonfarm background. The son-father correlations—the
six involving each of the former variables and either X or V—are

---

4 Albert J. Reiss, Jr., *et al.*, *Occupations and Social Status*, New York: Free Press
of Glencoe, 1961, Chapters 6 and 7.

TABLE 8.3.   SIMPLE CORRELATIONS FOR FIVE STATUS VARIABLES, BY FARM BACK-
GROUND.   ABOVE DIAGONAL: FOR NONFARM BACKGROUND; BELOW DIAGONAL: FOR
FARM BACKGROUND

Variable	Variable				
	Y	W	U	X	V
Y: Respondent's occ. status, 1962	...	.532	.595	.368	.296
W: First job status	.417	...	.536	.375	.316
U: Respondent's education	.476	.402	...	.413	.422
X: Father's occ. status	...[a]	...	...	...	.520
V: Father's education	.212	.174	.396	...	...

[a]Correlations involving X not computed for men with farm background.

somewhat lowered when men with farm background are excluded.
Even so, the greatest difference is about .04. We surmise that in studying a population wholly nonfarm in origin we should expect X, in
particular, to have a somewhat slighter influence than in the previous
results for all men. Yet the over-all pattern of the path coefficients
should not be greatly different.

We must be careful in comparing the correlations for men with
farm background with either those in the other half of Table 8.3 or
those in Table 5.1. This subpopulation is selected in such a way that
father's occupational status is virtually a constant. Correlations involving X are meaningless in this case, and the remaining correlations
are really tantamount to *partial* correlations with X held constant.
For this reason we should fully expect them to be lower than those
for men of nonfarm background, and the data bear out this expectation.

When we turn to the multiple relations, therefore, we should compare equations for men with nonfarm background containing X as
an independent variable with equations for men with farm background containing the same variables other than X. Such comparisons
in Table 8.4 suggest that (1) father's education has a greater net
influence on respondent's education in the farm-background population; (2) respondent's education has less influence on first-job status
in this population than among men with nonfarm origins—father's
education having a negligible direct effect in both populations; and
(3) both education and first job have slightly lesser net effects on 1962
occupational status in the farm-background population than in the
other population.

Although the net regression coefficients in Table 8.4 can be thus
compared, the coefficients of determination are not comparable. In
the upper panel (nonfarm background) R^2 is the squared multiple
correlation coefficient. In the lower panel (farm background) R^2 is

TABLE 8.4.   PARTIAL REGRESSION COEFFICIENTS IN STANDARD FORM (BETA COEFFICIENTS) AND COEFFICIENTS OF DETERMINATION FOR SPECIFIED COMBINATIONS OF VARIABLES, BY FARM BACKGROUND

Background and Dependent Variable[a]	Independent Variables[a]				Coefficient of Determination (R^2)
	W	U	X	V	
Nonfarm background					
U	...	...	.265	.285	.23
W	...	.450	.170	.037	.32
W	...	.460	.186	...	.32
Y	.279	.411	.103	-.019	.43
Y	.278	.407	.095	...	.43
Y	.298	.435	...	...	.42
Farm background					
U	...	...	...	.396	.16
W	...	.395	...	.018	.16
Y	.269	.358	...	.024	.29
Y	.269	.368	...	...	.29

[a]V: Father's education.
  X: Father's occ. status.
  U: Respondent's education.
  W: First job status.
  Y: 1962 occ. status.

tantamount to a squared multiple-partial coefficient, since X is virtually held constant in its calculation. We may, however, calculate multiple-partial coefficients for the nonfarm-background population for comparative purposes. We find $r^2_{UV.X} = .07$ for nonfarm-background men, as compared with $r^2_{UV} = .16$ for farm background; $R^2_{W(UV).X} = .21$ among the former and $R^2_{W(UV)} = .16$ among the latter; and $R^2_{Y(WU).X} = .33$ for men with nonfarm background, whereas $R^2_{Y(WU)} = .29$ for men with farm background.

The interpretation of these and the foregoing differences is not wholly obvious, but we have some suggestions that go only a little beyond the data. Controlling X (father's occupation) in the nonfarm-origin population is formally somewhat like looking at a population in which X is controlled by selecting a group in which occupational status is nearly constant. In reality, however, although the *occupational* status of farmers may be more or less constant, their *economic* status may vary widely in relation to such well-known factors as region, type of farming, and size of farm. It is possible, therefore, that V (father's education) reflects such economic variation in the farm-background population to a greater extent than in the nonfarm-background population. Or, to put it another way, controlling X in the latter leaves less residual economic variation than in the farm-background population.

A different sort of problem is involved in interpreting the lesser response of W (first job) to U (education) in the farm-background population. We know that very substantial numbers of farm-reared youth report farm labor as their first regular employment even though most of them ultimately found nonfarm pursuits. No doubt many of them began to work on the farm at an early age, and our assumption that U precedes W (discussed in Chapter 5) may be especially vulnerable for this group.

In regard to the determinants of Y (1962 occupational status) the differences in results for the two populations are not really great enough to call for elaborate explanation. There is, nevertheless, a somewhat delicate problem of interpretation when we come to translate the results thus far summarized into a statement about differential achievement of men from the two types of background. For this purpose we must consider differences in mean scores in the two populations and convert the standardized regressions into raw-score form.

In gross terms, there is little question about the differential in achievement of the two groups. The mean of Y (occupational status in 1962) is 40.1 for men with nonfarm background, 26.2 for men with farm background. The corresponding means of W (first job) are 28.7 and 17.2. The differential in educational attainment amounts to about one rung on the educational ladder, or two years of schooling, with means of 4.73 for men with nonfarm background and 3.60 for those with farm origins. But such differences could conceivably reflect nothing more than the fact that farm origin implies that the family background was one of low socioeconomic status. How may we take this initial handicap into account in assessing subsequent achievement?

Consider first the respondent's educational attainment. Expressing our regressions in raw-score form, we have

$$\hat{U}_F = .457V + 2.50 \qquad \text{(farm background)},$$

and

$$\hat{U}_N = .254V + .0196X + 3.23 \qquad \text{(nonfarm background)}.$$

As in the standardized form, the net effect for V is somewhat greater among men with farm origins. But the intercept (constant term) is higher for men with nonfarm background. To equate the two groups for father's occupation we must assign a value to X in the second equation that is presumed to be equivalent to the occupational status of farm fathers. If we were to credit the results of occupational prestige surveys, such a value would be about 50, and we should have

$$\hat{U}_N = .254V + 4.21.$$

Despite the steeper slope in the farm-background equation, this regression line would lie higher on the graph over the entire possible range of V, 0 to 8. The difference in $\hat{U}$ by background would be greatest when $V = 0$, amounting to $4.21 - 2.50 = 1.7$ steps on the education scale. At the upper limit of V the difference would be only 0.1. At the mean of V in the general population we should find a difference of 0.8. Imputing a high status to farm occupations, therefore, leads us to estimate a quite appreciable disadvantage for farm-background men in terms of educational achievement, particularly for men whose fathers had little education.

Modifying our assumption so that farm occupations are scored on the socioeconomic scale, we find that the mean of X is 13.4 in the farm background population. Equalizing the two populations on this basis, we obtain

$$\hat{U}_N = .254V + 3.49.$$

Now we discover that the two regression lines cross at a value of V just short of 5. Interpreted literally, this implies that farm background is a disadvantage (albeit a decreasing one, with increasing values of V) up to and including levels of father's education of one to three years of high school. It actually becomes an advantage if the father was a high-school graduate or attended college. We really must not take this result too seriously. Only 9 per cent of the farm-background men are in the region of V-scores where such an advantage would apply. We place a very severe strain on our assumption of linearity by reading this result literally. A more relevant calculation is the magnitude of the difference, $\hat{U}_N - \hat{U}_F$, when V for both groups is set equal to the mean for the farm group. This works out at 0.6, just over half a step on the education scale. A final alternative calculation is one in which we force the two lines to have a common slope but allow their intercepts to differ, the common slope being the average within-group slope. The relevant comparison here is the difference in intercepts, which comes out at 0.4—similar in order of magnitude to the estimate just given, both representing about one year of schooling.

Despite some ambiguity about what may have been true for the men whose fathers were exceptionally well-educated, for the bulk of the cases it seems that farm background was an educational handicap, though a rather lesser one than would appear from a simple comparison of means in the two populations. If someone insists that the index used here underestimates the occupational status of farm fathers, he will have to agree, as a consequence, that we have also underestimated the educational handicap of farm background.

It does not seem worthwhile to display the results for first job (W) in such detail. Proceeding in the same fashion as above, we note that the observed mean difference in the two populations is 11.5 points on the occupational status scale, in favor of men with nonfarm origins. Equalizing backgrounds, and considering the estimated values, $\hat{W}$, for men with education at the mean for farm-background men, this difference is no greater than 1.5. For men who were high-school graduates it is 4.5. If we force the two regressions to have common (average) slopes the constant difference in the respective values of $\hat{W}$ is 1.1, a nearly trivial difference on this scale (which has more than ten times the range of the educational score). If men originating on farms get a poorer start on their careers it is in large measure because of their lower educational attainment and the low occupational status of their fathers.

Finally, to study differentials in occupational achievement as of 1962, we compare the two regressions:

$$\hat{Y}_F = .368W + 4.49U + 3.66$$

$$\hat{Y}_N = .319W + 5.96U + .69 \qquad \text{(with } X = 13.4).$$

Contrary to the results for standardized regressions, W (first job) has a somewhat greater net effect for men with farm origins. The former, expressed in standard deviation units, takes account of the fact that the variation in first-job status among these men—many of whom begin as farm laborers—is quite restricted. The present version shows that those men who do manage to find a first job above the typical level gain thereby a considerable advantage in terms of subsequent occupational prospects.

Given the interaction with background, the comparison of the two populations cannot be wholly unequivocal. To be realistic we should consider the prospective achievement for a combination of U and W that is not unlikely to be observed in both populations. For example, a man with farm origin who only graduated from elementary school ($U = 3$) and whose first job was farm wage worker ($W = 6$) should expect, on the basis of the foregoing equations, an occupational status score in 1962 of 19.3. With the same education and a first job with the same score as farm wage worker, the nonfarm-background worker is expected to score 20.4 on Y. To take another example, suppose the nonfarm-background man's education and first job were at the mean of U and W for farm-background men. He should then expect a current occupational status score of 27.6, as against the mean of 26.1 for farm-background men. This difference of 1.5 points may almost be considered negligible, in comparison with the difference of 14.0 (40.1 — 26.1) in the actually observed means of nonfarm- and farm-background men. Finally, if we elect to average out the apparent interactions, we find a difference in intercepts—the net difference due to background and not to education, first job, and father's occupational status score—of only 0.9.

Despite any qualifications, therefore, it is evident that the discrepancy between the two populations in current occupational status is largely a product of their difference in initial socioeconomic status and education. The residual difference is too small to make it worthwhile to postulate appreciable effects of discrimination in the job market against men with farm background or handicaps due to the problem of assimilation to the urban environment. As before, this conclusion would change if we decided that our convention for scoring socioeconomic status of farm occupations was greatly in error. But the justification for making such a change would entail some tortuous reasoning. Perhaps it is best to assume that our score is realistic, which it seems to be, as far as can be judged from the evidence of patterns of status achievement.

As a final comment, we observe that the exclusion of men with farm background would produce fairly little alteration of the path coefficients in Figure 5.1, as can be verified by comparing the upper panel of Table 8.4 with Table 5.2 (Chapter 5). It is true, in terms of sheer manpower, that the farm sector has supplied disproportionate numbers of workers to the manual levels of the nonfarm sector. Yet this movement, in one sense, has really not constituted an exception to the general pattern of stratification, except as farm origin has been slightly more of an educational handicap than origin at a comparably low socioeconomic level in the nonfarm sector.

OCCUPATIONAL DIFFERENTIALS BY SIZE OF COMMUNITY

The preceding analysis suggests that men originating on farms are indeed disadvantaged by the low socioeconomic status of their origins and by an educational handicap not wholly attributable to their level of origin as such. Their subsequent occupational achievement, on the other hand, does not seem to reflect any sizable additional handi-

cap of farm origin beyond what can be attributed to these two circumstances. In short there is no vicious circle of cumulative handicaps, as
there is for Negroes.

Besides the qualifications that must be placed on these conclusions
for reasons already stated, the analysis is gross in that it deals with
just the two undifferentiated aggregates: all men with nonfarm background and all men whose fathers were in farm occupations. Moreover, no distinction was made, except in terms of the occupational
status score, between men originating on farms who continued in farm
pursuits and those who moved into the nonfarm sector. More refined
comparisons can be made by classifying men with farm and nonfarm
background according to place of residence in 1962. In this way we
may examine the outcome of competition between the two groups
when the opportunity structures within which they compete are
roughly equated.

As was noted above, the mean difference by background in 1962
occupational status is 14.0 points on the Y scale in favor of men with
nonfarm origins. If we compute the mean difference by size of place
we find that it is likewise 14.0 points in urbanized areas of over one
million inhabitants; 8.9 in urbanized areas of 250,000 to one million;
9.9 in urbanized areas of 50,000 to 250,000; 7.3 in other urban places
(2,500 to 50,000); 10.4 in rural nonfarm areas; and 6.1 among rural
farm residents. It may seem odd that none of the differences for a
size-of-place category exceeds the difference of 14 points in the whole
population. The explanation is that men with nonfarm background
are found in disproportionate numbers in large places, where values
of Y are high, whereas men with farm background are concentrated in
small places and rural areas, where prevailing levels of Y are low. The
implicit weighting by size of place, therefore, works to the disadvantage of men with farm background in aggregate comparisons.

It appears from the foregoing data that the largest cities are the
least favorable environment for men with farm background, relative
to men with nonfarm origins. This observation must be qualified,
however, by recognizing that in this class of communities the factor of
race confounds the comparisons. In urbanized areas of one million or
larger, 31 per cent of the OCG men with farm background are nonwhite, whereas the percentage is no higher than 17 in any other size
class.

Unfortunately our tabulations are not sufficiently detailed to permit
a thorough study of the possible interaction of farm background with
size of community. The best guess on the evidence available—taking
account of the initial socioeconomic and educational handicap and

the possibly confounding factor of color—is that farm background as such is not an obstacle to occupational achievement. This conclusion does not agree with results previously obtained for a small sample of Chicago men.[5] Hence it must be left an open question whether in very large cities there are obstacles to achievement for men with farm background not attributable to low socioeconomic status of origin and lack of education. In the remainder of the country, at any rate, we conjecture that men with farm background compete on at least even terms with those having comparably poor nonfarm origins.

The issue, in any event, is rapidly becoming one of primarily historical interest. Cohorts entering the labor force in the future will include diminishing minorities of men with farm background; and the persistence into the second generation of farm migrants of any disadvantage stemming directly from their parents' farm experience seems likely to be slight, if perceptible at all.

[5] Otis Dudley Duncan and Robert W. Hodge, "Education and Occupational Mobility," *American Journal of Sociology*, **68**(1963), 629-644.

CHAPTER 9

Kinship and Careers

The family into which a man is born exerts a significant influence on his occupational life, ascribing a status to him at birth that influences his chances for achieving any other status later in his career. The socio-economic level of the family defines class origins, whose influence on subsequent educational and occupational attainment has already been discussed. To be sure, his family's station in life does not predetermine a man's status as an adult in a class society, such as ours, in which there is a considerable degree of occupational and social mobility. Indeed, it is in the very nature of a class structure that a man's status is not ascribed to him completely on the basis of the family into which he was born, as in a caste system, but rests primarily on his achievements. These achievements, however, are strongly influenced by class differences among parental families. Characteristics of the family of orientation other than its socioeconomic status also have implications for occupational life. Thus a man's career chances are affected by the size of his parental family, by his position among his siblings and relations with them, and by the educational climate in his home.

This chapter is devoted to the influences exerted by various aspects of the structure of the parental family and a man's position in it on his subsequent career. Continuing with the general theme of the nexus between ascribed and achieved status, we now turn to the study of the relationships between family and occupational life. After dealing with the significance of the family of orientation, we shall examine in the following two chapters the significance of the family of procreation, with special emphasis on homogamy and fertility. The independent variables of central concern in this chapter are number of siblings, sibling position, role relations among siblings, and climate of the parental family.

The family in which a child grows up serves as a prime source of social as well as economic support for him. Both types of support might be expected to affect his educational and occupational development. A major reason for the importance for careers of economic support is that it greatly facilitates acquiring an advanced education. Higher education is expensive, even in these days of community colleges and scholarships. Financial sacrifices are demanded from parents for tuition, room and board, clothes, or merely continued support of a grown child at home while he attends a local college.[1] Even the completion of free secondary education puts a financial strain on the family, because it means that a teenager, instead of beginning to help support his younger siblings, continues to draw on his parents' resources. This creates hardships for poor families, especially if they are large.

In addition to economic support the family of orientation provides the child with diverse forms of social support, which range from such subtle factors as furnishing thought patterns and role models and having many books available at home to such explicit ones as encouraging children to study and helping them if they have trouble. It is from his parents that a child acquires a cognitive structure and linguistic patterns, which serve as basic equipment in the competition for occupational success.[2] The achievement orientation that disposes the man to strive to better himself is acquired by the child largely in his parental family. Conditions in the family of orientation tend to determine both whether the child develops the socialized anxiety that drives him to succeed and whether he receives the socio-emotional support to cope with this anxiety without becoming debilitated by it.

The actual influence exerted by emotional support on achievement is a subject of much speculation, but there is little systematic evidence. Nevertheless it seems reasonable to assume that differences in family structure affect social as well as economic support. Thus the number of siblings of a boy and his position among them affect the amount of money parents on a given economic level can spend on his education and on assisting him in other ways in his career, although parents with the same resources vary, of course, in respect to how large a proportion of their total resources they devote to the advancement of their children. The amount of social support and attention a boy receives from his parents and the degree to which these are supple-

[1] See James Davis, *Stipends and Spouses;* Chicago: Univer. of Chicago Press, 1962, pp. 35-49.

[2] See Roger Brown, *Social Psychology,* New York: Free Press, 1965, esp. pp. 306-349.

mented by supportive siblings also depend undoubtedly on the number of his siblings, their sex, and his position among them, though it is not entirely clear in what ways. For example, it is not evident *a priori* whether the greater amount of time and attention parents of one or two children can devote to them outweighs in significance for social support the integrative bonds in a peer group of siblings that the child in a larger family enjoys. Indeed we do not even know for certain whether children in small families receive more support from their parents than those in large ones, or whether children in large families receive more support from their siblings than those in small ones. Moreover, the significance of supportive family ties for occupational life is by no means self-evident. We do not know whether supportive behavior of parents furthers subsequent independent achievement by creating security or rather impedes it by creating overdependence. Although we cannot predict the specific influence of family support on occupational life we shall attempt to infer the intervening processes through which family structure affects occupational success; for example, whether economic or psychological factors are involved, and what role education plays.

Most of the analysis is based on answers to the following question, which was coded to indicate the effects of (1) number of siblings, (2) birth order, and (3) whether or not a man had an older brother:

> Number of brothers and sisters
> (Count those born alive but no longer living, as well as those alive now. Also include stepbrothers and sisters and children adopted by your parents.)
> a. How many sisters did you have? . . . . ———
>   or ☐ None
> b. How many of these sisters were older than you (born earlier)? . . . . ———
> c. How many brothers did you have? . . . . ———
>   or ☐ None
> d. How many of these brothers were older than you (born earlier)? . . . . ———

In tabulating the responses to this question, a classification error was made that affects the meaning of some categories used in the analysis. Men with exactly 10 siblings were inadvertently tabulated as "no response." Thus "4 or more siblings" refers to men with "4 or more siblings, except 10 siblings" and "no response" means "no response or 10 siblings." Actually the majority (72 per cent) in this latter category are men with 10 siblings.

The analysis of the influence of the family educational climate on occupational achievement and mobility, which follows the treatment of family size and birth order, relies on the education of the oldest brother as a rough indication of this climate.

SIZE OF PARENTAL FAMILY

Occupational achievement is clearly related to the number of siblings in the family in which a man grew up. Men from small families —those who have less than four siblings—achieve on the average considerably higher occupational status than men from large families with at least five children. The first two columns of Table 9.1 present 1962 occupational status by family size and birth order in deviations from the mean status for the total population (36.3). These columns show that a small family of orientation is associated with higher achievement, regardless of sibling position, and whether or not a child has an older brother, with the differences between men from small and men from large families ranging from 7.7 to 10.4 points. These differences do not necessarily reveal an adverse influence of large families on occupational life, however, since they may be due to the fact that people in lower socioeconomic strata tend to have more children and that their children tend to achieve lower occupational status than people in higher strata. Indeed, the mean occupational status of fathers of men from small families is considerably higher (32.9) than that of fathers of men from large ones (21.2).

Nevertheless, the great differences in occupational achievement between sons from small families and sons from large families are not primarily accounted for by the differences in socioeconomic status between small and large families. When father's occupational status is controlled, in columns 3 and 4 of Table 9.1, men from small families continue to manifest higher occupational achievement than men from large ones. The residual differences, however, are reduced to 3.6 points for youngest children and 6.0 points for oldest ones, with middle children intermediate (and those without older brothers profiting more from birth into a small family than those with one). These data indicate that the advantage of coming from a small family is greater for older than for younger siblings, a recurrent pattern that will have to be explained.

It should be noted what holding constant father's occupational status does and what it does not do in this analysis. It does eliminate the spurious effect on occupational achievements that is due to the tendency of higher socioeconomic strata to have both smaller families and more successful sons than lower strata, thus isolating the actual

TABLE 9.1. 1962 OCC. STATUS AND FIRST JOB, BY FAMILY SIZE AND SIBLING POSITION (IN DEVIATIONS FROM THE GRAND MEAN)

| | 1962 Occ. Status | | | | First Job | | | |
| | No Controls | | Father's Occ. Controlled | | No Controls | | Father's Education and Occ. Controlled | |
Sibling Position	3 Siblings or Less (1)	4 or more Siblings[a] (2)	3 Siblings or Less (3)	4 or More Siblings[a] (4)	3 Siblings or Less (5)	4 or More Siblings[a] (6)	3 Siblings or Less (7)	4 or More Siblings[a] (8)
Only child	7.1	---	4.1	---	7.8	---	4.3	---
Oldest child	6.2	-4.2	3.3	-2.7	5.0	-3.3	2.0	-1.5
Middle child								
No older brother	3.0	-5.8	1.6	-4.0	2.8	-4.9	1.3	-2.9
With older brother	2.2	-5.5	1.0	-3.1	1.1	-4.8	.0	-2.3
Youngest child	6.2	-2.0	3.8	.2	5.3	-2.1	2.7	.2
Grand mean		36.3				25.5		

[a]Except 10 siblings.

influence of family size on son's career. However, it does not eliminate differences in economic resources available for training sons, because fathers in the same economic position have less resources to devote to the training of each child if they have many than if they have few. Hence the effects in columns 3 and 4 net of father's status show that small families actually produce more successful sons than large ones, though they do not show that this influence is independent of the financial resources available for the training of each child.

Only children constitute a special case of family size. In one sense the only child is the first child in a particularly small family. But since the trauma of having younger siblings is not experienced by the only child, the one-child family represents a distinct family structure, different from other small as well as from large families. The occupational achievements of only children are greater than those of men from small families, regardless of the birth order of the latter, as shown in the top row of Table 9.1. This finding confirms the principle that the fewer the number of siblings, the better are a man's occupational chances. But occupational achievement does not appear to be a simple linear function of number of siblings, for differences in status between the only child and either the oldest or the youngest from small families are slight—much less than those between men with few and men with many siblings. The superiority of only children, then, appears to be not as great as one might expect, given the greater resources their parents can devote to raising and educating them.

Men with few siblings start their careers on higher levels and advance farther than do men with many siblings. Columns 5 and 6 in Table 9.1 show that the first jobs of men from small families, regardless of their sibling position, are consistently superior to those of men from large families; the differences range roughly from six to eight points. The superiority of the career beginnings of sons of small families persists in attenuated form when social origins (both father's education and occupation) are controlled, as is evident in the last two columns of Table 9.1. The introduction of career beginnings as a statistical control does not wipe out the differences in occupational achievement between men with few and men with many siblings (tabulation not shown). The tendency of men from small families to start their careers on higher levels than those from large ones does not account for the former's higher subsequent occupational achievements.

Only children enjoy a considerable head start in their careers. Their first jobs are clearly superior to those of either oldest children (by 2.8 points) or youngest children (by 2.5 points) in small families, and those of children in middle positions or from large families lag still further behind. The higher career beginnings of only children remain in evidence when social origins are controlled, as can be seen in the last two columns of Table 9.1. The initial career advantage of the only child is probably due to the greater resources his parents can make available for his schooling, as he does not have to share these resources with brothers and sisters. The high educational attainments of only children, which are revealed by the data in Table 9.2, support this interpretation.

In contrast to their starting points the subsequent careers of only children are not much superior to those of oldest or younger children with few siblings, the difference (either without controls or with father's occupation controlled) being in no case as great as 1.0. This incommensurate difference in destinations, given the one in origins, seems to reflect a failure on the part of only children to take full advantage of the head start in their careers, which may possibly be indicative of some psychological handicap to which growing up without siblings exposes a child. Perhaps the only child has special risks as well as special opportunities.[3] An alternative possibility, however, is that a demographic factor introduces an age bias that may account for the differences between only children and the rest. A disproportionate share of only children were born during the depression or World War II and were thus still young in 1962. (Specifically, 43 per cent of only and 35 per cent of other children were under 34 in 1962.) Hence their higher educational attainment may be partially a function of time trends in the United States, and their relatively low 1962 status a function of their comparative youth. Indeed controlling age reduces the differences between only children and others.

Multiple classification analysis, on which the findings in Table 9.1 and 9.2 are based, assumes that there is no interaction of the classificatory variable with the two correlated scalar ones. With a sample the size of the present one, of course, even very small interactions are statistically significant. However, the regression slopes of son's on father's occupational status differ little between categories in the family classification, and there are no consistent variations either with family size or with sibling position. Thus the assumptions made in using multiple-classification analysis are justified. The case of the relation-

3 It is interesting that the correlation between father's and son's occupational status is lower for only children than for any of the other eight categories. Besides, only children have the highest rates of both long-distance upward and downward mobility. Whereas 24.8 per cent of all men are upwardly mobile from their origins more than 25 points, 28.5 per cent of only children are. Similarly, whereas only 22 per cent of the total population is downwardly mobile more than 5 points, 26 per cent of only children are.

ship between first job and 1962 occupational status is not so clear. Whereas no noteworthy interaction by birth order is evident, there are some consistent though slight variations in the slopes by family size, with those for men from small families being steeper (ranging between .59 and .63) than those for men from large families (between .53 and .58).[4] Although men from small families have more successful careers than those from large ones, their careers are more closely dependent on the level on which they were started, albeit a relatively high level.

The significance of career beginnings for later achievement directs attention to the role of education as a mediator between family structure and occupational success. Parental resources are typically required to obtain an advanced education, which is of prime importance for occupational achievement in our society. The child who goes to school beyond the legal minimum age uses up parental resources, if only by continuing to depend on their economic support instead of beginning to contribute to the support of the family. A higher education makes particularly great demands on the financial resources of the parental family, for it generally requires substantial economic support for extended periods. Three-quarters of the college students in 1959 were partly and one-quarter were fully supported by their parents, and even among graduate students (in the arts and sciences) 22 per cent expect financial support from parents.[5] Parents remain an important source of financial support for higher education in the United States, notwithstanding the increasing numbers of scholarships, fellowships, and part-time employment. The greater the number of children in a family, the greater the strain on its financial resources, and the less the resources available for each, within a given range of family income. In an age in which the inheritance of a business, a farm, or a professional practice has become increasingly rare, a major channel through which affluent parents can transmit their superior status to their sons is by providing them with an advanced education. But many children restrict a family's ability to do so, just as they limit the property each child can inherit.

As might be expected, given the necessity to spread financial resources for education over more offspring the greater their number, family size has a pronounced influence on educational attainment. Columns 1 and 2 of Table 9.2 show that men from small families enjoy an educational advantage over men from large families regard-

---

[4] Estimates based on the nonfarm population alone.

[5] Herman P. Miller, *Rich Man, Poor Man,* New York: Crowell, 1965, p. 162; and Davis, *op. cit.,* pp. 178-179.

TABLE 9.2. EDUCATION AND 1962 OCC., BY FAMILY SIZE AND SIBLING POSITION (IN DEVIATIONS FROM THE GRAND MEAN)

| | Education | | | | 1962 Occ. Status, Own Education and Father's Occ. Controlled | |
| | No Controls | | Father's Occ. Controlled | | | |
Sibling Position	3 Siblings or Less (1)	4 or More Siblings[a] (2)	3 Siblings or Less (3)	4 or More Siblings[a] (4)	3 Siblings or Less (5)	4 or More Siblings[a] (6)
Only child	.80	...	.55	...	.1	...
Oldest child	.71	-.46	.47	-.33	.3	-.5
Middle child						
No older brother	.33	-.61	.22	-.46	.5	-1.0
With older brother	.27	-.60	.16	-.40	.1	-.5
Youngest child	.58	-.20	.39	-.01	1.2	.5
Grand mean	4.43				36.3	

[a] Except 10 siblings.

less of sibling position. When these educational scores are translated into years of schooling, the average education of men with three or fewer siblings is high-school graduation, whereas that of men from larger families is nearly two years less. In other words, the average man from a large family has dropped out of school at about what is now the legal minimum age, whereas the average man from a small family has gone on to graduate from high school. These differences persist, though in an attenuated form, when social origins are controlled in columns 3 and 4 of Table 9.2. Boys in small families advance further in school than boys in large ones from the same occupational level, independent of sibling position and of having an older brother, with the differences amounting to between three-quarters and one and one-half years of schooling in favor of men with few siblings.

As a matter of fact, a small family not only raises the mean educational attainments of sons but also the likelihood that they proceed with their education at most stages, though not all. Table 9.3 presents the proportion of men in each category of the family variable who continued their education from one level to the next. Column 2 indicates the proportion who graduated from elementary school (eighth grade); column 3 shows the proportion of these who went on to high school. Of these freshmen in high school, the proportion who finished it is found in column 4. The remaining three columns similarly indicate the proportion of high-school graduates who went to college; the proportion of those with some college experience who graduated; and the proportion of college graduates who pursued graduate training. Of course the size of the sample on which these continuation rates are based declines as one moves from left to right in the table; and one of the proportions in the last column represents less than 100,000 population (less than 25 sample cases). It is not easy to read a table of this type quickly, but an extra minute is worth the trouble. The dominant pattern in this table is that the rates are higher for men with few than for men with many siblings *up to college graduation,* regardless of birth order or position as oldest son (compare adjacent rows). On each of these educational levels, furthermore, the proportion of only children who continue to the next level is greater than that for any other category. Thus the fewer the number of siblings a boy has, the greater are his chances of continuing his education on every level up to college graduation.

A large family is an economic handicap, but once this handicap is overcome it may turn into an advantage. Sons in large families are doubly disadvantaged. They not only tend to have low-status parents, who usually have no tradition of going to college or even graduating

TABLE 9.3. PER CENT CONTINUING THEIR EDUCATION FROM ONE LEVEL TO NEXT, BY FAMILY SIZE AND SIBLING POSITION

Family Size Sibling Position	Population (in Thousands)	Elementary Graduate	Eighth Grade to Some High School	Some High School to High School Graduation	High-School Graduation to Some College	Some College to College Graduation	College Graduation to Graduate School
Only child	2,920	92.6	93.1	84.1	56.0	57.5	46.0
Oldest child							
Small family[a]	7,073	93.7	91.6	81.7	54.9	52.1	43.3
Large family[b]	3,038	80.1	76.6	64.9	38.2	48.1	47.3
Middle child with No older brother							
Small family[a]	2,251	89.7	89.9	75.4	48.4	49.6	41.3
Large family[b]	2,667	77.6	75.9	63.9	34.0	37.2	41.7[c]
Middle child with Older brother							
Small family[a]	3,080	98.0	88.8	78.3	46.0	49.8	38.2
Large family[b]	12,639	77.8	75.4	62.7	34.4	42.5	40.7
Youngest child							
Small family[a]	6,230	91.9	90.8	81.1	52.0	57.0	35.8
Large family[b]	3,191	83.9	83.0	69.5	34.5	52.7	41.3
All Classes	44,984	84.9	84.0	73.6	45.8	51.2	41.1

[a]Three or fewer siblings.
[b]Four or more siblings, except ten siblings.
[c]Estimated population in cell is 53,000 persons; in all others, it is at least 100,000.

from high school, and who have meager total financial resources, but they also must share the total parental resources with more siblings than children from small families on the same socioeconomic level. Those sons of large families who overcome their handicap and graduate from college, however, are more likely than men from small families to proceed to graduate or professional school. The proportion of college graduates who complete at least one year of postgraduate work is higher for men from large than those from small families in all four possible comparisons, in sharp contrast to the differences in all 20 comparisons pertaining to earlier educational stages. Although the differences are small and the number of cases is not sufficient to make them statistically significant, the consistency of the pattern for all sibling positions creates some confidence in it.

Difficulties do not, of course, increase the likelihood of success; on the contrary, they decrease it. The select few who succeed in overcoming the difficulties, however, appear to have a greater chance of further success than men who never were faced with them. It is not easy for men from large families to remain in school and graduate from college, but those of them who do meet this challenge are more likely to succeed in attaining the highest educational levels than are college graduates who did not have to pass through so rigorous a screening process. This finding is parallel to the one reported in Chapter 7 concerning the sons of immigrants. Men who had to surmount the obstacles posed by a disadvantaged ethnic background in order to obtain a college education, just as those initially disadvantaged by a large family, are better equipped to continue their education in graduate school than men who never confronted such challenges.

Frequently the analysis has revealed that the influence of other determinants of ultimate occupational achievement is mediated by education. Here again the higher educational attainments of men from small families largely account for their greater chances of occupational success. When both education and father's status are controlled, as in the last two columns of Table 9.2, the differences in achievement between men with few and men with many siblings almost completely disappear. The small residual differences that do remain average less than one point on the occupational scale (between .6 and 1.5). The superiority of the only child over all others is entirely the result of the educational advantages enjoyed by him, as a comparison of the first with the other rows in column 5 makes evident.

In brief, the superior occupational achievements of men from small families are essentially due to their superior education. Once education is taken into account, the man with few siblings is hardly superior in occupational status to the man from a large family. The addition of other factors as controls, such as first job or ethnic background, has little further effect as the differences are already so small. Family size affects the chances of occupational success of sons primarily because it affects their education.

SIBLING POSITION

The position a boy occupies among his siblings also influences his career as an adult.[6] In general, children in the extreme positions are the most successful. The first two columns of Table 9.1, read vertically, show that oldest and youngest children (as well as only children) achieve higher occupational status than middle children, whether they were raised in large or in small families. Controlling father's occupation in columns 3 and 4 does not alter the pattern, though the differences are reduced. Thus regardless of social origins, family size, or the existence of an older brother, middle children have less successful careers than the first-born and the last-born. Youngest children appear to have an occupational advantage over oldest ones in large families, though not in small ones. This advantage of youngest over first-born children persists when father's occupational status is controlled (column 4). We shall see, however, that the additional control of educational attainment substantially reduces the status superiority of sons in the two extreme sibling positions as well as the difference between them. In other words, the chief advantage enjoyed by men born either first or last, as well as by only children, is their better education.

The same pattern of differences revealed by 1962 occupation can be observed in regard to status of first job in columns 5 through 8 of Table 9.1. Neither in small nor in large families does the middle child typically start his career on as high a level as the first-born or last-born. Though there is very little difference in first jobs between oldest and youngest children in small families, the youngest children in large families do begin their careers slightly higher (1.2 points) than the oldest children in large families, and this difference somewhat increases when father's education and occupation are controlled (to 1.7 points).

The first-born son in a society with a tradition of primogeniture that has not entirely been forgotten gains special advantages, since his parents are often particularly eager for him to succeed. Moreover first-born children themselves are more likely to accept the values of

---

[6] It should be remembered that we are not comparing men with their own siblings but with men of different sibling positions in other families.

the adult community early[7] and hence to put a premium on occupational achievement. The youngest child also derives special benefits from his position, because he tends to be the beloved "Benjamin" of the family, because seniority may by this time have raised the father's income, and because the parents no longer have to economize for the sake of younger children. Being relieved of the worry about feeding and clothing younger children and setting aside funds for their education is undoubtedly most important for large families with their strained resources. This is reflected in the greater advantage the last-born in large families have over older siblings. Middle children, lacking a distinctive position, suffer by comparison with the oldest and the youngest.

Knowing that the most powerful influence on occupational status is educational attainment, we would expect oldest and youngest children to be better educated than their middle siblings. The data in Table 9.2 confirm this expectation for both small and large families (columns 1 and 2). The differences are not large, amounting to only two-thirds of a year of schooling, but they persist virtually undiminished when social origins are controlled (columns 3 and 4). Youngest children are somewhat better educated than oldest ones in large though not in small families; this calls attention to the same interaction effect already noted in respect to occupational achievements.

Sibling position affects education at every stage in the educational process, as indicated by the data on percentage continuing their education from one level to the next in Table 9.3. The influence of sibling position is consistent, so that on each level, for both large and small families, middle children, whether or not they are first sons, are less likely to continue their schooling to the next level than are either oldest or youngest children. There are only three exceptions to this conclusion in the 48 possible comparisons in the table. All three of these refer to the lesser likelihood of youngest children than middle ones to proceed from college graduation to graduate school.[8] These exceptions themselves conform to another tendency previously observed: that those men who have overcome initial handicaps are more

[7] See Irving Harris, *The Promised Seed,* New York: Free Press, 1964, a very suggestive discussion of the way in which differences in the interpersonal relations between first and later sons produce differences in their personalities and consequently differences in their achievements. Harris maintains that his theory pertains only to type of achievement, not to degree of success (personal communication).

[8] Only the two exceptions pertaining to small families exceed 1 per cent. The proportion who continue from college to graduate school among middle children who are first sons exceeds that among youngest children in *large families* by a mere .4 per cent, which constitutes the third exception.

likely than those never confronted by them to progress to further achievements. Because middle children have less chance to graduate from college than others, those who do are a more highly select group of potential achievers, and hence they are relatively more likely to continue to the most advanced educational level. In this case the initially disadvantaged group of middle children later surpasses only one of the two advantaged groups, youngest children, whereas the other, oldest children, remains superior.

In small families first-born children achieve consistently higher rates of continuation at each educational level than do the last-born, the only exception being college graduation, when youngest children are favored. In large families, by contrast, youngest children are more likely than oldest to continue their education, except that oldest are more likely to go from high school to college and, if they graduate, to pursue graduate training. Again we observe that the last-born child benefits most in large families.

The educational advantage enjoyed by children in extreme sibling positions accounts for the occupational superiority they achieve over middle children. Controlling educational attainment as well as social origin (columns 5 and 6 of Table 9.2) virtually nullifies the influence of sibling position on occupational status, just as it nearly nullifies the influence of family size on status. The only minor exception is that the last-born, in both small and large families, are slightly superior in occupational achievement to men in other sibling positions.

Parents are apparently more successful in encouraging a child to pursue his education if he is the oldest or youngest than if his position is intermediate. Whether they do so intentionally or inadvertently cannot be determined by these data, nor can it be ascertained whether the process involves greater financial support, more socio-emotional support, the encouragement of more independence, or something else. Perhaps both the greater responsibilities oldest children have to assume and the greater socio-emotional support youngest ones generally receive from parents and siblings further academic achievement. It may be that the mere fact of occupying a distinctive position as first-born or as baby of the family directs a disproportionate amount of supportive attention to a child, which benefits his personality development in some way favorable to achievement. Possibly sibling rivalries are less acute for sons in these distinctive positions. The last-born, especially in large families, may gain additional advantages from the fact that parents no longer have to set aside economic resources for additional children and that older siblings are available to assist if the parents' support is inadequate. Whatever the underlying process,

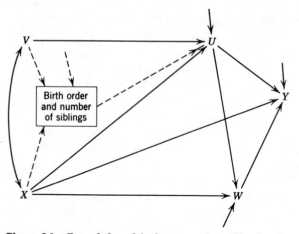

Figure 9.1. Extended model of process of stratification, including sibling classification. (*Note:* Dashed lines represent
hypothesized directions of influence, but cannot be given
numerical values in a path analysis because the sibling
classification is nonmetric.)

Code: *V:* father's education.
 X: father's occupation.
 U: respondent's education.
 W: respondent's first job, occupational SES.
 Y: respondent's occupational SES, March 1962.

the family situation of the oldest and the youngest child is more beneficial than that of a middle child for the development of a successful
man.[9]

A basic causal model of the process of stratification was presented in
Chapter 5, which may be extended to include the influence of family
of orientation on occupational achievement. Figure 9.1 represents an
attempt to introduce the combined variable "number of siblings and
birth order," which for convenience we shall refer to as the sibling
variable, into the previously discussed model. Birth order and number
of siblings are assumed to depend on social origins and to affect

[9] A problem arises in interpreting the differences between middle children and
children in extreme sibling positions as a result of the crude dichotomous control
of family size used here. In both the "small" and the "large" category of family
size used, a greater proportion of middle than either oldest or youngest children
come from relatively large families, since larger families have more middle but
no more oldest or youngest children than smaller ones. Hence some unknown
portion of the inferiority of middle children is due to the larger size of their
parental families, a variable we speak of as controlled, although the control is
only partial.

directly a man's educational attainment but only indirectly—via education—his first job and ultimate occupational achievement. Although the causal diagram resembles the one used for path analysis, we cannot give single numerical values to the quasi-paths leading from or to the sibling variable, because the latter is not a metrical variable but a manifold classification lacking even a single principle of ordering. We can, however, see if the data are consistent with this general arrangement, for example, by ascertaining whether the sibling classification has any bearing on occupational achievement apart from its effects on education. The procedure used for this purpose is to determine the percentage of the total sum of squares accounted for by a given variable or combination of variables. Considering the 1962 occupational status (Y) as the dependent variable, the relevant figures for percentage of sum of squares are:

Combination of variables[10]	Percentage of total sum of squares (Y)
Sibling	5.35
W, U	40.93
W, U, and Sibling	40.98

The sibling variable clearly influences occupational status, either directly or indirectly, for it accounts for more than 5 per cent of the total sum of squares in Y. Our causal model, however, posits two variables intervening between the sibling classification and Y. These two, first job and education $(W$ and $U)$, alone account for 40.93 per cent of the total sum of squares in Y. When the sibling variable is added to this combination, the percentage of total sum of squares accounted for rises only to 40.98, an increment of a mere .05 per cent. Evidently the entire effect of family size and sibling position on occupational achievement is mediated by education and first job, as previously noted and posited in the diagram, and the residual direct effect on 1962 occupation is negligible. The same procedure can be applied to examine how first job (W) is influenced by antecedent variables:

Combination of variables	Percentage of total sum of squares (W)
Sibling	5.69
U	32.73
U and Sibling	33.25

Again the sibling variable accounts for more than 5 per cent of the total sum of squares. Only one variable is assumed to intervene between

---

10 W refers to first job, U to education, and "Sibling" refers to the classification of family size and sibling position used throughout this chapter.

the sibling variable and first job (W), namely, education (U). The 32.73 per cent of the total sum of squares in W accounted for by U alone is increased only by $\frac{1}{2}$ per cent to 33.25 by the addition of the sibling variable. Thus most of the effect of family size and birth order on first job is mediated by education.

Moving farther to the left in Figure 9.1 and taking education as the dependent variable, we can ask how it is influenced by the sibling classification. The relevant percentages of sum of squares are:

Combination of variables	Percentage of total sum of squares (U)
Sibling	10.78
X (father's occupation)	19.86
V (father's education)	20.77
X and V	27.94
X and Sibling	24.42
V and Sibling	25.24
X, V, and Sibling	30.71

The effect of the sibling variable is substantial, nearly 11 per cent of the total sum of squares, and the causal diagram stipulates that this is a direct effect. Does the sibling classification entirely mediate the effects of the two variables lying behind it? The answer is clearly negative because each of these variables has a larger gross effect than the sibling variable and because each produces a substantial increment over the sibling variable alone, as is shown by the combinations "V and Sibling" and "X and Sibling." Comparing the three single variables with either of these two combinations makes it clear that direct paths from both X and V to education are called for, notwithstanding the sibling classification as an intervening variable. In other words, social origins influence occupational achievement not only by affecting family size and composition but also in ways that are independent of these family characteristics. On the other hand, the sibling variable clearly exerts an influence on education independent of that exerted by the two background variables, accounting for an additional 2.77 per cent of the total sum of squares $(30.71 - 27.94)$.

In sum an attempt has been made to place the multiple factor referring to the family of orientation into the causal model depicting the process of stratification that was developed earlier. Father's education and occupation influence the kind of family he establishes, and the characteristics of this family influence son's educational attainment. The impact of the parental family on occupational achievement seems to be entirely a result of its effect on education. By the nature of the sibling variable this model cannot distinguish between the influence of family size and of sibling position. It therefore cannot reveal how these two influences interact. This interaction effect and what it implies about the significance of family relations for occupational life are the topics to which we now turn.

THE STRUCTURE OF FAMILY RELATIONS

Number of siblings and sibling position interact in their effects on subsequent adult achievements, and this statistical interaction reflects something about the social interaction and role relations among siblings in a family. It has been noted repeatedly here that *youngest* children have special advantages in *large* families. This is the same as saying that *oldest* children have greater advantages in *small* families, for both statements refer to the fact that the influence of sibling position depends on family size.

The difference in 1962 occupational status between men from small and those from large families is greater for oldest children and for oldest sons who are not oldest children than for middle children with older brothers and for youngest children, as column 1 in Table 9.4

TABLE 9.4. DIFFERENCES BETWEEN MEN FROM SMALL FAMILIES[a] AND MEN FROM LARGE FAMILIES IN 1962 OCC. STATUS, EDUCATION, AND FIRST JOB, BY SIBLING POSITION

	1962 Occ. Status		Education		
Sibling Position	No Controls (1)	Father's Occ. Controlled (2)	No Controls (3)	Father's Occ. & Education Controlled (4)	First Job (No Controls) (5)
Oldest child	10.4	6.0	1.17	.65	8.3
Middle child					
No older brother	8.8	5.6	.94	.58	7.7
With older brother	7.7	4.1	.87	.42	5.9
Youngest child	8.2	3.6	.78	.23	7.4

[a] Small families are those with 4 or fewer children; large families, those with 5 or more, except 11, children.

shows. When social origins are controlled to eliminate the influence of fertility differentials associated with occupational status, the remaining status differences between small and large families, presented in column 2, are perfectly ranked by birth order. In brief, the advantage of a small family declines as sibling position moves away from that of first-born child. To express it in another way, the handicap of many siblings is reduced as birth order increases from first-born to last-born. The superiority of men from small over those from large families is greatest for oldest children and least for youngest ones. Having few rather than many siblings benefits the future careers of all boys, regardless of sibling position, but these benefits decline for successively later children.

The differences between the educational attainments of men from small and from large families reveal the same pattern, whether or not background factors (father's education and occupation) are controlled, as is apparent in columns 3 and 4 of Table 9.4. The educational superiority of men from small families steadily declines as one moves from oldest children to middle children without older brothers, middle children with older brothers, and youngest children. The differences between the first jobs of men with few and the men with many siblings (column 5) conform to the same pattern with one exception —middle sons with older brothers rank below youngest children.

This consistent pattern of differences may be explained in terms of the role relations among siblings in the family. The interpretation suggested is that older children assume responsibilities and must make sacrifices for younger ones, particularly when parental resources are inadequate. As younger sons are born parents tend to set aside resources—for building a larger house, buying more clothing, or paying college bills—that otherwise could have been devoted to the education of the older sons. Hence an older son is more disadvantaged by having many siblings than is a younger one. In families with few resources and many children, moreover, oldest children, and especially oldest sons, are under pressure early to assume some responsibility for and contribute to the support of younger ones. Under such pressures even the drive to achieve of an older son is likely to be channelled into endeavors to become financially independent and to assume the adult role of family supporter rather than into an interest in continuing to go to school. Contributing to the achievement of younger siblings becomes a substitute for the older son's own success. If there are several older siblings, they may join in helping to support a younger one in a large family and derive satisfaction from his success, which demonstrates to the world that "We Browns can be somebody too." Younger sons are undoubtedly not exposed to the same pressure to help siblings.

Since the more limited resources of large families are partly compensated by the help younger siblings receive from older ones, according to this interpretation, younger ones should be least disadvantaged by having many siblings. The data, as we have already seen, are consistent with this expectation. In brief, it is less of a disadvantage for a child's future success to have many older than to have many younger siblings. The explanation suggested for this finding is that role relations in the family require older siblings to assume some responsibility for and contribute to the development of younger ones. This is probably particularly true in large families, in which the resources of the parents are more likely to need supplementing, and in which the number of younger siblings an older child must help is greater. The result is the imbalance manifest in the observed interaction effect.

The question arises whether only older brothers contribute to the future success of younger brothers in large families, or whether older sisters have a similar beneficial effect on achievement. We can infer an answer to this question by comparing middle children with and without older brothers. If younger sons in large families derive special benefits only from older brothers and not from older sisters, it follows that middle children with older brothers are more successful than those without in large families, though not in small ones, whereas the absence of such differences would imply that older sisters as well as older brothers further the achievements of younger brothers in large families. The data reveal such differences, but their magnitude is extremely small, as can be seen by comparing rows 3 and 4 in adjacent columns of Tables 9.1 and 9.2. When social origins are controlled, having an older brother raises the mean occupational status of middle children .9 points in large families and lowers it .6 points in small ones. Similarly, the mean status of first jobs, controlled for social origins, of middle children is raised .6 points in large and lowered 1.3 points in small families by the existence of an older brother. The average educational attainment of middle children, controlled for father's status, is also higher in large families (by .06 points) and lower in small ones (by .06 points) if they have an older brother.

Although the differences are very small the pattern is so consistent, even when social origins are controlled, that one would have to conclude that younger boys in large families obtain special benefits from older brothers that older sisters do not provide, were it not for another factor that might have produced this pattern. There is a demographic difference between middle children with and and those without an older brother in our classification that affects the findings. Men with older brothers are more likely than those without to have a relatively large number of older siblings. The reason is that having an older brother is a more restrictive condition than having an older sibling, which means that men are most likely to have older brothers if they have many elder siblings. Hence the mean number of older siblings of men with older brothers must be greater than that of men without older brothers. We know already that older siblings lessen the handicap that a large family of orientation imposes. The slight superiority in achievements of large-family men with older brother over those without is probably attributable simply to their having more older siblings, brothers or sisters, who aid in their advancement. The most plausible conclusion, therefore, is that older brothers make no more contribution to the advancement of younger brothers in large families than older sisters do.

The finding that the average accomplishments of middle children without older brothers differ little from those of middle children with older brothers has another interesting implication. Middle children without older brothers are, of course, first sons. It is often assumed that oldest sons are more successful than younger ones, partly as a survival of the tradition of primogeniture. Indeed we found that sons who are oldest children attain higher educational levels and consequently have more successful careers than middle sons, though they are not superior to sons who are youngest children. However the finding that middle children without an older brother are not substantially more successful than those with one reveals that the career advantage of the oldest child who is a boy is the result of his being his parents' first child, not merely their first son.

FAMILY CLIMATE AND ACHIEVEMENT

Various aspects of the parental family influence the educational attainments, and through them the occupational achievements, of sons. The significance of family size, sibling position, and the role relations among siblings that are manifest in the interaction effect of size and position have been examined, but other characteristics of the family that are more difficult to measure than these surely also influence occupational achievement. It is of interest to ascertain whether differences in the family's "intellectual climate," as well as the structural characteristics investigated, affect the achievement of sons. Does an achievement motivation that induces sons to pursue their education and strive for success prevail in some families but not in others? Attitude surveys and psychological tests administered to all members of families combined with information on the later attainments of sons would yield data adequate to answer this question. Unfortunately no such data are available in this study. As a matter of fact these data could not even be collected for a sample like ours, since many members of the respondents' families are no longer living.

An admittedly second-best alternative to such data is to use the education of a man's eldest brother as a crude indication of the extent to which a family promotes achievement. Other conditions being equal, the education of a man's eldest brother can be assumed to reflect the extent to which learning and achievement are valued and encouraged in his family. To be sure, so does the respondent's own education, but it cannot be used as the independent measure of family climate, because it is to serve as the major dependent variable. Other conditions, of course, are not equal, because the education of the oldest son, just as that of other children, is known to be affected by the educational and occupational level of the father as well as by other background factors, notably color. The correlation between eldest brother's and own education primarily reflects the influence of these background factors on both and not simply the effect of one on the other. If background factors are controlled, however, brother's education does provide a rough indication of the degree to which the family climate furthers education and achievement. (Some conceptual problems encountered with such an indicator are discussed below.)

Not quite half (46 per cent) of the OCG sample reported the educational attainment of their oldest brothers. This information was obtained as a response to the following question: "Did any of your older brothers live to age 25? . . . If 'Yes,' . . . please indicate the highest grade of school the oldest brother completed." The bulk of the nonresponse on this question—about 48 per cent of the total sample—represents respondents who did not have an older brother who lived to age 25. About 3 per cent of the sample did not report number of siblings and birth order, or, if an older brother was reported, his education. The remaining 3 per cent of the sample represents a tabulating error: men with exactly 10 siblings were inadvertently tabulated as nonrespondents on number of siblings and birth order. This error is unfortunate, but there is no known reason why the omission of this small group should bias the analysis.[11]

As a preliminary, we examine whether brother's education affects achievement by determining the percentage of total sum of squares "explained" by it. Variations in eldest brother's education account for 11 per cent of the variance in 1962 occupational status. However when background factors—father's education, father's occupation, color, and region of residence—are controlled, the increment in percentage of total sum of squares produced by brother's education is a negligible $\frac{1}{4}$ per cent. The influence of eldest brother's education on the respondent's own education, in contrast, is not explained by these background factors. Brother's education alone accounts for fully 24 per cent of the total sum of squares. The portion of the total due to brother's education when social origins (father's occupation and education) are controlled is over 8 per cent, and it is still 5 per cent

11 Minor discrepancies between the data used here and those in the report of the Bureau of the Census, "Educational Change in a Generation: March 1962" (*Current Population Reports,* Series P-20, No. 132, September 1964) are presumably due to the correction of this error in the tabulations made for that report.

after color and region of residence as well as social origins have been taken into account.[12]

How conducive the family climate is to the pursuit of learning and high attainment, when measured by the education of oldest son, clearly influences the younger son's educational success. Detailed data are presented in columns 1 and 2 of Table 9.5. They show that the

TABLE 9.5. EDUCATIONAL ATTAINMENT NET OF FATHER'S OCC., FATHER'S EDUCATION, COLOR, AND REGION, BY FAMILY SIZE AND EDUCATION OF OLDEST BROTHER. (IN DEVIATIONS FROM THE GRAND MEAN)

Education of Oldest Brother	Education of Respondent (Net)		
	(1) 1 to 3 Siblings	(2) 4 or more Siblings	(3) Difference (1) - (2)
No older brother	.37	-.31	.68
Oldest brother completed			
0 to 7 years	-1.13	-1.12	-.01
8 years	-.65	-.54	-.11
High school, 1 to 3 years	.10	.03	.07
High school, 4 years	.34	.23	.11
College, 1 to 3 years	.80	.55	.25
College, 4 or more years	1.08	.70	.38

higher the education of eldest brother, controlling background factors, the higher are the average educational attainments of men, in both small and large families. Note that these controls mean, in effect, that men are compared whose fathers had the same education and occupation, whose color is the same, and who live in the same region. Even under these conditions the difference in educational attainments of men with the most- and those with the least-educated eldest brothers is more than four years of schooling in small families and more than three years in large families.

The educational climate in the family, as indicated by brother's education, has a pronounced impact on the schooling of sons. To be sure, our data do not permit us to specify precisely what conditions in the family constitute such a climate conducive to educational success. It may be that the oldest son acquired more education than is the norm in his family's social stratum, and so did the younger son, because the parents put strong emphasis on achievement and success. Alternatively, perhaps the parents were not particularly oriented toward education, but the oldest brother was, and he served as a role model for his younger brother. Indeed, there may be little explicit concern with achievement in the family. The data are compatible with the assumption that a child is more likely to succeed in school

[12] Detailed figures on which this summary is based are shown in Appendix H, Tables H.1, H.2, and H.3.

if his parents are relaxed and supportive than if they are very anxious about his success and continually push him toward greater achievements. The attempts of anxiously striving parents to implement their ambitions for their children may well be self-defeating. Whatever the specific mechanism at work, the findings indicate that families in which education is important, at least for some member, are more likely than other families with the same background characteristics to produce highly educated sons.

The impact of the family climate on the educational attainments of sons is more pronounced in small than in large families. The differences in education between respondents from small and from large families, controlling for background factors, are presented in column 3 of Table 9.5. The higher the brother's education, the greater the educational advantage of men with few siblings over those with many. If the eldest brother only went to elementary school the education of men from small families is not superior to that of men from large ones. If the eldest brother graduated from college, in contrast, small-family men have an average of three-quarters of a year more schooling than large-family men. The educational advantage accruing to boys by virtue of their being born into a small family is one year (.49 points on the educational scale) greater if their eldest brother is a college graduate than if he only graduated from grammar school.

This finding supports the previous suggestion that a family in which education is valued strengthens the motivation of sons to acquire much education. The positive correlation between brother's and own education when background factors are controlled was interpreted as revealing this influence of the educational climate of the family. An alternative interpretation of this correlation, however, is that better-educated older brothers can contribute more than less educated ones to the development and advancement of their younger brothers. We have seen that younger brothers derive more benefit from older ones in large families than in small ones. Thus the alternative interpretation implies that a well-educated oldest brother should further the educational attainments of younger siblings more in large than in small families. In fact, a well-educated eldest brother has just the opposite effect, improving the educational attainments of his siblings more in small families than in large ones. This fact makes the alternative interpretation less plausible and, by inference, the original one more so.

The explanation suggested by the new finding is that a favorable educational climate in the family affects the educational attainments of sons, at least in part, because it induces them or their parents to take advantage of the potential resources available for their education. When background factors are controlled the economic resources available for the education of each child are more limited in large than in small families. This advantage of the small family is utilized more fully the greater the education of the eldest son. The education of boys with poorly educated oldest brothers does not benefit at all from the less restricted resources of small families. The better educated the eldest brother is, the more the greater resources of small families are apparently taken advantage of to further the education of younger sons, as is indicated by the fact that the differences in education between small and large families increase with increasing education of the eldest brother. In other words, if the educational climate is not favorable to educational achievement it does not matter much whether a family's economic circumstances make it objectively easy to provide children with an education. It requires a positive orientation toward education to make available resources meaningful and relevant for actual educational attainment.

FORMALIZATION OF INTERPRETATIONS

The significance of family climate as manifest in the education of the eldest brother (variable Q) can be introduced into the formal causal model of the process of stratification.[13] A technical problem is that some of the correlations are available only for the total sample rather than exclusively for those men who report brother's education, but minor adjustments permit plausible estimates.[14] The relevant re-

[13] Oldest brother's education (Q) was not tabulated in quite so much detail as respondent's and father's education. For purposes of correlation analysis, the following scores were used:

Score	Education of oldest brother (Q)
1	Elementary, zero to seven years
3	Elementary, eight years
4	High School, one to three years
5	High School, four years
6	College, one to three years
7	College, four or more years

[14] Two correlations, r_{UV} and r_{YX}, are available for men reporting brother's education as well as for all men. In both cases the correlation for the former subpopulation is about .04 lower than for the whole population. There is a highly plausible explanation for this discrepancy. Men reporting brother's education are selected on number of siblings, a variable known to correlate with the several socioeconomic variables in the system. The question on brother's education eliminates all men with no siblings, a large fraction of those with one sibling (since that sibling could be female or younger than the respondent), a somewhat smaller but still sizable fraction of those with two siblings, and so on. By contrast, a high proportion of respondents from very large families will be able to report for an older brother. Thus any correlation for the subpopulation of men with older brothers is analogous to a *partial* correlation for the total population, with number

gressions are presented in Table 9.6.[15] One curious result apparent in this table is that eldest brother's education is somewhat more predictable from the two social-origin variables, father's occupation and father's education, than is the respondent's own education. This may indicate that the attainments of oldest sons are more closely tied to

TABLE 9.6. PARTIAL REGRESSION COEFFICIENTS IN STANDARD FORM (BETA COEFFICIENTS) AND COEFFICIENTS OF DETERMINATION FOR SPECIFIED COMBINATIONS OF VARIABLES, FOR MEN OF NONFARM BACKGROUND REPORTING OLDEST BROTHER'S EDUCATION

Dependent Variables[a]	Independent Variables[a]					
	W	U	Q	X	V	R^2
Q	...	...	...	.217	.358	.25
U	...	...	...	.245	.268	.19
U	...	...	.450	.147	.107	.35
W	...	.436	...	.163	...	.27
Y	.279	.382	...	.096	...	.38

[a]Y: Respondent's occ. status in 1962.
W: Occ. status of respondent's first job.
U: Respondent's education.
Q: Education of respondent's oldest brother.
X: Father's occ. status.
V: Father's education.

their background than are those of younger ones. On the other hand, it may simply reflect response error; specifically that the response on brother's education is contaminated by that on father's education. All of it is undoubtedly not a result of response error, because the correlation analysis reveals that the influence of father's occupation on son's is in fact greater for oldest than for other sons.

The model shown in Figure 9.2 represents the hypothesis that eldest brother's education is influenced by social origins and in turn influences respondent's education and through it his first job and 1962 occupation. The estimates of the path coefficients are taken from Table 9.6. The most interesting question about this model is whether it suffices to think of Q as affecting the respondent's first and 1962 occupation only by way of his education (U), or whether it is necessary to posit some other connection between Q and W or Q and Y. We are handicapped in approaching this question by the fact that no observed values of r_{WQ} are available, as this combination of variables was not tabulated. However, we do have r_{YQ}, and this allows a cogent, albeit indirect, examination of the problem.

of siblings held constant to some degree. The data indicate that an adjustment of —.04 would transform the correlations for the total population into reliable estimates for the subpopulation of men reporting brother's education.

[15] This analysis is based on men with nonfarm background only.

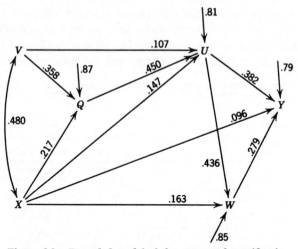

Figure 9.2. Extended model of the process of stratification, including brother's education as a determinant of respondent's education, for men with nonfarm background.

Code: *V:* father's education.
        X: father's occupational status.
        Q: oldest brother's education.
        U: respondent's education.
        W: status of respondent's first job.
        Y: respondent's occupational status in 1962.

If the model in Figure 9.2 is correct, then there is an implied value for r_{WQ}, to wit:

$$_c r_{WQ} = p_{WU} r_{UQ} + p_{WX} r_{QX}.$$

This calculation yields $_c r_{WQ} = .306$. The degree of accuracy of the model can now be tested by using this derived $_c r_{WQ}$ to compute the r_{YQ} implied by the model and comparing it with the observed r_{YQ}. Inserting the value obtained for $_c r_{WQ}$ into $_c r_{YQ} = p_{YU} r_{UQ} + p_{YX} r_{QX} + p_{YW} _c r_{WQ}$ yields a $_c r_{YQ}$ of .335. This compares quite satisfactorily with the observed value of .377, leaving a discrepancy of only .042. This result is in conformity with the earlier conclusion that brother's education affects respondent's occupational status only indirectly, via the positive association between the educational attainments of the two brothers.

At this point it is appropriate to reconsider the causal interpretation of the variable, brother's education. Earlier in this chapter the variable was described as a plausible indicator of the prevailing educational climate in the family, presumably influencing the educational outcome for both brothers. In the model presented in Figure 9.2, however, oldest brother's education (Q) is represented as having a direct influence on respondent's education. This representation is suitable for an interpretation stressing the oldest brother's function as a role model or one hypothesizing that the older brother may render financial or other assistance to his younger siblings.

Neither of these interpretations, of course, is required by the data. Both rest heavily on the assumed temporal priority of brother's education with respect to respondent's. If the OCG question had pertained to any brother, predesignated at random, interpretations relying on temporal priority would become less plausible. Yet we might still expect to find substantial interfraternal correlations. If so, the interpretation might well include reference to the family climate —subsuming a variety of factors favorable or unfavorable to schooling —as an antecedent to the educational attainments of *both* brothers.

Among such factors, in addition to father's education and occupation, would be race or ethnic classification, geographic location, and family size—to mention only some obvious conditions common to the family and shared by the two brothers. We may suspect, moreover, that the prevailing orientation toward learning and educational achievement in the family, though surely not independent of the foregoing background conditions, will not be perfectly correlated therewith. Such an orientation, however it may come to be established, could thus have an independent effect on the number of years the brothers remain in school. Finally, we should recognize that two brothers may resemble one another, albeit imperfectly, in traits that are relevant to perseverance in school, apart from the common influence of home conditions and the prevailing intellectual atmosphere.

These arguments suggest that the interpretation of brother's education as an indicator of family climate is not entirely straightforward. Let us consider how some of the foregoing complications will affect the conclusions drawn from a causal model.

To begin with, we know that the model in Figure 9.2 fails to reckon with all the significant factors in socioeconomic background. In the multiple classification analysis, V and X (father's education and occupation) alone account for only 25.14 per cent of the variation in respondent's education, U (from Appendix Table H.3, men with nonfarm background). When ethnic classification, regional location, and sibling pattern are included as additional background items (in the combination B, E, X, V) the figure rises to 29.99 per cent. We can represent this situation in a linear causal model in a somewhat artificial but nonetheless useful way. Suppose we assigned a composite background score, J, to the respondent based on his classification by ethnic category, regional location, number of siblings, father's occupation, and father's education, using as weights the net deviations obtained in the multiple classification analysis for the combination of factors B, E, X, and V. Such a composite score would then have a correlation with respondent's education (U) of .548, which is the square root of .2999, because this combination explains 29.99 per cent of the variation in U.

Now, suppose that the analysis is repeated for a sample consisting of one brother of each respondent, selected at random from the respondents' families. Let such a brother's educational attainment be denoted U' and his composite background score J'. Assume further that $r_{U'J'} = r_{UJ} = .548$. We do not know precisely what value we would find for $r_{JJ'}$ (the correlation between the two background scores). Presumably it would not be perfect, as the two brothers could not have the same sibling position, although they would have the same number of siblings; and father's occupation when one brother was age 16 need not be the same as when the other brother was that age. Yet it is quite likely that the two background scores would correlate highly, perhaps as much as .98. Hence, for simplicity, we shall take it that $r_{JJ'} = 1$, or merely that $J' = J$.

Now, if these assumptions are made and if (a) there are no other common causes of U' and U and (b) neither brother's education depends on that of the other, we can compute immediately that $r_{UU'} = (.548)^2 = .2999$. If it were found, in fact, that $r_{UU'}$ has a value similar to that observed for r_{QU} in the OCG data, .556, we could immediately reject this simple interpretation, which says that the correlation between the educational attainments of two brothers is solely due to the common home and family conditions measured in this study. The outcome of the analysis would be as shown in Model 9.3.1: the residual or partial correlation between U and U', taking account of common socioeconomic background, is .366. This residual correlation merely tells us that *something* other than common socioeconomic background (as here measured) must be producing a substantial correlation between the two brothers' educational attainments.

We next consider some alternative ways to represent the ways of thinking about this "something" that have been suggested by or implicit in the earlier discussion. In each instance we again assume that $r_{UU'} = .556$ and $r_{U'J} = r_{UJ} = .548$.

In Model 9.3.2 we introduce a hypothetical variable, H, which the reader may think of as the intellectual climate of the home, or the

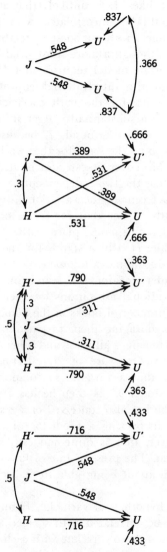

Model 9.3.1
Implies: $r_{UJ}^2 = .300$

Model 9.3.2
Implies: $r_{UH} = .648$
$R_{U(JH)}^2 = .557$

Model 9.3.3
Implies: $r_{UH} = .853$
$r_{UH'} = .488$
$R_{U(JH)}^2 = .868$

Model 9.3.4
Implies: $r_{UH} = .716$
$r_{UH'} = .358$
$R_{U(JH)}^2 = .812$

Figure 9.3. Alternative models for interpreting correlations among brothers' educational attainments (U and U'), composite socioeconomic background score (J), and hypothetical variables (H and H') described in the text. (All models assume $r_{UU'} = .556$ and $r_{UJ} = r_{U'J} = .548$.)

family's emphasis on learning, if he likes. It is unlikely that such a variable, if actually measured, would be uncorrelated with socioeconomic background. Here we assume a rather modest correlation of climate with background, $r_{HJ} = .3$, although a more substantial intercorrelation might be more realistic. The model requires that H and J in combination fully account for the interfraternal educational correlation, $r_{UU'} = .556$. When we solve for the path coefficients it turns out that climate, H, must have a substantially larger influence on son's education than socioeconomic background, J, because the respective path coefficients (assumed to be the same for the two brothers) are .531 for H and .389 for J. Moreover, it can also be deduced that $r_{UH} = .648$ and that the model has the two independent variables in combination accounting for 56 per cent of the variation in educational attainment (as compared with 30 per cent for socioeconomic background alone). It would seem that this model places rather severe demands on the unmeasured variable, H, which stands for the combination of factors antecedent to educational attainment collectively referred to as "climate." If the reader imagines a research in which parents are interviewed about educational aspirations for their children, attendance at PTA meetings, number of books in the home, aiding children in their homework, encouraging them to patronize the public library, and so on; and if he imagines all these and other likely indicators combined into a composite measure of "intellectual climate"; and, finally, if he supposes that a variable so compounded would perform like variable H in Model 9.3.2—then he has satisfied the assumptions of the model, but he has also conceived of a research that is uncommonly successful in discovering a predictor of educational attainment and one, moreover, that is quite modestly correlated with socioeconomic background. The present state of knowledge justifies no high degree of optimism about being able to realize such an enterprise.

In Model 9.3.3, we consider *two* hypothetical variables, H and H', each of which is again assumed to be correlated with socioeconomic background to the extent of .3, while the two correlate with each other only as much as .5. A variable that might possibly behave in this fashion is test intelligence, which has sometimes been found to be moderately related to socioeconomic status and to register an interfraternal correlation in the neighborhood of .5. We assume that respondent's intelligence directly affects only his own schooling, and that brother's intelligence affects only the brother's schooling, and that the model as described accounts for the observed correlation between the two measures of educational attainment. On these assumptions intelligence would have to be an exceptionally powerful predictor of educational outcome, for the path coefficient turns out to be $p_{UH} = p_{U'H'} = .790$, whereas the correlation is no less than $r_{UH} = r_{U'H'} = .853$. Such evidence as is known to us indicates that this is an unrealistically high value. Moreover, we may be skeptical of the extraordinarily high value of the coefficient of determination, $R^2_{U(JH)} = .868$, implying that the model accounts for five-sixths of the variation in the educational attainment of each brother. The assumption of such a high degree of determination makes this model appear even less realistic than the model focusing on educational climate.

The interesting feature of Model 9.3.3 is that the residual correlation between schooling of the two brothers not attributable to socioeconomic background is taken to be the result of a trait on which the brothers are similar but by no means identical, contrary to the situation in which we are postulating a condition common to all in the home. The same feature is again present in Model 9.3.4, but H and H' are here assumed to be uncorrelated with socioeconomic background. To identify a variable operating in just this way would be entirely speculative, but we might suppose that some trait of temperament, determined by heredity and thus virtually uncorrelated with socioeconomic environment, could perhaps be influencing the desires of the respective brothers to remain in school. The implications of this model are not greatly different from those of Model 9.3.3. Here, the path coefficient and the correlation for H (or H') are the same, in consequence of the assumption of zero correlation between H and J. Thus $r_{UH} = p_{UH} = .716$; and, in combination, H and J must account for 81 per cent of the variation in U (or U') to satisfy the assumption that the correlation between U and U' is exhausted by these variables. Once more we may perhaps be skeptical of the possibility that a "temperamental" variable of this degree of importance as a factor in schooling will soon be identified in empirical research.

In this discussion with models that are explicitly speculative—it would be presumptuous to call them merely "conjectural"—our purpose is to indicate that no simplistic assumption about the reasons for the interfraternal correlation in educational outcome is likely to prove correct. Each such assumption that we have entertained carries implications that strain our credulity. In fact we might almost claim to have demonstrated that not "intellectual climate" alone, not "intelligence" alone, and not "temperament" alone can account for the degree of resemblance in the educational attainment of two brothers that we actually observe.

On the other hand, something must account for it. No doubt a research undertaken to resolve this particular problem would be well advised to consider variables like all three of those on which we have speculated (not to mention still others that may come to mind). Although the correlation for brother's education that we initially observed, and which prompted this lengthy discussion, may have seemed none too high at .556, it turns out that it is high enough to make it worthwhile to address some considerable effort to explaining it. It will be no surprise if the ultimate explanation combines aspects of all the interpretive models we have entertained.

CONCLUSIONS

The structure of the parental family has been seen to affect the future careers of sons in a variety of ways. Most of the influences of family structure are mediated by education, the direc effects of either family size or sibling position on occupational acᵤievements being negligible. The proverbial large happy family is not conducive to occupational success. The task of raising many children evidently strains parental resources, with the result that the advantages of a higher education go predominantly to men with few siblings. Men from small families are more likely than men from large ones to continue their education on every level up to college graduation. However, college graduates from large families, many of whom had to overcome more serious obstacles than those most small-family boys had to face, are more likely to go on to graduate work.

Not only the size of the parental family but also a son's position in it exerts an influence on his subsequent career. In general the attainments of first-born and last-born children are superior to those of children in intermediate positions. The advantage or disadvantage associated with a given sibling position depends to some extent, however, on family size. Whereas there is little difference between the achievements of oldest and youngest children in small families, youngest sons are somewhat more successful than oldest in large families. In other words, sibling position and number of siblings interact in their effects on achievement.

The role relations among siblings in different family structures make the future success of an older child particularly dependent on being from a small family, since the differences in attainments between men with few and men with many siblings are greater for older than for younger sons. Older brothers are often called on to sacrifice their own occupational prospects and assume responsibility for younger siblings. The assistance older brothers furnish younger ones introduces a certain asymmetry into the influence of number of siblings on education. This asymmetry may be expressed by saying that having younger siblings is more disadvantageous than having older ones. Older brothers, therefore, are more handicapped by large families than are younger ones, for whom the disadvantage of having to share parental resources with many siblings is mitigated by the contribution older siblings make to their welfare and by having few younger siblings to help.

Eldest brother's education can be considered to indicate the educational climate in the parental family, specifically, how conducive the climate is to learning and achievement. The family climate, as indicated by oldest son's education, affects the educational attainments of younger sons even when background factors known also to affect education are controlled. Moreover, the educational advantage provided by small families, on whose resources fewer children make demands, is greater for men in families where education is important than for others. The implication is that a positive orientation to education in the family affects educational attainment, and through it occupational chances, by providing inducements to take full advantage of potential resources for obtaining an education, such as the greater resources available in small families. Without such an orientation the objective advantages of the small family are of little benefit. In short, it is the pertinent value orientation that activates potential economic resources and makes them serve as means for achievement and success.

The linear causal model of the process of stratification presented in Chapter 5 can be extended to represent alternative interpretations of the way in which the correlation between respondent's and brother's education arises. The possible mechanisms here are numerous, and it is difficult to rule out any one of them in the present state of our empirical knowledge. However, it does appear that treating brother's education *exclusively* as an indicator of the prevailing intellectual orientation or climate in the family of orientation—if we are to assume that such a factor or composite of factors is measurable in principle—is an overinterpretation of the data. In addition to the socioeconomic conditions of the family that we have measured in this research and the factors, whatever they may be, that comprise the family climate favoring or discouraging education, an adequate model will doubtlessly have to consider intellectual and motivational variables on which two brothers are likely to be moderately similar but not identical.

In sum, family size not only affects future chances of success by determining the resources available for the education of each child, but it also interacts with other conditions in the family to influence educational attainments and, thereby, occupational success. The careers of all men benefit from having few siblings, but those of oldest sons benefit more than those of younger ones. Older sons in large families appear to make sacrifices and assume responsibilities for younger ones. The resulting benefits that accrue to younger sons in large families compensate in part for the more limited resources available for any child if there are many. Hence younger sons are least disadvantaged by having many siblings. The educational benefits a small family is capable of providing, however, do not tend to be realized unless its climate is favorable to education, since a positive orientation to education is what induces parents and children to implement educational ambitions by drawing on potential resources, including the greater resources available in small families.

Although nearly the entire influence of the structure and climate of the parental family on occupational life is transmitted by education, this makes it no less important. The family into which a man is born exerts a profound influence on his career, because his occupational life is conditioned by his education, and his education depends to a considerable extent on his family.

CHAPTER 10

Marriage and Occupational Status

Several distinct questions arise in considering how patterns of marriage and the dissolution of marriage may be related to occupational achievement. First, we may look at the career from the standpoint of the family of orientation, inquiring whether a man who grew up in a home lacking one or both parents is handicapped in his career as compared with the man whose parents' marriage remained intact until he reached adolescence. Second, the contracting of a marriage by the man himself and the subsequent rupture of that marriage are contingencies that may have some bearing on his occupational success. Considering not just marital status alone but the characteristics of the spouse raises the third question: how much of the variation in men's occupational achievement may be attributed to differences in the status of the women they marry? The answer to this question turns out to depend heavily on the degree of assortative mating or homogamy. Hence our final inquiry has to do with the relationship between characteristics of husband and wife as of the time they marry.

BROKEN FAMILIES

The OCG question on this subject was, "Were you living with both your parents most of the time up to age 16? . . . If 'No,' . . . who was the head of your family?" (The respondent could check father, mother, other male, or other female.) Very nearly five-sixths of the respondents answered "yes" and are presumed to have lived in intact families at least through early adolescence. Not quite 4 per cent lived with father only, 9 per cent with mother only, 3 per cent in a family in which a man other than the father was the head, and 1 per cent in a family with another female as head. Almost 1 per cent failed to answer the question.

Given the overwhelming predominance of intact family background, we cannot expect this factor to produce any major variation in achieved status in the population at large, even if some categories of persons from broken homes are severely handicapped by the experience of family disruption. The analytical problem will be to see how such handicaps, if any, are transmitted in the process of stratification.

From the standpoint of causal analysis, the position of this variable is somewhat ambiguous. There is little question of its being causally prior to the three measures of achievement: education, first job, and occupational status in 1962. Whether it may be classified as either antecedent or subsequent to the measures of socioeconomic background—father's education and occupation—is another matter. On theoretical grounds we might wish to entertain the notion of reciprocal causation: a son born to parents of low status is in greater risk of losing one of them, particularly through separation, than a child born to affluence. In the other direction, the death of a parent or a breach of the parents' marriage may deplete the resources available to the child, in effect lowering the socioeconomic status of his background.

Another complication arises from the way the question was used in relation to the items on father's status. The questions on father's occupation and education carried this instruction, "If you were not living with your father, please answer for person checked [as head of your family]." To consider the possible impact of this instruction, we need to look at the pattern of nonresponse on the items involved (see Table 10.1). Although the instruction requested the respondent to

TABLE 10.1.   PER CENT NONRESPONSE TO OCG QUESTIONS ON FATHER'S OCC. AND EDUCATION, BY TYPE OF FAMILY IN WHICH RESPONDENT GREW UP

Type of Family	Total	Father's Occ. Not Reported	Father's Education Not Reported
All types	44,984	8.3	11.3
Both parents	37,087	3.6	9.4
Father only	1,167	7.1	19.1
Mother only	4,019	42.7	17.6
Other male head	1,403	9.9	17.7
Other female head	530	42.5	28.3
Not stated	326	63.8	64.7

report an occupation for the family head, whoever this might have been, about two-fifths of those with mother or another female as head were unable to make such a report. Thus the information we have on "father's occupation" actually pertains to a male head in 93 per cent of the cases, to a female head or unspecified person in 7 per cent. Although nonresponse on "father's education" was somewhat higher over-all, it was not so unevenly distributed by type of family.

In the multiple-classification analysis, "father's occupation not reported" and "father's education not reported" were simply treated as distinct categories in the respective classifications. This means that a disproportionate number of the NA's on these variables consist of respondents from broken families—about two-thirds of the NA's on father's occupation (64.5 per cent) and one-third of the NA's on father's education (31.9 per cent). When we look at net coefficients for type of family, we may, as a consequence, be holding constant too much. That is, we are in danger of attributing the effect of broken family to one of the two socioeconomic background items. Some care must be taken to avoid a conclusion based on statistical artifact. Fortunately, this problem arises only in connection with analyses in which educational attainment of respondent is the dependent variable. When first job or 1962 occupational status is at issue the problem can be by-passed, as will become apparent shortly.

Figure 10.1 represents the causal interpretation suggested on an extension of our basic model (Chapter 5) to include type of family as a background variable. For reasons given above it does not seem advisable to regard type of family as either antecedent or subsequent to father's education and occupation. Hence it is merely shown as being correlated with these variables. Following the pattern explained in Chapter 4, we may consider the relevant proportions of total sums of squares attributed to combinations of classifications in the multiple-classification analysis. These are shown, first, for the population of all men 20 to 64 years old and, second, for the subpopulation of men with nonfarm origins.

With 1962 occupational status (Y) as the dependent variable, we have the following results:

Combination of variables	Per cent of total $SS(Y)$	
	All	NF background
Family type	.69	1.54
W, U	40.93	40.26
W, U, and family type	41.00	40.48
W, U, X	41.93	41.14
W, U, X, and family type	41.98	41.26

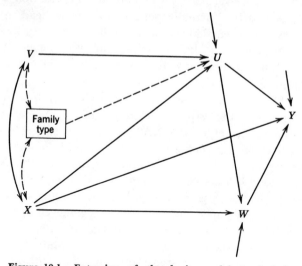

Figure 10.1. Extension of the basic model to include type of family as a background variable. (*Note:* Dashed lines represent hypothesized causal relationships or associations, but cannot be quantified with path coefficients or correlations, since family type is not a metric variable.)

Code: *V:* father's education.
         X: father's occupational status.
         U: respondent's education.
         W: respondent's first job, occupational status.
         Y: respondent's occupational status in 1962.

We are not surprised that family type has such a small gross relationship to occupational achievement. At least in the population with nonfarm background, however, the relationship is large enough to be worth considering. Our causal model suggests that education (*U*) and first job (*W*) are intervening variables. When these are entered into the multiple-classification analysis, the increment for family type in the combination *W, U,* and family type over the combination *W, U* is quite negligible: .07 per cent of total sum of squares in the total population, .22 in the population of nonfarm background. Finally the combinations involving *X* (father's occupation) suggest that a direct path from *X* to *Y* is needed, even when the correlation of *X* with family type is taken into account: the increment for *X* in each comparison is about 1 per cent of total *SS*.

Taking first-job status (*W*) as the dependent variable, the conclusion suggested by the figures below is much the same:

Combination	Per cent of total $SS(W)$	
	All	NF background
Family type	.34	.79
U	32.73	31.18
U and family type	32.80	31.34
U, X	35.86	33.61
U, X, and family type	35.89	33.71

Family type affords so small an increment over either U or the U, X combination as to render it negligible in terms of direct effect on W. Indeed its gross effect is already so small that we would be tempted to disregard it in any case.

Thus the effect, such as it is, of family type on occupational achievement is almost wholly transmitted via education. We must now examine whether effects of family type on education can be distinguished from those of the other two background variables. Here are the relevant summary figures:

Combination	Per cent of total $SS(U)$	
	All	NF background
Family type	1.11	1.94
X, V	27.94	25.14
X, V, and family type	28.22	25.39

By itself family type accounts for a larger proportion of the total sum of squares in U than in either W or Y. Its incremental contribution to the combination X, V is, however, rather unimpressive: .28 in the total population, .25 in the population with nonfarm background.

The introductory discussion warned, however, that such a result should not be accepted too hastily, inasmuch as the overlap of family type with the other two variables—which is what reduces its net contribution to explained sum of squares—may be artifactually enhanced by instructions given to respondents and by analytical procedures for handling these variables. This possibility cannot be readily explored in terms of explained sums of squares. We must examine the pattern of effects suggested by the multiple classification analysis. Table 10.2 reveals that this pattern is quite clear: any type of broken home handicaps a youth in regard to his educational attainment. To appreciate the order of magnitude of this effect, we must recall that the scoring of education is on a scale such that one point represents about two years of school. Except for the small group of respondents not stating family type, none of the effects approaches a full point on this scale. It is possible that the net effects are underestimated, insofar

TABLE 10.2. EFFECTS OF TYPE OF FAMILY ON EDUCATIONAL ATTAINMENT

	All Men		Men with Nonfarm Background	
Type of Family	No Controls (1)	Controlling Father's Education (V) and Occ. (X) (2)	No Controls (3)	Controlling Father's Education (V) and Occ. (X) (4)
Both parents	.08	.05	.11	.04
Father only	-.41	-.22	-.34	-.19
Mother only	-.28	-.20	-.44	-.15
Other male head	-.37	-.18	-.35	-.22
Other female head	-.62	-.32	-.73	-.29
Not stated	-1.03	-.43	-1.14	-.33
Mean all men	4.43	4.43	4.74	4.74

as the multiple classification analysis attributes some of the handicap of not having a father to the categories of father's occupation and education unknown in the X and V variables. For the "father only" and "other male head" types, however, the proportions not reporting father's occupation and education are not unduly high. Yet the net effects for these, as for the other categories of family type, are appreciably reduced by comparison with the gross effects.

Apparently we must conclude that a background of living in a broken family or with parents with disrupted marriages has some adverse effect on educational attainment, partially because of its association with socioeconomic background factors but partially for other reasons—assuming that socioeconomic influences are adequately indexed by our two measures thereof. The educational handicap is, in turn, translated into poorer than average occupational achievement, but there is little or no direct effect of rearing in a broken family on occupational success apart from this.

It is of passing interest, finally, that there is some evidence for intergenerational transmission of a liability for marital disruption. We consider the 1962 marital status of OCG men, excluding the widowed and the single, and identify those classified as married once, spouse present, as living in an intact first marriage. The remainder—the divorced, those married more than once, and those currently married but with the spouse absent—may be assumed to have experienced disruption of the first marriage. (It may be only a temporary disruption in the case of the "spouse absent" category.) The proportion of men with disrupted marriages is 15.6 per cent among those who lived with both parents, but 20.8 per cent among those coming from any type of broken home. Whether this effect holds up net of background or intervening socioeconomic circumstances that might be conducive to marital disruption cannot be readily ascertained from our tabulations.

MARITAL STATUS AS A CAREER CONTINGENCY

Turning to the respondent's own experience with marriage, our initial conceptual problem is to decide how marital status should be treated in an analysis of the process of stratification. Perhaps the most relevant consideration is that a classification by current marital status refers to events that occurred at some nonspecific time in the past. Ever-married men entered that status during their late teens or at some more advanced age. Those among them classified as married once, spouse present, have apparently undergone no subsequent change of status (although periods of separation from spouse may have intervened between marriage and 1962 without being recorded in the classification). At least two intervening events have occurred for men classified as married more than once, spouse present—disruption of at least one prior marriage and contracting of a new one. Of the widowed, divorced, and separated men (the last being grouped with "other" spouse-absent husbands), we can only say that at least one disruption of a marriage has occurred. Finally, the never-married—assuming their status to be correctly reported—have undergone no change in marital status at any time.

None of these events is dated, and none can be unequivocally ordered with respect to either (a) completion of schooling or (b) entry into first job. For a majority of men we may perhaps assume that marriage follows these two occasions, though this is certainly not true for a substantial minority. No doubt an even larger proportion of the instances of marriage disruption occur after educational attainment and first job status has been determined. As a first approximation, therefore, the causal ordering of Figure 10.2 is suggested as a framework for interpreting the relationships between marital status and occupational achievement.

This interpretation regards marital status as a "career contingency" —if a man marries or if his marriage is disrupted this may have a positive or negative effect on his subsequent occupational achievement. Of course the problem of causation is not really resolved, for it is possible that marriage or marriage disruption does not as such affect men's careers but rather that these events occur, with disproportionate frequency, to men who for other reasons are likely to achieve above or below average occupational status. The "selection" hypothe-

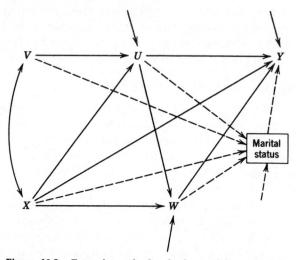

Figure 10.2. Extension of the basic model to include marital status as an intervening factor in the process of stratification. (*Note:* Dashed lines represent hypothesized causal relationships, but cannot be quantified with path coefficients, since marital status is not a metric variable.)

Code: *V:* father's education.
     X: father's occupational status.
     U: respondent's education.
     W: respondent's first job, occupational status.
     Y: respondent's occupational status in 1962.

sis, here as elsewhere, is a serious rival to the "causation" hypothesis. We can, however, carry out some statistical analysis designed to control for certain possible bases of selection. Thus Figure 10.2 implies that marital status has some net effect on occupational status, independent of its other measured determinants (*W*, *U*, and *X*, as well as *V*, indirectly). The following analysis is intended to ascertain whether this is a justified conclusion.

As in the preceding section, we consider whether the net contribution of the factor under study to total sum of squares (*SS*) accounted for is large enough to make it worthwhile discussing that factor's direct effect. Here, in view of the interpretation of marital status as a contingency intervening between education and first job status, on the one hand, and 1962 occupational status, on the other, we need only investigate the contribution of marital status to the "explanation" of variation in *Y*. The following summary presents the proportions of sums of squares due to the indicated combinations of variables in three populations—all men 20 to 64 years old, those with nonfarm background, and those whose fathers were in farm occupations:

Combination of variables	All	Per cent of total $SS(Y)$	
		Nonfarm	Farm
Marital status	1.25	1.28	1.37
U, W	40.93	40.26	28.13
U, W, X	41.93	41.14	—
U, W, marital status	41.95	41.29	28.88
U, W, X, marital status	42.95	42.19	—

We should not, of course, expect a major contribution to explained SS from marital status, since three-fourths of the men are in the same category of that classification. Its gross effects, however, are unmistakable, as over 1 per cent of total SS is accounted for by marital status alone. For all men and for men with nonfarm background, the increment due to marital status, in the combination U, W, X, marital status as compared with U, W, X, remains no less than 1 per cent. For men with farm background (father's occupation being held constant by the definition of the population), the increment due to marital status in combination with U and W is no larger than ¾ per cent, but this is still a reliable and not wholly negligible contribution.

To study the pattern of these effects refer to Table 10.3. In terms of gross effects the only clearly favorable category of marital status is married (in first marriage), wife present. The net effects, however, suggest a favorable influence of remarriage and widowhood as well. The divorced, separated, and never-married exhibit lower occupational achievements than other men. This conclusion stands however we resolve the issue of direction of causation. It is possible that lack of occupational success is a prelude to the disruption of a marriage or, on the other hand, that such a disruption has a disorganizing effect on the occupational career. Our data do not permit a decision on which of these mechanisms—if not both—is responsible for the net association of marital status with occupational achievement. The otherwise plausible interpretation that wives have a beneficial influence on careers is made quite questionable by the finding that widowers are as successful, taking into account background variables, as married men.

The results, of course, contain no surprise for sociologists, who have long been aware that married men are somewhat insulated from such forms of personal failure as delinquency and suicide. We have shown here, however, that the association of marriage with occupational

TABLE 10.3. EFFECTS OF MARITAL STATUS ON 1962 OCC. STATUS

Population and Marital Status	Number (Thousands)	1962 Occ. Status	
		No Controls	Controlling Education, First Job, Father's Occ.[a]
ALL MEN			
Married, spouse present			
In first marriage	31,075	1.6	1.2
Previously married	4,499	-1.6	.8
Widowed	558	-4.1	1.3
Divorced	1,027	-4.4	-1.6
Married, spouse absent	1,085	-8.9	-4.1
Never married	6,739	-3.9	-5.3
Mean for total	44,984	36.3	36.3
MEN WITH NONFARM BACKGROUND			
Married, spouse present			
In first marriage	22,532	1.7	1.3
Previously married	3,245	-2.1	.3
Widowed	369	-3.8	.8
Divorced	743	-4.2	-1.4
Married, spouse absent	765	-9.4	-4.1
Never married	5,229	-3.7	-5.2
Mean for total	32,879	40.1	40.1
MEN WITH FARM BACKGROUND			
Married, spouse present			
In first marriage	8,546	1.2	.6
Previously married	1,255	.4	1.9
Widowed	189	-.7	3.7
Divorced	284	-4.2	-1.8
Married, spouse absent	322	-5.7	-2.9
Never married	1,511	-5.1	-4.5
Mean for total	12,105	27.3	27.3

[a]Father's occ. not included as a control variable for men with farm background, since this population is defined on the basis of father's occ.

achievement is not readily explained away by a combination of obviously relevant background variables and prior achievements. The net effect of marital status is by no means pronounced. We may, moreover, have overestimated it slightly by failing to include a control on age (in particular, this may account for the especially unfavorable effect of remaining single, because the single men are concentrated in the age interval 20 to 24). Nevertheless, it seems clear that contracting a marriage and maintaining it intact are favorable signs for the occupational career.

MAKING A GOOD MATCH

If there is any proposition that is popularly accepted as an axiom of social mobility, it is that a man "on his way up" is well advised to make a good marriage. No doubt he is. The proposition to be examined here is that the kind of marriage a man contracts will affect the level of his occupational achievement. Specifically, we wish to raise the question of *how much* difference the marriage makes. As will become evident, the analysis is somewhat formidable, yet the interpretation cannot be wholly unequivocal in the end.

In this analysis we shall be concerned only with *white* respondents who were living with their spouses in March 1962. The respondents are classified by age of the wife in 1962 into eight five-year intervals from 22–26 to 57–61. Hence there are eight parallel analyses for that many cohorts. We have already observed in the preceding section that men living with their wives in 1962 were a somewhat select group in respect to occupational status, as compared with the widowed, divorced, separated, and single men.

As a base line for comparisons, we show in the first panel of Table 10.4 (Model I) the results of calculations like those reported in previous summaries of the regression analysis. Respondent's occupational status in 1962 is assumed to be influenced by the status of his

TABLE 10.4. PATH COEFFICIENTS FOR VARIABLES AFFECTING OCC. STATUS IN 1962, DERIVED FROM THREE ALTERNATIVE MODELS, FOR WHITE OCG RESPONDENTS LIVING WITH WIVES 22 TO 61 YEARS OF AGE, BY AGE OF WIFE

Independent Variables	Age of Wife							
	22–26	27–31	32–36	37–41	42–46	47–51	52–56	57–61
MODEL I[a]								
Respondent's first job	.323	.258	.219	.206	.219	.208	.220	.259
Respondent's education	.437	.484	.488	.437	.444	.435	.375	.363
Father's occ. status	.034	.096	.105	.108	.086	.130	.098	.172
Multiple R-squared	.472	.518	.477	.399	.398	.423	.339	.415
MODEL II[a]								
Respondent's first job	.310	.242	.210	.195	.212	.200	.209	.254
Respondent's education	.395	.419	.448	.389	.399	.390	.308	.319
Father's occ. status	.022	.081	.095	.091	.072	.119	.076	.150
Wife's education	.053	.069	.044	.068	.052	.076	.091	042
Wife's father's occ. status	.055	.101	.064	.069	.063	.028	.081	.074
Multiple R-squared	.476	.531	.483	.408	.404	.428	.351	.421
MODEL III[a]								
Respondent's first job	.260	.166	.165	.122	.149	.119	.132	.215
Respondent's education	.376	.408	.440	.359	.382	.348	.283	.302
Father's occ. status	-.031	-.018	.038	.037	.015	.111	.007	.081
Hypothetical factor (H)	.306	.394	.292	.339	.307	.320	.355	.310
Multiple R-squared	.476	.531	.483	.408	.404	.428	.351	.421

[a]See Figure 10.3.

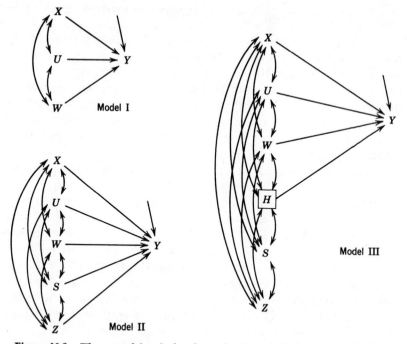

Figure 10.3. Three models of the determination of husband's occupational status in 1962.

Code: Y: husband's occupational status, 1962.
      X: husband's father's occupational status.
      U: husband's educational attainment.
      W: occupational status of husband's first job.
      S: wife's educational attainment.
      Z: wife's father's occupational status.
      H: hypothetical variable, unspecified characteristic of husband.

first job, his educational attainment, and the status of his father's occupation, as shown in Figure 10.3. The patterns are much like those already described in Chapter 5 and need no further discussion.

In the second panel we consider Model II, which incorporates two additional determinants of 1962 occupational status, wife's education and her father's occupational status. In estimating the path coefficients for these five variables we must, of course, take into account their intercorrelations. It is noted in the next section that the correlation between the occupational statuses of the spouses' fathers varies between .25 and .37 for the eight age groups, with most values being very close to .3. Moreover, the educational attainment of the wife is correlated with that of the husband about .6 (variation over cohorts being from .55 to .63).

With assortative mating this pronounced we cannot expect the net effects of the wife's characteristics on husband's occupational status to be substantial. In fact, none of the R^2 values for the five-variable model exceeds the corresponding one for the three-variable model (omitting wife's characteristics) by more than .013. From this point of view the kind of marriage match a man makes does not loom large as a predictor of his occupational success. Of course we are here taking assortative mating as given. This process guarantees that most men will have mated in a way that is appropriate to their backgrounds or their qualifications for occupational achievement.

The same result is seen in the path coefficients for wife's education and father-in-law's occupational status in Table 10.4. There is some fluctuation over age groups, but in order of magnitude these are comparable to the path for the occupational status of the respondent's own father. Most of these coefficients have standard errors in the neighborhood of .02 to .04. Hence a few of them, individually, might not be statistically significant. However, the consistently positive values over eight age groups virtually rule out "chance" as an explanation for their differences from zero. Small though the paths are for the wife's characteristics, there can be no doubt of their reality, assuming the correctness of the model. In brief, a man's occupational status is about as much related to that of his father-in-law as to that of his own father.

Model II is, in fact, only one possible interpretation of the observations. We wish to call attention to another that is quite conceivable, though no independent evidence supporting it is at hand. We might reason that the list of respondent's characteristics taken as determinants of occupational status is far from exhaustive. It would be easy to make an *a priori* case for several additional determinants: motivation, intellectual ability, age at marriage (possibly an indicator of the "deferred gratification syndrome"), and so on. Most of the items that come readily to mind would probably be correlated with variables that we have measured—not only the husband's characteristics but also those of the wife. Hence we should entertain the possibility that inclusion of one or more additional variables could alter the pattern of path coefficients we have estimated from the data at hand. There is no way to be sure how the result would come out, but we can illustrate one possible result (see Figure 10.3, Model III).

Assume a hypothetical variable H to represent any one or a combination of characteristics of the husband we have not measured in this study. By placing some arbitrary but not unreasonable conditions on H and observing how it then operates in Model III we wish to ascertain whether our data are compatible with an interpretation requiring that occupational achievement be accounted for entirely by characteristics of the husband and not at all, in any direct fashion, by those of the wife. Let Y be the dependent variable, X, U, and W the measured characteristics of the husband, and S and Z the measured characteristics of the wife. We know $(5)(4)/2 = 10$ intercorrelations of the measured independent variables and five correlations of the dependent variable with each of the independent variables. We can write five equations corresponding to the latter, including H as a sixth independent variable:

$$r_{YX} = p_{YX} + p_{YU}r_{UX} + p_{YW}r_{WX} + p_{YH}r_{XH}$$
$$r_{YU} = p_{YX}r_{UX} + p_{YU} + p_{YW}r_{UW} + p_{YH}r_{UH}$$
$$r_{YW} = p_{YX}r_{XW} + p_{YU}r_{UW} + p_{YW} + p_{YH}r_{WH}$$
$$r_{YS} = p_{YX}r_{XS} + p_{YU}r_{US} + p_{YW}r_{WS} + p_{YH}r_{SH}$$
$$r_{YZ} = p_{YX}r_{XZ} + p_{YU}r_{UZ} + p_{YW}r_{WZ} + p_{YH}r_{ZH}$$

This system does not include p_{YS} and p_{YZ}, because in this illustration we are assuming that H operates in such a way as to make them zero. Our five equations, therefore, contain four paths to be estimated and five correlations ($r_{XH}, \ldots, r_{ZH}$) that are unknown, for a total of nine unknowns. We reduce the number of unknowns to six by assuming

$$r_{UH} = r_{WH} = r_{SH} \quad \text{and} \quad r_{XH} = r_{ZH}$$

(that is, H correlates the same with the three measures pertaining directly to the spouses and also the same with the two measures pertaining to the two fathers). For the sixth condition required to obtain an explicit solution, let us suppose that $R^2_{Y(XUWH)} = R^2_{Y(XUWSZ)}$; that is, we assume that inclusion of H increases predictability over the three-variable model to just exactly the same extent that the five-variable model improves over the 3-variable model. These arbitrary assumptions need cause no anxiety if we bear in mind that the entire calculation is hypothetical. The foregoing condition can be spelled out algebraically:

$$R^2_{Y(XUWH)} = p_{YX}r_{YX} + p_{YU}r_{YU} + p_{YW}r_{YW} + p_{YH}r_{YH},$$

where

$$r_{YH} = p_{YH} + p_{YX}r_{XH} + p_{YU}r_{UH} + p_{YW}r_{WH},$$

and where $R^2_{Y(XUWH)}$ is given the value obtained for $R^2_{Y(XUWSZ)}$ with Model II.

The solution for the six unknowns is straightforward, albeit a bit tedious. The results are shown for Model III in the bottom panel of Table 10.4. What is perhaps most interesting about them is that H emerges as a relatively important determinant of Y. The paths, p_{YH}, for the eight age groups range from .29 to .39, and the correlations, r_{YH}, from .53 to .65, which makes H nearly as important as respondent's education. Although these magnitudes are not trivial, it is perfectly possible that some variable not measured (or a combination of such variables) could behave in somewhat the fashion postulated for H. It turns out, incidentally, that the two distinct values assumed for the intercorrelations of H with the remaining independent variables vary between .3 and .5 over the age groups. These are not at all implausible values for such characteristics of the husband as his occupational abilities, class identification, and achievement motivation.

We conclude: (1) Because of assortative mating, knowing the two characteristics of the wife that we measured adds little to the accuracy with which we can predict the respondent's occupational status on the basis of the three characteristics measured for the respondent. (2) The net, or direct, effects of these characteristics of the wife, though they are modest in magnitude, cannot be dismissed as chance findings. (3) It is quite possible, however, that they would disappear in a system of variables including one or more strategic characteristics of the husband that we failed to measure in this study.

The third conclusion is, of course, the kind of logical *caveat* that should be implicit in any statement of findings based on regression analysis of observational data. Here we have made it not only explicit but also plausible. (It might have happened, for example, that the implied path coefficients or correlations involving H were implausible, which would have required rejection of the alternative interpretation provided by Model III.)

Another possible reservation concerning our conclusion arises from the fact that we have not considered the interaction of husband's and wife's characteristics with respect to the husband's subsequent occupational achievement. Although the wife's characteristics have little net effect in an additive model, it may be argued that pronounced discrepancies between, say, the educational levels of the spouses produce a distinctive effect on the husband's occupational status. The force of this reservation is diminished, however, by the very fact of pronounced assortative mating. It is a statistical truism that two highly correlated variables seldom have large interaction effects. Even if such effects were noted for the extreme cases of husband–wife discrepancy (and this is only a hypothetical possibility, not supported by any available evidence), the rarity of such cases guarantees that the variation in occupational status attributable to interaction would be slight.

Lest there be misunderstanding, it should be emphasized that none of our conclusions implies that patterns of mate selection are an insignificant part of the process of stratification. Rather, the force of these conclusions is to push the analysis back to the prior phase of assortative mating itself. Instead of focusing on what making a good match does for a man's career, we should be looking for an explanation of how matches get made.

ASSORTATIVE MATING[1]

The previous section brought out the importance of assortative mating in the context of estimating the contribution of variation in the wife's characteristics to variation in the husband's achievement. The topic has a wider interest, as is suggested by the proliferation of sociological inquiries on mate selection[2] and the significant role assigned to assortative mating in theories of human genetics.[3] In the literature on occupational mobility most of the major national studies have included material on the topic, and Geiger, in particular, considered it at length.[4]

Our analysis falls into two major parts: first, a detailed examination of the cross-classification of the occupations of the fathers of the husband and wife; and, second, a more compact treatment of assortment by occupational origin in relation to other characteristics of the spouses.

The basic data on parental occupations are given in Appendix Table J10.1. The first task, readily accomplished, is to demonstrate the occurrence of assortment with respect to occupational background. By assortative mating, of course, we merely mean some systematic departure from random mating. Such a departure might, in theory, involve a greater number of pronounced discrepancies between characteristics of husband and wife than would occur by chance. In regard to socioeconomic characteristics, however, this type of negative assort-

---

[1] Much of this section and the next is based on two papers by Bruce L. Warren, "A Multiple Variable Approach to the Assortative Mating Phenomenon" *Eugenics Quarterly*, 13(1966), 285-290; and "Assortative Mating: a Review of the Literature and Some New Findings" (1964, unpublished).

[2] See the review of literature in Alain Girard, *Le choix du conjoint*, Cahier No. 44, Institut national d'études démographiques (Paris: Presses Universitaires de France, 1964).

[3] J. N. Spuhler, "Empirical Studies on Quantitative Human Genetics," in *The Use of Vital and Health Statistics for Genetic and Radiation Studies*, New York: United Nations, 1962.

[4] Theodor Geiger, *Soziale Umschichtungen in einer Dänischen Mittelstadt*, Acta Jutlandica, XXIII, Copenhagen: Ejnar Munksgaard, 1951.

ment is seldom observed. We find, instead, homogamy; that is, spouses tend to resemble each other more closely than would be the case under random rating.

Table 10.5 takes as the norm of comparison the model of independence, and the observed frequencies of husband's father's occupation by wife's father's occupation are shown as relative departures from this chance model. That is, if O_{ij} is the observed frequency of couples in which the husband originated in occupation group i and the wife in group j, and E_{ij} is the corresponding frequency expected on the hypothesis of independence, the relative departure is defined as $(O_{ij} - E_{ij})/E_{ij}$ or $(O_{ij}/E_{ij}) - 1$, which is the quantity entered in Table 10.5. (This value plus 1 is identical with the index of association used in Chapter 2.) Positive values indicate that the combinations of backgrounds occur with greater than chance frequency; negative values indicate that they occur with less than chance frequency. If random mating were in effect the values would all be near zero.

In Table 10.5 the nonfarm occupations are in rank order by socioeconomic status, except that the aggregate of sales occupations should perhaps be placed above self-employed MOP (essentially proprietors). In fact the index of occupational status differs very little for the three lowest white-collar occupations, so that the question of rank here is perhaps moot. Accepting the ranking as given, it is apparent at once that assortment with respect to occupational background takes the form of a tendency toward homogamy, or greater similarity between spouses than would be expected by chance. All diagonal cells have positive entries, as do a number of other cells relatively close to the diagonal.

The suggestion advanced in Chapter 2 concerning class boundaries may be re-examined with these data. The hypothesis concerns a disjunction between white-collar and manual occupations—between categories (6) and (7)—and one between manual and farm occupations—between (10) and (11). The argument calls for a pattern of class endogamy, so that positive departures should appear in the three large diagonal blocks outlined in the lower half of Table 10.5, and negative departures elsewhere. To facilitate inspection, exceptions to this pattern are identified with the symbol "O" in the bottom half of the table.

It sometimes happens that corresponding cells above and below the diagonal have different signs, though the low frequency of such inconsistencies is surprising in view of the fact that the cell frequencies have substantial sampling errors. In studying exceptions to the endogamous pattern, therefore, we may well confine attention to cells in

TABLE 10.5. ASSORTATIVE MATING WITH RESPECT TO FATHER'S OCC., FOR OCG COUPLES IN WHICH WIFE WAS 22 TO 61 YEARS OLD IN MARCH, 1962: RELATIVE DEPARTURES FROM FREQUENCIES EXPECTED ON THE HYPOTHESIS OF INDEPENDENCE, (OBSERVED − EXPECTED)/EXPECTED

Husband's Father's Occ.	Wife's Father's Occ. (see stub)											
	(1)	(2)	(3)	(4)	(5)	(6)	(7)	(8)	(9)	(10)	(11)	(12)
(1) Prof., S-E	1.92	1.42	1.28	1.31	1.09	.61	−.06	−.57	−.25	−.77	−.44	−.80
(2) Prof., sal.	2.06	1.44	1.22	.86	.38	.27	.07	−.27	.05	−.60	−.56	−.75
(3) MOP, sal.	1.45	.58	1.60	.54	.86	1.10	−.07	−.17	.35	−.51	−.53	−.93
(4) MOP, S-E	1.55	.48	.24	1.12	.53	.24	−.03	−.17	.22	−.47	−.36	−.80
(5) Sales	.44	.41	.77	.59	1.59	.47	.16	−.27	.20	−.28	−.56	−.38
(6) Clerical	.61	.39	.40	.49	.61	.05	.09	−.20	.48	−.08	−.40	−.16
(7) Crafts	−.28	.15	.12	−.07	−.07	.24	.40	.15	.05	.08	−.42	−.41
(8) Operatives	−.46	−.26	−.35	−.21	−.04	−.11	.18	.74	.05	.12	−.45	−.29
(9) Service	−.10	−.22	−.33	−.04	−.17	.35	.36	−.07	.79	.19	−.48	−.24
(10) Laborers	−.22	−.27	−.54	−.38	−.09	.03	−.14	.26	.24	1.81	−.42	1.04
(11) Farmers	−.60	−.48	−.46	−.42	−.54	−.49	−.41	−.34	−.41	−.23	1.12	.15
(12) Farm labor	−.41	−.39	−.55	−.65	−.33	−.46	−.20	−.19	−.21	.71	−.11	7.43

Analysis of Pattern[a]

	(1)	(2)	(3)	(4)	(5)	(6)	(7)	(8)	(9)	(10)	(11)	(12)
(1) Prof., S-E	⋮	⋮	⋮	⋮	⋮	⋮	⋮	⋮	⋮	⋮	⋮	⋮
(2) Prof., sal.	⋮	⋮	⋮	⋮	⋮	⋮	0	⋮	0	⋮	⋮	⋮
(3) MOP, sal.	⋮	⋮	⋮	⋮	⋮	⋮	X	⋮	0	⋮	⋮	⋮
(4) MOP, S-E	⋮	⋮	X,0	⋮	⋮	⋮	X,0	⋮	X,0	⋮	⋮	⋮
(5) Sales	⋮	⋮	⋮	⋮	X	⋮	0	⋮	0	⋮	⋮	⋮
(6) Clerical	⋮	⋮	⋮	⋮	⋮	⋮	⋮	⋮	⋮	X	⋮	⋮
(7) Crafts	⋮	0	X,0	⋮	X	0	⋮	⋮	⋮	⋮	⋮	⋮
(8) Operatives	⋮	⋮	⋮	⋮	⋮	⋮	⋮	⋮	X	⋮	⋮	⋮
(9) Service	⋮	0	⋮	⋮	X	⋮	⋮	X,0	⋮	⋮	⋮	⋮
(10) Laborers	⋮	⋮	⋮	⋮	⋮	X,0	⋮	⋮	⋮	⋮	⋮	0
(11) Farmers	⋮	⋮	⋮	⋮	⋮	⋮	⋮	⋮	⋮	⋮	X,0	⋮
(12) Farm Labor	⋮	⋮	⋮	⋮	⋮	⋮	⋮	⋮	⋮	⋮	X,0	X

[a] Lines represent hypothesized class boundaries.   0: Exceptions to class endogamy.   X: Asymmetry of sign pattern.

which the exception occurs consistently. This is the case for seven pairs of cells (out of the 66 possible pairs). Marriages between offspring of craftsmen and offspring of two of the white-collar groups—salaried professional and clerical—exceed chance frequency, contrary to the hypothesis of class endogamy. Similar exceptions apply to marriages of offspring of service workers with offspring of four white-collar occupations: salaried professional, both groups of MOP, and clerical. Finally, marriages involving the combination of backgrounds of farm laborer with nonfarm laborer occur with greater than chance frequency across the manual-farm boundary.

Unfortunately, we lack a criterion for the number of exceptions required for the rejection of the hypothesis of class boundaries. If the hypothesis is not rejected outright, it should certainly be qualified by the recognition that service occupations are in an anomalous position. If, for the sake of argument, we changed the rank of service workers so that this occupation fell between clerical and craft workers, it would present exceptions whether it was grouped with the white-collar or with the manual pursuits. It is true, of course, that the classification of service occupations is problematic. Their educational and income levels justify grouping them with the manual pursuits. The work context of many of the specific service occupations, however, is an office or business establishment, and their situation therein is not greatly different from that of the lower white-collar occupations. Such a context, moreover, offers a wider range of opportunities for contact with higher status occupations than are open to the typical manual worker.

A final comment on Table 10.5 concerns its general appearance of symmetry. We should not expect a perfectly symmetrical table, both because the data are subject to sampling errors and because the marginal distributions (see Table J10.1) are not identical. The lack of coincidence of the marginal distributions of husbands and wives by occupational origin arises, in part, from the fact that they are drawn from different birth cohorts. There is also the awkward circumstance that we are lacking data for about 15 per cent of the eligible couples because of nonreporting of father's occupation by one or both spouses. Despite the distortions that may have been produced in the data for these reasons, a strong tendency toward symmetry is evident at least in the sign pattern of the relative departures. Only five of the 66 pairs of cells in corresponding positions across the diagonal exhibit discrepant signs (see lower half of Table 10.5). There are perhaps some systematic departures from symmetry in regard to magnitudes rather than signs. If so, these should be reflected in the further analysis of these data to which we now proceed.

In Table 10.6 the index of dissimilarity is used in the way previously explained in Chapter 2. We consider the dissimilarity of occupations of wife's origin (her father's occupational status) with respect to their distributions by husband's origin; and, conversely, the dissimilarity of occupations of husband's origin with respect to their distributions by wife's origin. The two sets of indices are given, respectively, above and below the diagonal of Table 10.6. If the basic frequency table were perfectly symmetrical, the two parts of Table 10.6 would, of course, be identical. Evidently they are not identical. Yet there is a very high correlation between the two sets of "distances." Both sets exhibit a general tendency for distance to increase the further apart two occupations are in status rank order; but both also show similar departures from this general tendency. In line with the observation already made, a number of these departures concern the service occupations. In addition, the indices for the two farm occupations do not fall into a neat pattern.

As in the previous work with mobility tables (Chapter 2), we are led to consider whether a formal analysis of the pattern of distances clarifies the interpretation. Again, we rely on the Guttman-Lingoes smallest-space program. In a one-dimensional space the data identified as set A in Table 10.7 have a coefficient of alienation of .127; the two-dimensional solution reduces this to .050. Nearly identical results are obtained for set B: a coefficient of alienation of .126 for the one-dimensional solution and .060 for the two-dimensional. We accept the two-dimensional solutions presented in Table 10.7 as the basis for further discussion. The scale values are arbitrary, and the solution has been subjected to a plane rotation, so that the first dimension is defined by the straight line between self-employed professional and nonfarm laborers. The rotation and the transformation of scales are, of course, intended merely to effect a convenience in presentation and interpretation. The essential properties of the solution are not thereby affected.

Broad similarities between the two sets of solution values reflect the general tendency toward symmetry of the assortative mating table already discerned. There is a very high correlation between the first-dimension values for set A and those for set B. Indeed, omitting the farm occupations, this correlation is nearly perfect, except for one occupation: salaried professional. This has a rather lower value in the set A solution than in the solution for set B, and a surprisingly low value for set A in the light of the status score for this occupation, to which we refer shortly. The solutions for the two sets are not fully

TABLE 10.6. INDICES OF DISSIMILARITY BETWEEN PAIRS OF OCCUPATIONS IN TABLE OF ASSORTATIVE MATING BY PARENTAL OCC. ABOVE DIAGONAL: DISSIMILARITY BETWEEN WIFE'S FATHER'S OCC. GROUPS WITH RESPECT TO HUSBAND'S FATHER'S OCC.; BELOW DIAGONAL: DISSIMILARITY BETWEEN HUSBAND'S FATHER'S OCC. GROUPS WITH RESPECT TO WIFE'S FATHER'S OCC.

Occ.	(1)	(2)	(3)	(4)	(5)	(6)	(7)	(8)	(9)	(10)	(11)	(12)
(1) Prof., S-E	...	15.9	17.2	14.1	17.9	22.0	31.3	37.5	26.6	42.3	48.9	51.0
(2) Prof., sal.	10.7	...	6.8	8.6	11.8	8.8	15.7	23.2	13.2	28.1	45.5	45.5
(3) MOP, sal.	13.8	10.4	...	11.4	14.3	9.7	18.4	26.5	15.3	30.7	45.9	47.6
(4) MOP, S-E	13.5	10.9	10.1	...	11.0	14.0	19.4	26.1	14.7	30.4	44.4	45.0
(5) Sales	17.8	11.1	10.8	13.1	...	11.3	18.9	24.8	13.9	29.6	46.8	45.7
(6) Clerical	19.8	13.6	12.1	8.5	9.0	...	10.7	19.5	10.0	24.4	45.9	44.1
(7) Crafts	29.8	22.7	22.8	18.6	18.1	13.8	...	13.0	9.2	18.9	43.0	42.2
(8) Operatives	36.0	28.5	28.6	25.2	23.8	19.5	11.0	...	14.9	16.2	41.2	38.0
(9) Service	28.9	20.8	19.5	18.1	15.2	11.4	6.7	15.7	...	18.5	43.0	40.1
(10) Laborers	38.4	33.9	30.4	27.2	30.2	23.4	17.8	16.7	21.6	...	39.1	27.8
(11) Farmers	49.5	47.4	46.5	41.6	44.5	39.2	40.6	41.1	41.8	39.6	...	33.3
(12) Farm labor	45.0	41.6	39.2	34.2	38.6	31.1	31.2	31.6	31.7	23.6	33.4	...

Occ. (see stub)

TABLE 10.7. OCC. STATUS SCORES AND TWO-DIMENSIONAL GUTTMAN-LINGOES SOLUTIONS FOR THE INDICES OF DISSIMILARITY IN TABLE 10.6

Occ.	Occ. Status Score[a]	Guttman-Lingoes Solution[b]			
		Set (A)		Set (B)	
		First Dimension	Second Dimension	First Dimension	Second Dimension
Prof., S-E	84	77	8	77	15
Prof., sal.	73	59	7	68	7
MOP, sal.	68	63	6	63	12
MOP, S-E	47	62	10	56	17
Sales	49	59	0	55	5
Clerical	45	55	4	49	15
Crafts	31	45	4	34	7
Operatives	18	38	14	23	0
Service	17	48	7	39	2
Laborers	7	30	8	15	15
Farmers	14	15	52	24	83
Farm laborers	9	0	16	0	40

[a] From Reiss, Occupations and Social Status, op. cit., Table VII-4, supplemented by crude estimates for the distinction between self-employed and salaried professional and MOP.

[b] Set (A) refers to indices above the diagonal in Table 10.6, Set (B) to indices below the diagonal in Table 10.6.

consistent in their placement of farm occupations on the first dimension. Reference back to the original indexes of dissimilarity indicates why this is so. In set B farmers are in all instances farther from nonfarm occupations than are farm laborers, but in set A there are several exceptions to this pattern.

Apart from the two farm occupations, both solutions show very slight variation on the second dimension, and there is little correlation between the two. There is agreement between them, however, in regard to the high value for farmers on the second dimension. Apparently in both solutions the second dimension functions primarily to represent the fact that farm occupations are distant from all other occupations and do not really fit into a unidimensional ranking very well.

It seems apparent that the first dimension in both solutions is essentially the socioeconomic status ordering of the occupations. Hence the first column of Table 10.7 shows the status scores, and in Figure 10.4 each set of first-dimension values is plotted against the scores. The chart reveals that the first dimension in both solutions has a straight-line relationship to the status score, with certain interesting

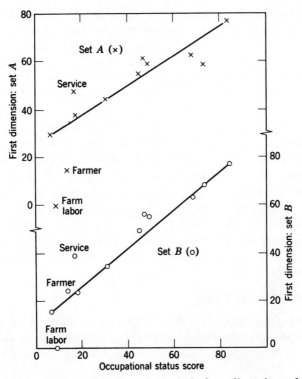

Figure 10.4. Relationship of rotated first dimension of Guttman-Lingoes solution to occupational status score (based on data shown in Table 10.7). (*Note:* The lines connect points for self-employed professional and nonfarm laborers; they are not least-squares regression lines.)

exceptions. In set *A* neither farm occupation fits on this line, and in set *B* the value for farm laborers is rather lower than would be expected from its status score. In addition, both solutions yield a considerably higher value for service occupations than a straight-line relationship would suggest.

The case for a "class" effect in assortative mating that goes beyond the socioeconomic effect is perhaps strengthened by these observations on the farm occupations. Marriage across the farm–nonfarm boundary, of course, encounters the obstacle of spatial separation as well as that of social distance. The result for service occupations invites other kinds of speculation. It may be that the status score is somewhat misleading in the present context. The score was originally determined for all economically active males in the 1950 labor force, including both very young and very old men. There are certain service occupations with pronounced patterns of age grading, and some of these may not be proportionately represented in data on the fathers of persons who were 16 years old. Another consideration previously noted is that many service occupations involve more regular contact with white-collar persons than other manual pursuits. Thus the opportunity for out-marriage from the manual level may be enhanced for children of service workers.

There are some other discernible departures from a straight-line relationship of first-dimension values to occupational status. These, however, do not have any obvious explanation. Moreover, we should not overemphasize such deviations at the expense of the strong evidence that the major pattern of assortative mating by occupational background consists in the tendency toward status homogamy. Although this result was not unexpected it is perhaps surprising that it should show up so unequivocally. We are encouraged to pursue the problem of assortative mating with an approach that relies solely on the correlation of occupational status scores.

EDUCATIONAL HOMOGAMY

One way of summarizing the results just reviewed is to state that they indicate an appreciable correlation between the status of the wife's father's occupation and the status of the husband's father's occupation. However, the analysis was designed to reveal the pattern of the association, not to obtain a single summary figure for its order of magnitude. For the latter purpose we make use of data in which the parental occupations, initially coded in detailed categories, are scored on the index of occupational status. With such data it may be determined that the correlation is approximately .3. In Table 10.8 the correlation is shown in column 3 for each of eight white cohorts and five nonwhite cohorts. The data for whites fluctuate, though not very widely, around a value of .3; the results for nonwhites, ranging between .11 and .37, are more erratic, which is not surprising in view of the small samples of nonwhites.

Table 10.8 confirms that there is appreciable assortment with respect to parental occupational status, but it also shows a much closer approach to homogamy in the educational attainment of the spouses themselves (column 2). For the white cohorts assortative mating with respect to education of bride and groom is well represented by a correlation of about .6, and the individual cohort correlations deviate little from this central tendency. Most of the nonwhite cohorts show a comparably high value, despite more marked fluctuations in the correlations.

TABLE 10.8. SIMPLE AND PARTIAL CORRELATIONS BETWEEN SELECTED CHARACTERISTICS OF SPOUSES, BY COLOR AND AGE OF WIFE

Color and Age of Wife	Number of Couples[a] (Thousands) (1)	Years of School Completed (2)	Father's Occ. Status (3)	Number of Siblings (4)	Father's Occ. Status, Holding Constant--	
					Education (5)	5 Variables[b] (6)
WHITE						
22 to 26	3,726	.63	.31	.21	.16	.12
27 to 31	4,077	.61	.27	.17	.10	.09
32 to 36	4,685	.59	.25	.19	.10	.07
37 to 41	4,907	.55	.31	.17	.18	.15
42 to 46	4,311	.62	.30	.20	.18	.16
47 to 51	3,785	.60	.29	.16	.14	.11
52 to 56	2,810	.60	.32	.15	.21	.17
57 to 61	1,846	.63	.37	.18	.25	.20
NONWHITE						
22 to 26	393	.52	.30	-.02		
27 to 31	417	.62	.21	.07		
32 to 36	473	.70	.37	.20	(not computed)	
37 to 41	458	.39	.16	.13		
42 to 61	984	.62	.11	.01		

[a]Includes couples not reporting on certain variables.
[b]Educational attainment and number of siblings of both spouses, and status of husband's first job.

One other characteristic of the spouses may be studied in the same way, the respective number of siblings of husband and wife. Here we observe a correlation approaching .2 for each of the white cohorts, although the correlations for nonwhites are not at all consistent.

The three series of correlations demonstrate that assortative mating occurs for more than one social characteristic, but that the degree of assortment (or magnitude of the correlation) varies considerably from one characteristic to another. This kind of variation has been previously noted in the literature, where coefficients for a considerable number of anthropometric and psychometric traits are reported. Variations of this kind invite one to theorize in terms of a hierarchy of traits or characteristics, ranging from those evidencing pronounced tendencies toward homogamy to those in which there is an apparently reliable but nonetheless very low degree of assortment. The need for a theory of mate selection accounting for this hierarchic pattern is evident; unfortunately, we are not in a position to offer especially cogent considerations toward such a theory. The following observations are only suggestive of a line of conjecture and further inquiry.

Many writers have emphasized the role of spatial propinquity in mate selection. If marriage presumes prior social contact (neglecting betrothals arranged by parents in nonwestern societies or by computers in the West), and if spatial proximity is at least a limiting factor in determining the chances for such contact, it would indeed make sense to regard propinquity as a significant condition in mate selection. From studies of residential patterns, we know that people living close to one another in space tend to be alike in socioeconomic characteristics. Hence a choice of mate solely on the basis of propinquity would give rise to some assortative mating by socioeconomic variables.

In American society, where coeducational structures prevail, the school may be thought of as a spatial context offering even greater possibilities for relevant contact than residential areas.[5] The age-grading of pupils guarantees that persons attending school will be acquainted with a considerable number of potential mates. It is no news to educators that secondary schools and colleges function in considerable measure as marriage markets. The attrition of enrollment with advancing age, moreover, tends to remove eligibles from this particular market. Hence persons continuing education to a given level are more likely to find mates among others at that level than among those leaving school earlier. The contracting of a marriage is itself a frequent occasion for termination of schooling by either or both parties.

There are, therefore, good reasons for appreciable assortment by education quite apart from elements of more or less conscious choice. The latter are not to be disregarded, nonetheless. Although persons seeking mates may not explicitly rate eligibles in terms of years of schooling, similarity of educational experience may be entailed in some measure by matching on the basis of temperamental and intellectual compatibility or congeniality of tastes and orientations.

It does not seem difficult, therefore, to make a case for educational attainment as a more or less direct basis of assortment. Let us grant for the argument that it does in fact function in this way. But since education is associated with a number of factors in each mate's background, apparent assortment with respect to these background factors would thereby be generated indirectly. Indeed, we could entertain as a null hypothesis that the correlation between background factors, such as the respective fathers' occupations, can be completely accounted for on the basis of assortment by educational attainment and the correlation of education with the background factors.

It should be noted that this line of argument reverses the direction

5 See Albert Lewis Rhodes, Albert J. Reiss, Jr., and Otis Dudley Duncan, "Occupational Segregation in a Metropolitan School System," *American Journal of Sociology*, 70(1965), 682-694, and "Erratum," *American Journal of Sociology*, 71 (1965), 131.

of causation that we have heretofore assumed in discussing the development of careers. We reasoned earlier from the premise that educational attainment depends on family background. Now we are suggesting that, *from the point of view of the marriage,* rather than from the point of view of the individuals contracting it, the combination of background variables formed by the marriage depends on the combination of educational levels.

After all, marriage in our society is not arranged by parents on the basis of suitable background characteristics and family connections, as it used to be in the past, but it results largely from a romantic emotional involvement of the future marriage partners themselves. Dating and courtship patterns lead to romantic involvements, and young people get married because they have fallen deeply in love. Family connections do not *directly* influence such emotional involvements, but the personality characteristics, acquired tastes, and styles of life of the partners themselves *do,* and the clearest indication of these individual differences available in our data is education, quite aside from the previously noted significance of educational level for providing opportunities for social contacts at the time of courtship. From the standpoint of the marriage, therefore, whatever homogamy in respect to family background exists may be merely incidental to the homogamy in respect to the personal attributes of the partners themselves, as manifest in our data on educational homogamy.

In terms of these considerations it seems appropriate to consider the partial correlation between occupational backgrounds of the spouses, holding constant their educational attainment. On the null hypothesis this correlation would be zero, a result compatible with the argument that assortment takes place directly on educational attainment but only indirectly on the basis of background. Results of such a calculation for the white cohorts are shown in the next-to-last column of Table 10.8. Clearly, the correlation for parental occupational status is reduced when assortment by education is taken into account. Equally clearly, however, it does not disappear. Whereas the simple correlations approximate .3, the partials generally drop to around .2 or a bit lower.

An extension of this approach is based on a somewhat more elaborate assumption. Suppose that assortment takes place directly on several current characteristics of the spouses, whatever they may be. These in turn bring to the marriages thus formed their associations with background factors, indirectly inducing assortment with respect to the latter. For illustration, we have considered two characteristics of the wife—educational attainment and number of siblings—and three characteristics of the husband—these two plus status of first job, because first job may be more or less proximate in time to the marriage. Taking account of the intercorrelations of all these five variables as well as their correlations with the parental occupational statuses, we may compute the partial correlation for parental status, holding constant the five variables describing the spouses' characteristics. These partials are exhibited in the last column of Table 10.8. There is only a slight further reduction of the correlation for fathers' occupational statuses, which remains unmistakable.

This exercise can hardly be regarded as supplying crucial evidence for the kind of theory being suggested, as the characteristics under examination do not exhaust the obvious possibilities for variables on which we might assume that assortment is relatively "direct." If, nevertheless, we take these results and the reasoning leading to them at face value, we should conclude that mate assortment occurs primarily with respect to education, and that assortment with respect to social origins plays only a secondary role, though one that is by no means insignificant. Such a conclusion tends to modify the emphasis usually placed on the role of marriage in social mobility. The impression from the literature is that the marriage market is so structured as to assure homogamy in regard to social origins. Our results, it can be argued, tend to make such homogamy in considerable measure a by-product of assortative mating on the achieved statuses (educational attainment, in particular) of the spouses themselves. We feel justified in recommending that this point of view be explored systematically in future studies more sharply focused on mate selection than this one could be.

At the same time, the possibilities of the traditional argument have hardly been exhausted. From the long-range perspective of family institutions and the stratification system, the persistence of homogamy by social origins is of considerable significance. Given romantic love as the primary basis of marriage in our value system, the only way parents can encourage their children to marry spouses with the proper family background, and thus the only way for perpetuating the family's position in the social order, is by placing their children into an environment largely populated by prospective mates with suitable family connections. Parents typically accomplish this by living in distinctive neighborhoods, by necessity in the case of the poorer strata and by deliberate design in that of the wealthier ones, and sending their children to appropriate schools and colleges. The restrictions on opportunities for falling in love thereby imposed permit family background to exert some indirect influence on mate selection even if it is directly influenced primarily by the personal characteristics of the mates themselves. Romantic love weakens the hold of social origins on mate selection, but ecological segration in neighborhoods and schools indirectly restores some power over marriage to social origins.

CONCLUSIONS

Some of the results reported in this chapter depart little from what might be expected on hypotheses generally accepted in the sociological literature. We have, however, been able to specify and support them a little more clearly than is sometimes the case. We found that being reared in a broken family is a handicap for subsequent status achievement. Virtually the entire amount of this handicap, however, can be attributed to the educational disadvantage that such rearing confers. We noted, secondly, that our data are compatible with the supposition that marriage per se—contracting a marriage and protecting it from disruption—is an asset, if a comparatively minor one, for an occupational career. This effect, moreover, is not readily explained entirely by the favorable socioeconomic selection of men remaining married to the date of the survey.

The findings reported later in the chapter are perhaps a little more surprising. At any rate, we have ventured interpretations that are not quite so standard. Considering the question of how important are the characteristics of the wife for the husband's occupational success, we found that making a good match is perhaps less important than one might have guessed from the folklore on marriage as a channel of mobility for men. In fact, it is perfectly possible that a more complete understanding of the husband's characteristics that produce success and failure would reduce the apparent role of the wife's characteristics to nil.

The key to this interpretation is that assortative mating results in a rather high correlation between characteristics of husband and wife. Hence the wife's education and her socioeconomic background can make little *independent* contribution to variation in husband's achievement. Recognizing this relevance of assortative mating for the process of stratification suggests the desirability of investigating assortative mating as a phenomenon in its own right and of attempting to construct a theory accounting for the patterns of assortment observed. Here again, our suggestion seems to run counter to some of the prevailing thinking on the subject. We showed that assortment is much more pronounced with regard to the education of the spouses themselves than with respect to their social origins. If educational assortment can be rationalized in terms of the factors of propinquity and compatibility, it becomes plausible to think of assortment as occurring directly and primarily on the basis of schooling and personal characteristics of the mates, and only secondarily and indirectly on the basis of the occupational status of the parental generation. The test of this theory seemingly requires attention to a greater range of variables representing different degrees of assortment than has been possible here and the development of models designed to account for the hierarchical patterns that such variables may present.

CHAPTER 11

Differential Fertility and Occupational Mobility

Most of this study is concerned with status achievement or social mobility as a dependent variable. Theories of mobility, however, also stress a number of hypothesized consequences of mobility, both for whole societies and for individuals or particular strata within societies.[1] The OCG survey was not designed to yield much information about such consequences. Only one variable, the cumulative fertility of couples classified by kind or degree of mobility, was selected for examination on this point of view. The treatment of even this one topic must be far from definitive, but it may nonetheless be suggestive as a mode of attack on the problem of imputing consequences to mobility within a population.

Some preliminary observations on the phenomenon of differential fertility are needed to put the analysis into perspective.

HISTORICAL BACKGROUND

A long-term decline in the birth rates has been noted in all the now highly developed Western countries. The time at which this trend originated probably differed considerably among such countries, but it was clearly under way in most of them by the last quarter of the nineteenth century. Estimates of the pattern of timing vary in reliability according to the adequacy of historical data. Moreover, the problem of dating the trend harbors unsuspected complexities that

---

[1] Pitirim Sorokin, *Social Mobility*, New York: Harper, 1927, pp. 493-546; Morris Janowitz, "Some Consequencies of Social Mobility in the United States," *Transactions of the Third World Congress of Sociology*, London: International Sociological Association, 1956, Vol. 3, 191-201.

come to light when refined demographic measures, rather than the conventional crude birth rate, are examined.[2] In any event, as the fact of decreasing natality became inescapably obvious, demographers initiated inquiries into its causes. These efforts yielded, after about 1900, a growing body of firm evidence that socioeconomic strata were not contributing equally to the changes in aggregate fertility rates. Instead, the higher strata in virtually all countries were coming to produce much smaller numbers of offspring, on the average, than the lower strata.

There was a strong tendency, when this fact came to light, to interpret both differential fertility (variation between strata) and declining fertility to variation or change in physiological reproductive capacity ("fecundity" in the technical vocabulary of the demographer). This view was gradually superseded, however, when the facts about fertility change and differentials were shown to be compatible with an alternative explanation, one couched in terms of the spreading practice of deliberate limitation of family size by means of contraceptive practice. In modern studies convincing direct evidence in favor of this explanation has been forthcoming.[3] Although the evidence on family planning serves to define more precisely the phenomenon to be explained, it does not in itself constitute a satisfying explanation. The problem now becomes that of specifying the conditions, presumably personal or social, that give rise to increasing but differential practice of family limitation.

Theories accepting this formulation appeared early, among them a proposition about "social capillarity" to be mentioned later in this chapter. No single theory, however, has been able to muster strong supporting evidence, and in the current state of affairs investigators are preoccupied with the patient testing of a number of specific hypotheses.

In the meantime the phenomena under study have continued to evolve. As the demographic transition has run its course, fertility has ceased to move uniformly downward and some countries like the United States have undergone a prolonged "baby boom." The present disposition of population analysts seems to be to acknowledge the possibility that each cohort of women (or of married couples) adjusts

2 N. B. Ryder, "Problems of Trend Determination During a Transition in Fertility," *Milbank Memorial Fund Quarterly*, 34(1956), 5-21.

3 E. Lewis-Faning, *Report on an Enquiry into Family Limitation and Its Influence on Human Fertility During the Past Fifty Years*, "Papers of the Royal Commission on Population," Vol. I, London: HMSO, 1949; and Ronald Freedman, P. K. Whelpton, and A. A. Campbell, *Family Planning, Sterility, and Population Growth*, New York: McGraw-Hill, 1959.

its current and ultimate fertility levels to fairly short-run conditions. Hence cohorts separated by only a few years of historical experience may have rather different aggregate fertility, reach their ultimate level of natality performance via distinct temporal patterns of childbearing, and manifest considerable variation in the kind and degree of differential reproduction. It is thought, for example, that the "baby boom" involved a coincidence of economic conditions becoming favorable as a consequence of "Kuznets cycles" so that cohorts ready to initiate childbearing at the end of World War II were encouraged to have larger families than their immediate predecessors and to advance their childbearing cycles rapidly.[4] Subsequent cohorts may well respond differently to altered circumstances. Fertility dynamics can no longer be described neatly with a simple formula—declining trend with differential natality inversely related to socioeconomic status. For the time being, apparently, we must rest our hopes less on the chance of hitting on a general theory of fertility than on an *analytical strategy* that is sensitive to historical shifts in patterns of family-formation and family-building from period to period. These observations are offered not so much as insights meriting reflective consideration but rather as qualifications on the generality of the results presented below. These results, as it will appear, pertain to a very special set of cohorts whose experience may or may not have much bearing on the understanding of the behavior of cohorts located elsewhere in the stream of history.

Perhaps the best way to substantiate this point is to look at differentials in cumulative fertility in a sequence of cohorts with respect to a single socioeconomic variable: educational attainment of women. In many ways, education is the most satisfactory variable for analyses of differentials in completed fertility, as it is typically determinate at or near the beginning of the child-bearing period. Variables like husband's occupation or income, by contrast, are typically ascertained as of the survey date and may not accurately represent relevant conditions during the preceding years while childbearing was actually under way.

Table 11.1 provides a highly compressed summary of intercohort comparisons with respect to differential fertility. The measure of fertility is children ever born for all women (although subsequent analysis in this chapter is limited to married women living with husbands). The measure of the degree of differential fertility is the linear regression coefficient of number of children on number of years of school completed. Although there are some interesting departures from

[4] Richard A. Easterlin, *The Baby Boom in Historical Perspective*, "Occasional Paper No. 79," New York: National Bureau of Economic Research, 1962.

TABLE 11.1. REGRESSION OF CUMULATIVE TOTAL FERTILITY ON EDUCATIONAL ATTAINMENT FOR SELECTED COHORTS OF NATIVE WHITE WOMEN, 1940, AND WHITE WOMEN, 1950 AND 1960, FOR THE UNITED STATES (ITEMS IN PARENTHESES ARE FOR WOMEN UNDER 45 YEARS OLD)

Birth Year of Cohorts	Native White Women, 1940	White Women	
		1950	1960
MEAN NUMBER OF CHILDREN EVER BORN			
1925 to 1929	...	...	(2.40)
1920 to 1924	...	...	(2.47)
1915 to 1919[a]	...	(1.86)	(2.36)
1910 to 1914[a]	...	(2.04)	2.20
1905 to 1909[a]	(1.64)	(2.14)	2.14
1900 to 1904[a]	(2.11)	2.26	2.24
1895 to 1899	(2.42)	2.46	2.46 ⟩ 2.52[b]
1890 to 1894	2.61	2.70	...
1885 to 1889	2.69	...	...
1875 to 1884	2.85	...	...
1865 to 1874	3.10	...	...
REGRESSION OF NUMBER OF CHILDREN EVER BORN ON YEARS OF SCHOOL COMPLETED			
1925 to 1929	...	...	(-.091)
1920 to 1924	...	...	(-.095)
1915 to 1919[a]	...	(-.125)	(-.110)
1910 to 1914[a]	...	(-.155)	-.135
1905 to 1909[a]	(-.182)	(-.182)	
1900 to 1904[a]	(-.218)	-.217	-.199[b]
1895 to 1899	(-.232)	-.226	
1890 to 1894	-.238	-.250	
1885 to 1889	-.241	...	...
1875 to 1884	-.251	...	...
1865 to 1874	-.248	...	...

[a]Birth years of cohorts included in OCG analysis.
[b]Women 50 years old and over in 1960 (education data not available by age intervals within this group).

SOURCE: 16th Census of the United States: 1940. Population. Differential Fertility, "Women by Number of Children Ever Born" (Washington: Government Printing Office, 1945), Table 49; 1950 United States Census of Population, Special Report. P-E, No. 5C, "Fertility" (Washington: Government Printing Office, 1955), Table 20; United States Census of Population: 1960; Subject Report PC(2)-3A, "Women by Number of Children Ever Born" (Washington: Government Printing Office, 1964), Tables 1 and 25.

linearity for certain cohorts this regression is quite useful as a single index of the extent to which fertility differs among educational strata. Cohorts are identified by year of birth and the data are further labelled by the census year in which information on cumulative fertility was collected. Figures are shown for white women only (or, in 1940, native white women).

The top half of Table 11.1 documents the long-term downward trend in fertility. Women in the earliest cohorts represented in these data bore an average of slightly more than three children each. A generation later, aggregate natality amounted to only 2.5 children per woman. The lowest value of completed fertility was reached by the birth cohorts of 1905 to 1909, who were in their twenties in the depth of the Depression and 50 to 54 years old in 1960. For these cohorts, the number of children ever born was only 2.14 per woman. The rise in fertility of subsequent cohorts is revealed in the 1960 column of Table 11.1. As of that date women in the 1920 to 1924 cohorts had borne an average of 2.47 children (equal to the ultimate performance of the 1895 to 1899 cohorts), even though their cycle of childbearing was not yet finished. The 1925 to 1929 cohorts, beginning their child-bearing in the midst of the baby boom, had already borne more children by age 30 to 34 (as of 1960) than the 1900 to 1914 cohorts by the end of their childbearing period. It is apparent, therefore, that the latter cohorts, which are dealt with in terms of OCG data subsequently, fall in the trough of a curve of declining followed by increasing fertility.

In parallel with the declining trend of fertility, the lower half of Table 11.1 shows a more or less continuous attenuation of the magnitude of differentials by education. For the earlier cohorts each increment of one year of schooling was accompanied by a decrement of one-fourth of a child in terms of the ultimate ratio of children ever born to women completing the childbearing period. For the most recent cohorts this effect has shrunk to one-eighth or one-tenth of a child. Although the cohorts born after 1910 have raised their aggregate fertility as compared with the 1905 to 1909 cohorts, they have shown no tendency to restore the earlier pattern of differential fertility by education. The OCG cohorts, therefore, apparently stood near the end of a transition period during which this form of differential fertility was in process of vanishing.

The OCG data themselves afford some basis for extrapolating this trend toward the diminution of educational differentials. The couples in the survey in which the wives belonged to the 1900 to 1919 cohorts were classified by farm–nonfarm residence and background (Table 11.2). If either the husband or the wife in a couple living in a nonfarm residence reported father's occupation as farmer or farm laborer, the couple was characterized as having "farm background." The lower panel of Table 11.2 shows that differential fertility by education was very slight for nonfarm couples with nonfarm background. It was comparatively strong, however, for couples with farm background living in nonfarm residences, as it was for those still living on farms. The OCG data show[5] that 51 per cent of the couples in which the wife

5 Otis Dudley Duncan, "Farm Background and Differential Fertility," *Demography*, 2(1965), 240-249.

TABLE 11.2. MEAN NUMBER OF CHILDREN EVER BORN, BY FARM RESIDENCE AND
BACKGROUND OF COUPLE AND EDUCATIONAL ATTAINMENT OF WIFE, FOR WIVES 42 TO 61
YEARS OLD IN MARCH, 1962, LIVING WITH HUSBANDS IN OCG SAMPLE

| Years of School Completed By Wife | Total | Nonfarm Residence | | Farm Residence |
		Nonfarm Background	Farm Background[a]	
NUMBER OF COUPLES (THOUSANDS)				
Total	13,733	7,435	5,005	1,293
Elementary				
0 to 4	525	126	291	108
5 to 7	1,466	563	687	216
8	2,431	1,154	970	307
High school				
1 to 3	2,662	1,523	945	194
4	4,326	2,688	1,364	274
College				
1 to 3	1,366	752	487	127
4 or more	957	629	261	67
CHILDREN EVER BORN PER WIFE				
Total	2.45	2.21	2.58	3.34
Elementary				
0 to 4	3.96	2.30	4.24	5.15
5 to 7	3.07	2.39	3.39	3.85
8	2.71	2.43	2.77	3.53
High school				
1 to 3	2.47	2.38	2.46	3.26
4	2.11	2.09	2.02	2.70
College				
1 to 3	2.14	1.99	2.24	2.62
4 or more	1.98	1.98	1.91	2.18

[a]Husband and/or wife reported father's occ. as farmer or farm laborer.

belonged to the 1900 to 1904 cohort were nonfarm residents with
nonfarm background; the percentage was 72 for couples in which the
wives belonged to the 1935 to 1939 cohort. Thus the sector in which
differential fertility is of relatively minor importance is a rapidly
growing one.

Looking at the matter in a slightly different way, Table 11.2 suggests
that fertility appreciably higher than the general average of 2.45 births
per wife is to be found only among couples with *both* farm background (including farm residents) and educational attainment below
the level of high-school graduation. With these characteristics—and
especially this combination of characteristics—becoming less and less
frequent with each succeeding cohort there is reason to expect the

classic pattern of differential fertility to become more and more difficult to detect.

The OCG data on the 1900 to 1919 cohorts, in sum, are especially interesting in that they represent experience at the end of a long period of fertility decline during which an established pattern of differential fertility was in process of dissolution. Their special interest in this historical perspective, however, may render these data somewhat unsuitable as a basis for understanding what was happening at the time the mobility hypothesis was formulated or for anticipating what is likely to happen in the next few decades. With this *caveat* stated we may proceed to a review of the mobility hypothesis, and to some analysis of the OCG data in the light of this hypothesis.

THE MOBILITY HYPOTHESIS

The name usually cited in connection with the early history of the mobility hypothesis is that of Arsène Dumont, who at the turn of the century called attention to the phenomenon of *capillarité sociale,* observing that "just as a column of liquid has to be thin in order to rise under the force of capillarity, so a family must be small in order to rise in the social scale."[6]

It does not seem worthwhile to trace the fortunes of this and related ideas in detail. It is possible, however, to point up some issues that have arisen during several decades of discussion. It is important to distinguish between what may be called the "strong form" and the "weak form" of the mobility hypothesis. There is a contrast, as well, between theories stressing a set of presumed "bio-social" mechanisms producing a relationship between mobility and fertility and theories emphasizing various "psycho-social" mechanisms.

The strong form of the hypothesis asserts, in effect, that differential fertility by socioeconomic status, social class, or some similar type of variable is completely explained by social mobility. Classes with low average fertility are those into which individuals or couples with low fertility have moved, whereas classes with high average fertility are those whose ranks have been thinned of low-fertility couples or individuals. Thus, if it were possible to examine only those persons or marriages not undergoing mobility, no class differences in average number of births should appear. Although no student of the subject may have been willing to support so extreme a version of the strong

6 Quoted in Charles F. Westoff, "The Changing Focus of Differential Fertility Research: The Social Mobility Hypothesis" (1953), reprinted in J. J. Spengler and O. D. Duncan (Eds.), *Population Theory and Policy*, Glencoe, Ill.: Free Press, 1956, p. 404. See A. Dumont, *Dépopulation et Civilisation*, Paris: 1890.

hypothesis, Fisher verged upon it in stating two propositions that he emphasized by using them as subheadings within the chapter in which his position was developed: (1) "Infertility in all classes, irrespective of its cause, gains social promotion"; and (2) "Selection [is] the predominant cause of the inverted birth rate."[7] The qualification "predominant" preserved him from complete commitment to the strong hypothesis; other "causes," however, he did not discuss.

Fisher's argument for his first proposition is worth reproducing; the case has never been more felicitously presented:[8]

That the economic situation in all grades of modern societies is such as favours the social promotion of the less fertile is clear, from a number of familiar considerations. In the wealthiest class, the inherited property is for the most part divided among the natural heirs, and the wealth of the child is inversely proportioned to the number of the family to which he belongs. In the middle class the effect of the direct inheritance of wealth is also important; but the anxiety of the parent of a large family is increased by the expense of a first-class education, besides that of professional training, and by the need for capital in entering the professions to the best advantage. At a lower economic level social status depends less upon actually inherited capital than upon expenditure on housing, education, amusements, and dress; while the savings of the poor are depleted or exhausted, and their prospects of economic progress often crippled, by the necessity of sufficient food and clothing for their children.

Although Fisher's subsequent discussion dwells on the "decay of ruling classes" attributed to the promotion of the infertile into their ranks, this passage makes it clear that he expected the relationship between mobility and fertility to hold at all levels, not just in the case of elite strata. Moreover, if "selection" were indeed the "predominant cause of the inverted birth-rate," then persons other than those being selected for mobility should not manifest much in the way of class variation in fertility.

The weak form of the hypothesis is noncommittal on this point. It merely asserts that "social mobility, both in its subjective and objective dimensions, is directly related to fertility planning and inversely related to the size of the planned family—both relationships persisting within otherwise homogeneous socioeconomic groups."[9] This evidently leaves open the question whether there are socioeconomic differentials other than those attributable to mobility.

[7] R. A. Fisher, *The Genetical Theory of Natural Selection* (1929), 2nd rev. ed., New York: Dover Publications, 1958, Chapter 9.

[8] *Ibid.*, p. 252.

[9] Westoff, *op. cit.*, p. 404.

As to the other line of distinction between versions of the general hypothesis, we need not be surprised that the "bio-social" account of the mechanism has been put forward largely by students of heredity, whereas "psycho-social" mechanisms have seemed a plausible alternative thereto in the thinking of social psychologists and sociologists.

Fisher argued that "not merely physiological infertility, but also the causes of low reproduction dependent from voluntary choice, such as celibacy, postponement of marriage, and birth limitation by married couples, are also strongly influenced by hereditary factors." In his account, therefore, an inherited tendency toward low fertility comes first, and "selection" operates in such a way that the naturally infertile are promoted. The alternative line of reasoning, reversing the direction of presumed causation, indicates how the disposition to be mobile may lead to voluntary limitation of family size. Westoff, for example, writes:[10]

Very briefly . . . the ideal-type of the couple either in the actual process of vertical mobility or effectively geared toward its anticipation probably has the following characteristics: a maintained rationality of behavior; intense competitive effort; careerism with its accompanying manipulation of personalities; psychologial insecurity of status with its attendant anxieties; and an increasing exhaustion of nervous and physical energies; in short, a pervasive success-orientation and all that is implied by it.

Or, as the United Nations experts wrote in their summary of opinion on this topic,[11]

The desire to improve one's position in the social scale has been stressed as an important motive for family limitation. . . . The effect of social mobility on fertility appears to be attributed in general to the fact that rearing children absorbs money, time, and effort which could otherwise be used to rise in the social scale. Social mobility is thus more feasible with one or two children than with a larger number.

The crucial question for the present investigation is this: on what empirical basis might a choice be made between the versions of the social mobility hypothesis, or on what empirical grounds can any version of it be regarded as sustained? It would seem that the strong hypothesis should be rejected if substantial socioeconomic differentiation in fertility is observed for persons or couples not subject to

10 Idem.
11 United Nations, Population Division, *The Determinants and Consequences of Population Trends*, New York: United Nations, 1953, p. 79.

mobility, particularly if the pattern of this differentiation resembles that observed among all couples or among the mobile alone. If non-mobile couples vary in fertility by social rank, then obviously such variation in the general population is not exclusively attributable to mobility. The weak hypothesis, by contrast, should be rejected if there is no appreciable variation in fertility properly attributable to mobility, whether or not differential fertility arising in some other way is in evidence. It is possible, of course, for a particular body of data to indicate rejection of both forms of the hypothesis.

A valid objection to these criteria should be acknowledged. It may be that it is not mobility as such—that is, the actual experience of social promotion or demotion—that produces differentials, but rather the mere aspiration or desire for mobility. To test this supposition, of course, one must be privy to the hopes and wishes of individuals, for the inference thereto from conventional types of demographic observation is tenuous and equivocal. It is true, however, that the statement of the weak hypothesis already quoted specifically refers to "social mobility, *both* in its subjective and objective dimensions" (emphasis supplied). Hence, if the subjective dimension is beyond the scope of an inquiry like the present one, it may still be of interest to see what can be said on the basis of selected measures of the objective dimension.

As to the issue between "bio-social" and "psycho-social" mechanisms, Fisher himself pointed to a means of investigating the matter even in the absence of definitive knowledge of the genetics of reproductive capacity or propensity:[12]

. . . on the theory that we have to do principally with heritable factors affecting fertility, the fertility of the upper social classes must be prevented from rising by the lower fertility of those whom social promotion brings into their ranks; the stream of demotion of the more fertile members of the upper classes being relatively a very feeble one. Consequently, the groups enjoying rapid social promotion should, on this theory be even less fertile than the classes to which they rise.

If, on the contrary, the important causes were any of those to be included under "social environment," we should confidently expect the families who rise in the social scale to carry with them some measure of the fertility of the classes from which they originated.

This is straightforward enough as a basis for designing an analysis. Unfortunately, some have sought to illuminate the problem by look-

---

12 Fisher, *op. cit.,* p. 254.

ing solely at elite groups, distinguishing those mobile into the elite from those born to this status, but neglecting to supply themselves with appropriate observations on the fertility of the strata whence those moving into the elite came. Indeed, it is not unfair to state that only one previous investigation, that of Berent,[13] both covered a sufficiently large sample to justify conclusions and employed an analytical design suited to the test Fisher proposed. Berent's data quite decisively indicate rejection of the strong hypothesis. When examined in the way suggested here, moreover, they afford no support for the weak hypothesis.[14] Indeed, it is the plausibility of the hypothesis rather than the quality of any supporting evidence that seems to account for its continuing appeal. Although no set of negative results can be definitive—because a different outcome might follow from studies in different populations or with alternative measures of mobility—it appears that at some point the burden of proof may fairly be shifted to the proponents of the hypothesis.

FERTILITY IN RELATION TO INTRAGENERATIONAL MOBILITY

The analysis of the OCG data is confined to couples in which the wife's period of childbearing was finished, or nearly so, by March 1962; it concerns the number of children ever born to wives 42 to 61 years old on that date, that is, wives who were members of the 1900 to 1919 birth cohorts. The study is thus limited to completed marital fertility. It excludes not only unmarried women and married women not living with their spouses but a few women in this age group married to men falling outside the age range of men in the OCG sample (20 to 64 years old).

Four occupational statuses were ascertained in the survey: the occupations of the wife's and the husband's fathers, that of the husband's first job, and his occupation in March 1962. Six pairs of statuses can be formed from these, but fertility data for combinations of broad occupations groups are available only for four. Hence we consider mobility from first job to 1962 occupation, from wife's father to husband's first job, from wife's father to 1962 occupation, and from husband's father to 1962 occupation. A rather coarse grouping of occupations was necessary to avoid the problem of low frequencies in many cells of the mobility tables. The so-called "broad" occupation groups used here are combinations of census major occupation groups:

13 Jerzy Berent, "Fertility and Social Mobility," *Population Studies*, 5(1952), 244-260.

14 Otis Dudley Duncan, "Methodological Issues in the Analysis of Social Mobility," in N. J. Smelser and S. M. Lipset (Eds.), *Social Structure and Social Mobility in Economic Development*, Chicago: Aldine, 1966.

Higher white-collar
  Professional, technical, and kindred workers
  Managers, officials, and proprietors, except farm
Lower white-collar
  Sales workers
  Clerical and kindred workers
Higher manual
  Craftsmen, foremen, and kindred workers
Lower manual
  Operatives and kindred workers
  Service workers
  Laborers, except farm
Farm
  Farmers and farm managers
  Farm laborers and foremen
Not stated
  Not in experienced civilian labor force (applies to 1962 occupation)
  Not reported (applies to first job, wife's father's occupation and
    husband's father's occupation)

The sample, including both white and nonwhite persons, is approximately 6,000 couples. Owing to the complex sample design, however, standard errors are somewhat larger than they would be for a simple random sample of this size.

The data with which we are working are quite voluminous. There are four mobility tables each with 36 cells (six origin statuses by six destination statuses, counting "not stated" as an occupation group). For each of these cells we know the number of couples and the aggregate number of children ever born to the wives. There are several ways in which these data could be summarized, and it is not evident that previous investigators have been entirely sure what procedure to follow in facing a comparable task. It turns out, moreover, that some apparently plausible procedures can lead to very misleading impressions. It will be necessary, therefore, to indicate the present analytical strategy explicitly. For illustration, the data on intragenerational mobility, husband's first job to occupation in 1962, are presented first.

The first panel of Table 11.3 shows the cross-classification of first jobs by current occupations. Evidently there was a considerable volume of intragenerational mobility. About five-eighths of the husbands were in an occupation group in 1962 that differed from the classification of their first jobs; about three-eighths were in the same broad occupation category (disregarding the men not stating one or both

TABLE 11.3. MEAN NUMBER OF CHILDREN EVER BORN PER WIFE, BY HUSBAND'S FIRST JOB AND 1962 OCC., FOR WIVES 42 TO 61 YEARS OLD IN MARCH 1962, LIVING WITH HUSBANDS IN OCG SAMPLE

First Job	All Couples	Occ. in 1962					
		White-Collar		Manual		Farm	Not stated[a]
		Higher	Lower	Higher	Lower		
Number of Couples (Thousands)							
All couples	13,771	3,778	1,418	2,894	3,719	1,109	853
Higher white-collar	1,038	777	88	54	60	24	35
Lower white-collar	2,584	1,093	606	314	402	38	131
Higher manual	1,184	372	64	482	200	18	53
Lower manual	5,742	1,161	513	1,432	2,050	185	401
Farm	2,796	282	116	508	882	806	202
Not stated	422	93	31	104	125	38	31
Children Ever Born Per Wife							
All couples	2.45	2.12	1.91	2.56	2.61	3.18	2.70
Higher white-collar	1.95	1.96	1.44	2.63	1.75	2.25	2.11
Lower white-collar	1.94	2.03	1.70	2.20	1.98	1.61	1.76
Higher manual	2.30	2.04	1.78	2.53	2.64	1.78	1.62
Lower manual	2.46	2.16	2.03	2.51	2.62	3.34	2.52
Farm	3.11	3.03	2.69	2.83	2.98	3.32	3.88
Not stated	2.50	1.63	2.81	3.07	2.24	2.42	3.97
Children Ever Born Per Wife, Calculated Values[b]							
Higher white-collar	...	1.92	1.70	2.18	2.18	2.45	2.30
Lower white-collar	...	1.89	1.68	2.16	2.16	2.43	2.27
Higher manual	...	2.14	1.93	2.40	2.40	2.68	2.52
Lower manual	...	2.28	2.06	2.54	2.54	2.81	2.66
Farm	...	2.80	2.59	3.07	3.07	3.34	3.18
Not stated	...	2.29	2.08	2.56	2.55	2.83	2.67
Children Ever Born Per Wife, Observed Minus Calculated							
Higher white-collar	...	.04	-.26	.45	-.43	-.20	-.19
Lower white-collar	...	.14	.02	.04	-.18	-.82	-.51
Higher manual	...	-.10	-.15	.13	.24	-.90	-.90
Lower manual	...	-.12	-.03	-.03	.08	.53	-.14
Farm	...	.23	.10	-.24	-.09	-.02	.70
Not stated	...	-.66	.73	.51	-.31	-.41	1.30

[a]Husband not in experienced civilian labor force.
[b]Based on results in Table 11.4, computed before rounding net effects to two decimal places.

occupations). It is apparent too that upward mobility predominated, since the higher white-collar and higher manual categories gained via mobility, whereas the lower white-collar and lower manual categories, as well as the farm groups, lost. The second panel of Table 11.3 shows mean completed fertility for couples in each of the 36 combinations of first job with current occupation. This is the raw information for the analysis, and results subsequently reported are simply concerned with the summary or reduction of this information.

There is obviously variation from cell to cell in mean fertility, and presumably not all this variation is due to sampling fluctuations. There is, then, some kind of association between "mobility" and fertility. The interpretation to be placed on this finding, however, depends a good deal on the *pattern* of variation. It is advisable, therefore, to make several systematic summaries of the data before venturing a substantive conclusion. In the first place, although fertility does vary over the several combinations of first job with current occupation that register mobility, there is also variation by occupation over the five categories of nonmobile couples. This may be seen by looking at the diagonal (upper left to lower right) cells in the second panel of Table 11.3.

We see at once that, whatever the relationship of fertility to mobility, *differential fertility by occupational status cannot be accounted for by occupational mobility solely.* In fact, if we compare the differentials along the diagonal with those along any row or any column of the table, it appears that occupational status makes at least as much difference for the nonmobile as does occupational mobility for any stratum of origin (first job) or destination (current occupation). For this particular body of data rejection of the mobility hypothesis in its strong form is unequivocally indicated.

The test of the weak form of the hypothesis is more complicated, and its rationale depends on what one is to regard as an "effect" of mobility. In this context mobility refers to the fact that the first job and the occupation in 1962 fall into different broad occupation groups. We have already discerned "occupation effects" not due to mobility by studying nonmobile couples. We now propose that such effects may also apply to mobile couples. If so, and if in estimating these we can simultaneously account for the fertility levels of the nonmobile couples, we shall assert that there is no "mobility effect" *per se,* except in the sense that mobile couples manifest differences from nonmobile in the same occupational class of origin (destination) because they are simultaneously influenced by their membership in a different class of destination (origin). Thus we are led to consider a model that may account for fertility variation among both mobile and nonmobile couples in such a way that there is no remainder to be attributed uniquely to the factor of mobility itself.

To be explicit, suppose there is an effect on fertility specific to each origin status and similarly an effect for each destination status, and that the two effects combine by simple addition. It is plausible to assume that there are separate effects for the two statuses because differential fertility is observed when couples are classified either by husband's first job or by current occupation (see the first column and first row in the second panel of Table 11.3). There is, however, some redundancy in this statement, for the two statuses are not independent. We require, therefore, a way of getting at the two sets of effects that takes account of the correlation between origin and destination status. The appropriate model is the additive multiple-classification model described in Chapter 4. Here, let

$$Y_{ija} = \overline{Y} + a_i + b_j + U_{ija},$$

where Y_{ija} is the number of children ever born to the αth wife whose husband's first job fell in group i and 1962 occupation in group j. $\overline{Y}$ is the grand mean fertility for all wives; a_i is the (net) effect on the wife's fertility due to membership in the ith origin class and b_j the (net) effect due to membership in the jth destination class. U_{ija} is then the amount by which the fertility of the αth couple deviates from the expected value,

$$\hat{Y}_{ij} = \overline{Y} + a_i + b_j.$$

The estimates of a_i and b_j are obtained on the least-squares criterion that $\Sigma_{i,j,a}\ U_{ija}^2$ be a minimum. An indication of the procedure for obtaining the solution on this criterion was given in Chapter 4. It should be noted that the net effects, a_i, come out as deviations from the grand mean, and their weighted sum (the weights being the frequencies of the several classes) is zero; the same applies to the net effects, b_j.

Table 11.4 records the solution values for the problem at hand. The net effects, a_i, are shown in the third column, and the b_j values are in the last column. The first two columns show for comparison the gross effects, that is, observed marginal means as deviations from

TABLE 11.4. EFFECTS OF HUSBAND'S FIRST JOB AND 1962 OCC. ON CHILDREN EVER BORN PER WIFE, AS ESTIMATED FROM ADDITIVE MODEL APPLIED TO DATA IN TABLE 11.3

Occ. Group	Gross Effects[a]		Net Effects[a]	
	First Job	1962 Occ.	First Job	1962 Occ.
Higher white-collar	-.49	-.32	-.36	-.17
Lower white-collar	-.50	-.53	-.38	-.38
Higher manual	-.14	.12	-.13	.09
Lower manual	.02	.17	.00	.09
Farm	.67	.74	.53	.37
Not stated	.06	.26	.02	.21

[a]Deviations from grand mean, 2.45.

the grand mean. The net effects are closer, in each instance, to zero than the gross effects, because part of the gross effect for each classification is due to its overlap or correlation with the other classification.

The expected value of children ever born per wife on the basis of the model is computed from the formula given above. These values appear in the third panel of Table 11.3. Before considering the closeness of fit of the calculated to the observed means, two elementary properties of the model should be noted. First, the model is, in mathematical parlance, a linear equation. This means that only first-degree terms occur in the equation and the terms are combined by addition or subtraction (not multiplication). It does *not* mean that the model assumes a straight-line relationship of the dependent variable to the occupation classes. In fact the model does not even assume a monotone relationship, because the order in which the classes are listed is irrelevant to the solution. Note, for example, that the net effects for the lower white-collar class have greater negative values than those for the higher white-collar class.

Second, the model explicitly assumes that the effect for class of origin (destination) is the same irrespective of the class of destination (origin). If there is some specific effect on fertility of moving from, say, farm origins to upper manual status that is not shared by other couples with farm origins or other couples with upper manual status, then the model ignores this specific effect. Indeed, as has already been stated, what is meant by a mobility effect on the point of view taken here is precisely some kind of specific effect of a particular set of origin-destination combinations that is not taken into account by a strictly additive model.

If, now, we compare the calculated values, $\hat{Y}_{ij}$, with the observed means, $\overline{Y}_{ij}$, for each origin-destination combination, we secure the set of deviations, $\overline{Y}_{ij} - \hat{Y}_{ij}$, shown as the bottom panel of Table 11.3. The model obviously does not achieve a perfect fit to the sample data, as not all the deviations are zero. In fact none of them is identically zero. We may observe, however, that all of the "large" deviations—those, say, outside the range $\pm.4$—occur in cells that the process of occupational mobility has left very thinly populated. The observations for these cells are, accordingly, subject to considerable sampling error. To decide whether all the deviations from the model are reasonably attributable to sampling error, we use the F-test for interaction in a two-way analysis of variance with disproportional subclass frequencies.[15] The reader should be warned that several of the assumptions of this test are not met with these data, and it is possible to make only a crude allowance for the inflation of standard errors due to the use of a complex sample design. There is some interest in the descriptive statistics computed for this test: the additive model accounts for some 4.3 per cent of the total sum of squares of number of children ever

[15] K. A. Brownlee, *Statistical Theory and Methodology in Science and Engineering*, New York: Wiley, 1960, Chapter 18.

born, whereas the observed means, $\overline{Y}_{ij}$, account for 5.3 per cent. Taking at face value the result of the analysis of variance, this increment is real: there is variation (beyond the amount reasonably attributed to sampling fluctuations) between the means of origin-destination combinations that is not reproduced by the additive model.

The indication is, therefore, that the additive model should be rejected as an hypothesis to account for the observed variation. If it is rejected, however, the problem immediately becomes: What alternative hypothesis are we to accept? From a purely statistical standpoint, we can fall back on the assertion that the observed $\overline{Y}_{ij}$ contain all the information involved in the analysis, whereas the computed values, $\hat{Y}_{ij}$, sacrifice some of this information. This is hardly a satisfactory situation in terms of the substantive interest that motivated the analysis. We wanted to say something about the effect of "mobility" that would be consistent with the data at hand.

One could, at this point, stop computing and start talking—this has to be done at some point, in any event. The talk, however, would become quite prolix, as we considered reasons why mobility from lower manual to higher white-collar is accompanied by higher fertility than movement from higher to lower white-collar, and so on. Surely, we would soon be tempted to consider hypotheses that offer some simplification, a simplification, preferably, that somehow incorporates the idea of pattern or type of mobility. In short, we are not satisfied to observe that significant deviations $\overline{Y}_{ij} - \hat{Y}_{ij}$ occur; it must be shown that these deviations are in some systematic way related to the notion of mobility.

Table 11.5 essays one interpretation of this requirement. It divides the sample into two parts, the mobile and the nonmobile (ignoring the unclassifiable cases). In the second column the mobile are classified by stratum of origin, and in the fourth column by stratum of destination. The middle column gives the stratum classification of the nonmobile. These groupings are suited to reveal the effect, if any, of the simple dichotomy, mobile vs. nonmobile. *Aggregate* fertility (second panel) for the two groups does show a difference, 2.50 children ever born per wife for the nonmobile, 2.39 for the mobile—a difference of 0.11. Before interpreting this difference we must determine whether it in fact reflects the influence of mobility itself.

Other differences are noted if the comparisons are made specific for origin status (comparing the second and third columns in the second panel of Table 11.5) or for destination (comparing the third and fourth columns). For example, mobile couples departing from higher

TABLE 11.5. MEAN NUMBER OF CHILDREN EVER BORN, BY OCC. LEVEL AND MOBILITY CLASSI-
FICATION, IN TERMS OF HUSBAND'S FIRST JOB AND OCC. IN 1962, FOR WIVES 42 TO 61 YEARS OLD
IN MARCH, 1962, LIVING WITH HUSBANDS IN OCG SAMPLE

Broad Occ. Group	All Couples, By Husband's First Job	Mobile, By Husband's First Job	Nonmobile, By Husband's First Job	Mobile, By Husband's 1962 Occ.	All Couples, By Husband's 1962 Occ.
NUMBER OF COUPLES (THOUSANDS)					
All groups	13,771	7,806	4,721	7,806	13,771
Higher white-collar	1,038	226	777	2,908	3,778
Lower white-collar	2,584	1,847	606	781	1,418
Higher manual	1,184	654	482	2,308	2,894
Lower manual	5,742	3,291	2,050	1,544	3,719
Farm	2,796	1,788	806	265	1,109
Not stated	422		1,244[a]		853
CHILDREN EVER BORN PER WIFE					
All groups	2.45	2.39	2.50	2.39	2.45
Higher white-collar	1.95	1.89	1.96	2.18	2.12
Lower white-collar	1.94	2.04	1.70	2.04	1.91
Higher manual	2.30	2.19	2.53	2.54	2.56
Lower manual	2.46	2.36	2.62	2.63	2.61
Farm	3.11	2.93	3.32	2.88	3.18
Not stated	2.50		2.60[a]		2.70
CHILDREN EVER BORN PER WIFE, COMPUTED VALUES					
All groups	2.45	2.41	2.45	2.41	2.45
Higher white-collar	1.95	2.03	1.92	2.17	2.12
Lower white-collar	1.94	2.01	1.68	2.09	1.91
Higher manual	2.30	2.21	2.40	2.60	2.56
Lower manual	2.46	2.39	2.54	2.71	2.61
Farm	3.11	3.00	3.34	2.72	3.18
Not stated	2.50		2.63[a]		2.70
CHILDREN EVER BORN PER WIFE, OBSERVED MINUS COMPUTED VALUES					
All groups	...	-.02	.05	-.02	...
Higher white-collar	...	-.14	.04	.01	...
Lower white-collar	...	.03	.02	-.05	...
Higher manual	...	-.02	.13	-.06	...
Lower manual	...	-.03	.08	-.08	...
Farm	...	-.07	-.02	.16	...
Not stated	...		-.03[a]		...

[a]Not classified by mobility; either first job or current occ., or both, not stated.

white-collar first jobs are observed to have slightly lower fertility than
nonmobile couples beginning at this level and remaining there,
whereas mobile couples moving into the higher white-collar positions
after beginning in some lower status have higher fertility than the
nonmobile higher white-collar couples. Indeed, the mobile couples
in every destination stratum but one have higher fertility than the
nonmobile, and the mobile couples in every origin stratum but one
have lower fertility than the nonmobile (second panel). The reader
may be tempted to place a substantive interpretation on this pattern

of observed differences, but such a temptation should be resisted, for they may represent nothing more than a simple weighting of additive origin and destination effects.

Mobile couples in the higher white-collar stratum in 1962 arrived there from a variety of lower statuses, most of which have higher fertility than do white-collar persons. If they brought with them something of the fertility patterns of their origin strata, therefore, we should find that they do indeed have higher fertility than the nonmobile higher white-collar couples (contrary to the Fisher hypothesis). Similarly, for every comparison between mobile and nonmobile couples, we should take into account the "mix" of origin (or destination) statuses when interpreting the fertility of couples in a given class of destination (or origin).

We fall back on calculations derived from the additive model. Let us take the computed values $\widehat{Y}_{ij}$ given for each cell of the origin-destination classification and convert this average to an absolute number of births by multiplying $n_{ij}\widehat{Y}_{ij}$, where n_{ij} is the number of couples in a cell. Now when we aggregate off-diagonal cells as in Table 11.5, we sum the "expected number of births," $n_{ij}\widehat{Y}_{ij}$, in the several cells being combined and at the same time sum the numbers of couples, n_{ij}. The quotient, $\Sigma^* n_{ij}\widehat{Y}_{ij}/\Sigma^* n_{ij}$ (where Σ^* means the summation is restricted to the particular combination of cells being aggregated into a mobility category), is shown in the third panel of Table 11.5, which presents the computed values of children ever born per wife for each mobility category. These computed values are the ones implied by, though not explicit in, the additive model. The point at issue, of course, is whether the model adequately reproduces the differentials by origin and destination strata and the differences between mobile and nonmobile couples in these strata. Hence the bottom panel of Table 11.5 shows deviations of the observed from the calculated means.

The deviations indicative of a mobility effect vary between —.14 and .16. These two largest deviations correspond to the two smallest frequencies in the population. No stratum-specific comparison of mobile with nonmobile couples produces a difference between their deviations as large as .2. For the aggregate of all nonmobile couples the deviation is .05 as compared with —.02 for all mobile couples; a mobility effect of .07 does not seem to require much discussion.

In sum, although the additive model cannot be accepted without reservation, it comes very close to predicting all the effects produced by a simple classification of couples as mobile or nonmobile. Given the results of the additive model, there appears to be no need to enrich the statement of conclusions with a summary of fertility variation by mobility categories.[16]

It may be, however, that the simple dichotomy of mobile and non-mobile is not well designed to capture the true effects of mobility. Hence Table 11.6 offers as an alternative the aggregation of the cou-

TABLE 11.6. MEAN NUMBER OF CHILDREN EVER BORN PER WIFE, BY TYPE OF MOBILITY, IN TERMS OF HUSBAND'S FIRST JOB AND 1962 OCC., FOR WIVES 42 TO 61 YEARS OLD IN MARCH, 1962, LIVING WITH HUSBANDS IN OCG SAMPLE

Type of Mobility	Number of Couples (Thousands)	Children Ever Born Per Wife		
		Observed	Computed	Observed Minus Computed
All types	13,771	2.44	...	...
Nonmobile, nonfarm	3,915	2.33	2.27	.06
Nonmobile, farm	806	3.32	3.34	-.02
Upward mobile, nonfarm	4,635	2.21	2.23	-.02
Downward mobile, nonfarm	1,118	2.14	2.17	-.03
Nonfarm to farm	265	2.88	2.72	.16
Farm to nonfarm	1,788	2.93	3.00	-.07
Not classified[a]	1,244	2.60	2.63	-.03

[a]Either first job or current occ., or both, not stated.

ples into the several types of mobility listed in the table stub. There are indeed some variations in mean fertility by type of mobility. Both upward and downward mobile couples within the nonfarm sector, for example, have slightly lower mean fertility than the nonmobile. Once again, however, we are led to inquire whether fertility variation by mobility type conveys information not already implicit in a model assuming only additive effects of origin and destination status. Therefore the values computed (as explained above) from the model and the deviations of observed means from them are shown as the last two columns. The only deviation of any possible substantive interest is the one that indicates a slightly higher (.16 higher, to be specific) mean fertility than expected for couples in which the husband moved from a nonfarm first job to a farm occupation in 1962. This was a rather infrequent type of mobility and our estimate of its effect, therefore, is subject to considerable sampling error. In short, neither the "mobility types" of Table 11.6 nor the mobility classification of Table 11.5 brings out substantial mobility effects in the sense of a mean fertility differing appreciably from the one predicted on the supposition of no specific effects of mobility.

[16] Hubert M. Blalock, Jr., has shown that the data that fit an additive model may also be compatible with an interaction model, but he adds, "if a simple additive model predicts almost as well to a given dependent variable as does this more complex theory, the additive model is to be preferred." ("The Identification Problem and Theory Building," *American Sociological Review*, 31, 1966, 61.)

Tables 11.5 and 11.6 do not, of course, exhaust the possibilities for categorizing couples in respect to mobility. If the reader wishes to try other combinations (as we shall in the last section of this chapter), Table 11.3 supplies the requisite raw materials. The bottom panel of that table, however, suggests that an account of the deviations from the additive model that uses mobility as an interpretive category will have to be stated in highly particularistic terms. The exercises already completed in Tables 11.5 and 11.6 suggest that there is no general effect of mobility apart from the circumstance that mobile couples reflect in their fertility record the influence of both their origin and their destination statuses. Thus despite some departures from a strictly additive model, the data do not fall into a pattern supporting in any substantial way the weak form of the mobility hypothesis.

FERTILITY IN RELATION TO INTERGENERATIONAL MOBILITY

The foregoing discussion was somewhat prolonged in order to illustrate adequately the point of view on which the analysis is based and to make clear what precautions are necessary if we are to distinguish between variations in fertility that are, in some specific sense, due to mobility and those that are more readily interpreted as resulting from a simple combination of the effects of the origin and destination statuses. Now that the pattern of analysis has been illustrated we can proceed more rapidly to summarize the results for the three remaining forms of mobility, all pertaining to intergenerational movements (wife's father's occupation to husband's first job, husband's father's occupation to husband's occupation in 1962, and wife's father's occupation to husband's occupation in 1962).

As before, the study of intergenerational mobility must begin by calculating the net effects for the additive model to provide a benchmark for detecting interactions, or departures of the observed means from the additive model. The results of this calculation, which are recorded in Appendix Table J.11.1, seem to require no discussion here, for the patterns of net effects are much like those already observed in our illustrative example.

Turning to the assessment of interactions, we can quickly dispose of one set of results, those concerning the combination of wife's father's occupation with husband's first job. The analysis of variance for these data, which are shown in Appendix Table J11.2, yields an insignificant sum of squares for interaction (the probability of the computed F-value exceeds 0.1). The additive model is wholly acceptable for these data, and neither the weak nor, *a fortiori*, the strong mobility hypothesis finds any support whatever. This particular combination of statuses, incidentally, defines the one form of mobility for which the mobility experience clearly preceded the completion of fertility. Each of the other three involves 1962 occupation as the destination status, and this status may have been first achieved at some time during or even entirely after the completion of the wife's childbearing period.

We must look more closely at the other two sets of results, pertaining respectively to mobility from husband's father's and wife's father's occupation to husband's occupation in 1962. The analysis of variance points to significant interactions; departures of the mean fertility in cells of these mobility tables from means expected on the additive model cannot be readily attributed to sampling fluctuations. Tables 11.7 and 11.8 show these departures. Certain of the larger deviations should be interpreted cautiously because of the small number of sample cases on which they are based. In some respects the patterns of deviations in the two cases are similar, in others different. Looking only at the signs of the deviations in the 25 cells not involving a "not

TABLE 11.7. MEAN NUMBER OF CHILDREN EVER BORN, BY HUSBAND'S FATHER'S OCC. AND HUSBAND'S 1962 OCC., FOR WIVES 42 TO 61 YEARS OLD IN MARCH, 1962, LIVING WITH HUSBANDS IN OCG SAMPLE

| | | Husband's Occ. in 1962 | | | | | |
| | All | White-Collar | | Manual | | | Not |
Husband's Father's Occ.	Couples	Higher	Lower	Higher	Lower	Farm	Stated[a]
NUMBER OF COUPLES (THOUSANDS)							
All couples	13,748[b]	3,777	1,412	2,886	3,710	1,109	854
Higher white-collar	2,006	1,071	296	254	270	36	79
Lower white-collar	830	377	141	117	124	18	53
Higher manual	2,304	659	291	632	517	32	173
Lower manual	2,924	642	311	675	1,060	58	178
Farm	4,542	758	270	932	1,352	911	319
Not stated	1,142	270	103	276	387	54	52
CHILDREN EVER BORN PER WIFE							
All couples	2.45	2.12	1.92	2.57	2.62	3.18	2.70
Higher white-collar	1.98	1.96	1.68	2.01	2.24	2.53	2.24
Lower white-collar	1.99	2.01	1.56	2.44	2.18	2.44	1.42
Higher manual	2.39	2.31	2.08	2.64	2.52	1.88	1.99
Lower manual	2.33	2.13	1.88	2.41	2.52	2.91	2.26
Farm	2.84	2.27	2.07	2.78	2.86	3.26	3.73
Not stated	2.46	2.04	2.38	2.61	2.55	3.54	2.35
OBSERVED MINUS CALCULATED MEANS							
Higher white-collar	...	.07	.01	-.22	-.02	-.12	-.11
Lower white-collar	...	.13	-.10	.22	-.07	-.20	-.93
Higher manual	...	.11	.10	.11	-.04	-1.08	-.67
Lower manual	...	.03	-.01	-.02	.05	.05	-.31
Farm	...	-.22	-.20	-.04	(-).00	.01	.77
Not stated	...	-.18	.38	.05	-.04	.55	-.34

[a]Husband not in experienced civilian labor force.
[b]Marginal and grand totals are sums of cell frequencies; totals vary between tabulations because of accumulated rounding errors.

TABLE 11.8.   MEAN NUMBER OF CHILDREN EVER BORN, BY WIFE'S FATHER'S OCC. AND HUSBAND'S 1962 OCC., FOR WIVES 42 TO 61 YEARS OLD IN MARCH, 1962, LIVING WITH HUSBANDS IN OCG SAMPLE

| | | Husband's Occ. in 1962 | | | | | |
| | | White-Collar | | Manual | | | |
Wife's Father's Occ.	All Couples	Higher	Lower	Higher	Lower	Farm	Not Stated[a]
NUMBER OF COUPLES (THOUSANDS)							
All couples	13,747[b]	3,779	1,413	2,891	3,710	1,106	848
Higher white-collar	2,077	936	296	317	324	70	134
Lower white-collar	805	362	117	157	100	26	43
Higher manual	2,270	684	272	600	544	50	120
Lower manual	3,138	713	321	729	1,092	89	194
Farm	4,146	805	291	820	1,154	793	283
Not stated	1,311	279	116	268	496	78	74
CHILDREN EVER BORN PER WIFE							
All couples	2.45	2.12	1.91	2.56	2.62	3.19	2.72
Higher white-collar	2.14	2.01	1.83	2.67	2.07	2.69	2.44
Lower white-collar	2.13	2.22	1.69	2.22	2.40	2.38	1.47
Higher manual	2.30	2.06	1.73	2.59	2.53	2.40	2.39
Lower manual	2.32	2.06	2.02	2.29	2.53	2.75	2.50
Farm	2.82	2.37	2.07	2.65	2.86	3.41	3.56
Not stated	2.53	1.97	2.03	3.06	2.73	2.73	1.91
OBSERVED MINUS CALCULATED MEANS							
Higher white-collar	...	.02	.06	.28	-.34	-.15	-.07
Lower white-collar	...	.25	-.08	-.16	.00	-.44	-1.03
Higher manual	...	-.01	-.13	.12	.03	-.52	-.20
Lower manual	...	.02	.19	-.15	.06	-.14	-.07
Farm	...	-.06	-.16	-.19	-.01	.12	.59
Not stated	...	-.25	.02	.43	.08	-.34	-.84

[a]Husband not in experienced civilian labor force.
[b]Marginal and grand totals are sums of cell frequencies; totals vary between tabulations because of accumulated rounding errors.

stated" category, there is consistency between the two tables in 17 and inconsistency in 8 cells.

Unfortunately, few clues to an interpretation of the departures from the additive model are found in Table 11.9, where mobile couples are alternatively classified by origin status and by current status and the results are compared with differentials for nonmobile couples. In each instance there is only one sizable departure from the values implied by the additive model. The few couples moving from nonfarm origins to 1962 farm occupations show a mean somewhat below that calculated from the model. Apparently, couples experiencing this rare type of mobility do not fully reflect the effect of their destination status in their childbearing performance. The salient conclusion from Table 11.9 is that nonmobile couples, like mobile ones, exhibit the pattern of differential fertility associated with their occupational position. Indeed, one gains the impression that the differentials are somewhat more pronounced for the nonmobile than

TABLE 11.9. DEVIATIONS OF OBSERVED NUMBER OF CHILDREN EVER BORN PER WIFE FROM VALUES CALCULATED FROM ADDITIVE MODEL, BY MOBILITY CLASSIFICATION, FOR WIVES 42 TO 61 YEARS OLD IN MARCH, 1962, LIVING WITH HUSBANDS IN OCG SAMPLE

| | | Occ. Group | | | | |
| | All | White-collar | | Manual | | |
Mobility Classification	Groups	Higher	Lower	Higher	Lower	Farm
HUSBAND'S FATHER'S OCC. TO HUSBAND'S 1962 OCC.						
Mobile, by origin status	-.03	-.07	.10	.03	(+).00	-.08
Nonmobile	.05	.07	-.10	.11	.05	.01
Mobile, by 1962 status	-.03	-.01	-.02	-.04	-.02	-.28
WIFE'S FATHER'S OCC. TO HUSBAND'S 1962 OCC.						
Mobile, by origin status	-.04	-.01	.08	-.03	-.03	-.09
Nonmobile	.07	.02	-.08	.12	.06	.12
Mobile, by 1962 status	-.04	.02	-.01	-.10	-.05	-.25

for the mobile couples, whether the latter are classified by their origin status or their destination status.

In Table 11.10, in which account is taken of the direction of mobility, we can see very little difference between the observed fertility of the aggregate of nonmobile nonfarm couples and that of either the downwardly or the upwardly mobile couples. Departures from values calculated from the additive model are hardly noteworthy, with the already mentioned exception of nonfarm-to-farm movers.

TABLE 11.10. DEVIATIONS OF OBSERVED NUMBER OF CHILDREN EVER BORN PER WIFE FROM VALUES CALCULATED FROM ADDITIVE MODEL, BY TYPE OF MOBILITY, FOR WIVES 42 TO 61 YEARS OLD IN MARCH, 1962, LIVING WITH HUSBANDS IN OCG SAMPLE

Type of Mobility	Husband's Father's Occ. to Husband's Occ. in 1962	Wife's Father's Occ. to Husband's Occ. in 1962
Nonmobile, nonfarm	.06	.06
Nonmobile, farm	.01	.12
Upward mobile, nonfarm	.05	.00
Downward mobile, nonfarm	-.04	.00
Nonfarm to farm	-.28	-.25
Farm to nonfarm	-.08	-.09

Despite the initial observation of significant interaction, these data offer little basis for substantive interpretations in terms of the effect of mobility on fertility. Direct comparison of mobile couples of various types with nonmobile couples seems to contribute little to an understanding of the evident, though not terribly marked, variation of fertility by occupational status. The strong hypothesis receives no support whatever from these data, whereas the weak hypothesis is supported only to the extent that its simplest rival—that of a strictly additive combination of effects of origin and destination statuses—is not wholly acceptable. No clear pattern of the sort one should expect if the weak hypothesis were sound emerges on detailed inspection of the departures from an additive model.

In all four sets of data we find significant net effects for both origin and destination class. Thus the expectation for mobile couples is that their fertility will combine the effects of class of origin with class of destination. This result, it should be noted, conforms perfectly with Fisher's criterion (quoted earlier) for recognizing causation due to "social environment," to wit, that "the families who rise in the social scale . . . carry with them some measure of the fertility of the classes from which they originated." This conclusion can be reached without recourse to the formalism of the additive model. Let us look again at the 25 observed means in the second panel of Table 11.3 (omitting the "not stated" row and column). Mobile couples may be compared with nonmobile at the class of origin and destination respectively. Thus we find for upward mobility from a lower white-collar first job to a higher white-collar occupation in 1962 a fertility of 2.03. This is higher than the fertility of nonmobile couples in both the origin class (1.70) and the destination class (1.96). We can make 10 such triangular comparisons for upwardly mobile and 10 for downwardly mobile couples. In Table 11.3 we find just one cell where upwardly mobile couples have this type of positive deviation (the example just given). There is likewise only one cell showing the opposite kind of deviation —fertility in the upwardly mobile group lower than either diagonal (nonmobile) value. In the remaining 8 cells for upwardly mobile couples the cell mean is intermediate between the diagonal values for class of origin and class of destination. In the 10 cells for downward mobility we find 3 with positive deviations, 4 with negative, and 3 intermediate.

Carrying out the same inspection for the three intergenerational mobility tables (11.7, 11.8, and J11.2), we find:

		Positive	Intermediate	Negative
Wife's father's occupation				
to husband's first job	Up	0	8	2
	Down	3	7	0
Husband's father's occ.				
to husband's 1962 occ.	Up	1	8	1
	Down	0	9	1
Wife's father's occ.				
to husband's 1962 occ.	Up	1	8	1
	Down	1	8	1

Evidently the prevailing pattern is that the fertility of mobile couples is intermediate between that of couples remaining in the class of origin and that of the nonmobile in the class of destination. This is especially consistent (in all four tables) for upwardly mobile couples, which is the category on which most discussion of the mobility hypothesis has focused. The pattern observed in these fertility data, then, conforms most nearly to what one of us has termed acculturation, for which this explanation has been offered:

. . . mobile persons are not well integrated in either social class. Without extensive and intimate social contacts, they do not have sufficient opportunity for complete acculturation to the values and style of life of the one group, nor do they continue to experience the full impact of the social constraints of the other. But both groups exert some influence over mobile individuals, since they have, or have had, social contacts with members of both. . . . Hence their behavior is expected to be intermediate between that of the two nonmobile classes.[17]

Whether the explanation in terms of socialization or influence of contacts is correct cannot be determined from the data at hand.

Whereas only shifts from one broad occupational group to another have been considered in the foregoing analysis, the mobility hypothesis can also be tested by using a different criterion of mobility, namely change in occupational status. For this purpose, each occupation is placed in one of ten intervals on the scale of occupational status: 0 to 9, 10 to 19, . . . , 90 and over. Merely as a convenience, these intervals are designated as ten "steps" on the occupational scale, and mobility is measured by the number of steps up or down from the occupational status of origin to that of destination. We have fertility data in relation to all six kinds of mobility defined by the four occupational statuses measured in the survey. One of these types pertains to intragenerational and the other five to intergenerational mobility. Again, the parameters of an additive model were estimated. Deviations from the values expected on this model were aggregated for cells representing different directions and degrees of mobility. Table 11.11 records these departures.

It is difficult to know just what to make of these results. We are looking specifically for evidence that mobility as such makes a difference once the estimated additive effects of origin and destination status are allowed for. Hence, in scanning the columns of figures, the eye

17 Peter M. Blau, "Social Mobility and Interpersonal Relations," *American Sociological Review*, 21(1956), p. 291.

TABLE 11.11. DEVIATIONS FROM ADDITIVE MODEL OF EFFECTS OF ORIGIN AND DESTINATION STATUSES, BY DISTANCE AND DIRECTION OF MOBILITY, FOR WIVES 42 TO 61 YEARS OLD IN MARCH, 1962, LIVING WITH HUSBANDS IN OCG SAMPLE

Distance and Direction of Mobility (Number of steps)	Husband's First Job to 1962 Occ.	Husband's Father's Occ. to:		Wife's Father's Occ. to:		
		Husband's 1962 Occ.	Husband's First Job	Husband's Father's Occ.	Husband's First Job	Husband's 1962 Occ.
OBSERVED MINUS COMPUTED CHILDREN EVER BORN PER WIFE						
Up: 6 to 9	-.29	-.27	-.12	-.21	.07	-.02
5	.09	.01	-.07	-.06	-.19	-.08
4	.05	.09	-.08	-.14	-.05	-.04
3	.04	-.17	.15	.02	.11	-.12
2	.09	.16	-.08	.03	-.04	-.03
1	-.01	.06	.00	-.09	-.20	.03
Stable: 0	.04	.01	.09	.08	.07	.05
Down: -1	.06	-.04	-.10	-.01	.01	.13
-2	-.16	.06	-.08	-.16	-.01	.09
-3	.07	.05	.06	.05	.02	.15
-4 to -9	-.40	-.23	-.08	-.02	.02	-.19
PER CENT DISTRIBUTION OF COUPLES[a]						
Up: 6 to 9	5.3	5.8	2.0	2.1	2.1	6.7
5	5.0	5.5	2.3	2.6	1.5	5.8
4	7.8	7.6	3.5	3.7	2.7	7.4
3	9.7	9.3	4.9	4.7	5.7	9.4
2	11.8	10.7	6.0	7.3	7.3	10.5
1	17.7	13.8	20.3	11.1	10.8	14.7
Stable: 0	27.7	26.6	33.8	37.9	28.1	23.3
Down: -1	8.2	10.2	10.4	10.3	19.9	10.1
-2	3.3	3.9	6.8	6.1	6.8	4.3
-3	2.0	3.1	4.6	5.4	5.4	2.8
-4 to -9	1.5	3.5	5.4	8.8	9.7	5.0
Total	100.0	100.0	100.0	100.0	100.0	100.0

[a]Based on cases for which both origin and destination status are reported.

tends to fix on discrepancies supporting this conclusion but to ignore those failing to do so. Two things seem clear, however. There is no general or pervasive effect of upward or downward mobility common to all kinds of occupational mobility and differing only by degree of mobility. Besides, if there is any substantial effect of mobility—as registered in a deviation greater than, say, 0.2—it is confined to the extremes of long-distance upward or downward mobility. Actually, in the six sets of figures there are but five deviations this large. None of them pertains to a category including as many as 6 per cent of the sample couples. If we take a more liberal criterion and regard deviations no greater than 0.1 as interesting, then we encounter problems of interpretation. Several of these are adjacent to deviations of opposite sign. It is difficult to explain why, for example, moving up two steps should produce an increment of .16, three steps an increment of −.17, and four steps an increment of .09 (second column of Table 11.11) in average fertility.

If any of the apparent mobility effects are real it is presumably the ones in the first two columns of Table 11.11 that are most interesting. In movement from either first job or husband's father's occupation to husband's 1962 occupation, both long-distance upward and long-distance downward mobility depress fertility. We may elaborate the multiple-classification model to provide alternative estimates of these effects. Let

$$Y_{hija} = \overline{Y} + a_i + b_j + m_h + U_{hija}$$

where m_h is a three-category classification ($h = 1,2,3$). A constant m_1 is estimated for long-distance downward mobility (-4 to -9 steps); m_2 for short-distance mobility or stability (-3 to 5 steps, and including cases with either origin or destination status unknown); and m_3 for long-distance upward mobility (6 to 9 steps).

When the solution for this model is obtained for the first two kinds of mobility in Table 11.11, the net effects for origin and destination (a_i and b_j) are much the same as in the previous no-interaction model. The solution also provides, however, the following estimates of effects for the mobility classification:

	m_1	m_2	m_3
Husband's first job to 1962 occupation	—.35	.03	—.40
Husband's father's occupation to 1962 occupation	—.18	.03	—.40

In both cases the additive model is slightly improved by including these mobility effects, ranging from —.2 to —.4 and applying to less than one-tenth of the population.

Although the earlier analysis with broad occupation groups failed to discover any apparent mobility effects of interest, the present analysis may have revealed some such effects, of a very special kind. They occur in connection with only two of the six possible kinds of mobility defined by comparisons of four occupational statuses. They pertain not to mobility in general but to extreme upward or downward mobility. The mobility hypothesis as it has been developed in the literature casts no light on either of the two circumstances, (a) that only two kinds of mobility reveal the effect, and (b) that the same effect—such as it is or appears to be—occurs for both upward and downward mobility. Indeed, *any* explanation of these findings will have to be a somewhat specialized one, because the bulk of the evidence indicates that the major consequence of mobility is simply that mobile couples have a completed family size intermediate between the averages pertaining to their respective origin and destination statuses.

CONDITIONS MODIFYING OCCUPATIONAL
DIFFERENTIALS IN FERTILITY

Earlier in this chapter attention was given briefly to the interaction of wife's education with farm background of the couple in the pattern of differential fertility. Having analyzed occupational differentials in some detail we may now inquire whether a similar result obtains in the case of the occupation variable. Table 11.12, confined to couples living in nonfarm residences, shows fertility differentials by occupational status and farm background in terms of both the husband's 1962 occupation and his first job.

TABLE 11.12. CHILDREN EVER BORN PER WIFE, BY SOCIOECONOMIC STATUS OF HUSBAND'S FIRST JOB AND 1962 OCC., BY FARM BACKGROUND OF COUPLE, FOR COUPLES LIVING IN NONFARM RESIDENCES IN MARCH, 1962, WIVES 42 TO 61 YEARS OLD

Item and Background of Couple	Occ. Status Score				
	0–9	10–19	20–39	40–59	60 and over
HUSBAND'S 1962 OCC.					
Number of couples (Thousands)[a]					
Nonfarm	489	1,211	1,546	1,579	2,191
Farm	592	1,255	1,098	920	785
Children ever born per wife					
Nonfarm	2.61	2.37	2.28	2.34	1.94
Farm	3.12	2.64	2.75	2.17	2.06
Difference	–.51	–.27	–.47	.17	–.12
HUSBAND'S FIRST JOB					
Number of couples (Thousands)[b]					
Nonfarm	1,394	1,762	2,072	1,223	761
Farm	1,665	1,761	772	378	274
Children ever born per wife					
Nonfarm	2.64	2.28	2.08	1.97	1.91
Farm	2.73	2.73	2.28	2.29	1.92
Difference	–.09	–.45	–.20	–.32	–.01

[a]Omits husbands not in experienced civilian labor force.
[b]Omits husbands not reporting first job.

In general fertility is negatively related to occupational status within both types of background. In terms of 1962 occupation the differential is more pronounced for couples with farm background (husband's or wife's father reported as farmer or farm laborer). At the lowest socioeconomic level farm background raises mean fertility 0.5 above the figure for couples with nonfarm background; at the highest level this difference is only 0.1.

In terms of first job background makes little or no difference at the extremes of the status scale. At intermediate statuses (10 to 59), however, farm background elevates fertility somewhat in comparison with fertility for couples with nonfarm background. Indeed, except for the very lowest interval of occupational status, differentials for first job are rather minor in the case of couples with nonfarm background.

These results, therefore, sustain the impression already gained that differential fertility is quite attenuated when the analysis is focused on the growing sector of couples with nonfarm background. Perhaps this is only another way of indicating the sphere of applicability of the mobility hypothesis. Movement to nonfarm residences from farm backgrounds is, of course, a form of social and occupational mobility. Such a move is accompanied by a reduction of fertility, as compared with that of persons remaining on farms. The amount of reduction, however, is directly related to the degree of upward mobility in the nonfarm sector. If the migrants from farms remain in low-status occupations or fail to obtain average or greater amounts of education their fertility remains high relative to other nonfarm residents. If they undergo upward mobility their fertility is sharply reduced, though not below the levels of persons with nonfarm origins enjoying comparable occupational achievement or educational attainment. The interaction of background with occupational status or educational attainment delineates a specific mobility effect of some considerable demographic importance, if we are willing to extrapolate. As was pointed out, smaller and smaller proportions of successive cohorts will have farm background as this source of movement into nonfarm areas nears exhaustion. In that event differential fertility on the classic pattern will cease to be manifest in any great degree, barring emergence of some new principle of differentiation. By the same token the mobility hypothesis, as traditionally discussed, may become more or less irrelevant.

This conclusion has, in a way, already been anticipated by demographers concerned with fertility analysis, insofar as their interest in conventional studies of differential fertility has waned considerably in recent years. Under contemporary conditions much more refined analysis will doubtlessly be required to discern significant variation in fertility by social status.

An interesting lead for such analysis has turned up in recently issued tabulations from the 1960 Census of Population. An illustrative excerpt from these tables is shown in Table 11.13. The data are limited to couples residing in urbanized areas, so that the proportions with farm background are doubtlessly rather small. The significant princi-

TABLE 11.13.   CHILDREN EVER BORN PER WOMAN, BY SOCIOECONOMIC CHARACTERISTICS OF HUSBAND, FOR WHITE WOMEN MARRIED ONCE AND HUSBAND PRESENT, BY AGE OF WOMAN AND WOMAN'S AGE AT MARRIAGE: U.S. URBANIZED AREAS, 1960 (DEVIATIONS FROM THE GRAND MEAN)

Subject	Age 35–44 Married at age –		Age 45–54 Married at age –	
	Under 22	22 and over	Under 22	22 and over
All women (grand mean)[a]	(2.73)	(2.17)	(2.57)	(1.75)
Husband's occ.				
Farm	.66	.20	.87	.36
Laborers, except farm	.51	-.01	.79	.20
Service workers	.07	-.09	.12	-.06
Operatives	.14	-.08	.22	.05
Craftsmen	.03	.00	.11	.03
Clerical and sales	-.19	-.06	-.32	-.14
MOP	-.12	.06	-.28	.01
Professional, technical, and kindred	-.12	.11	-.39	.03
Husband's education				
No high school	.26	-.08	.25	.04
High school, 1 to 4 years	-.07	-.05	-.17	-.06
College, 1 year or more	-.10	.12	-.38	.05
Income				
Under $2,000	.33	-.37	.37	-.12
$2–4,000	.21	-.27	.34	-.12
$4–7,000	-.01	-.10	.04	-.04
$7–10,000	-.05	.11	-.16	.01
$10,000 or more	-.05	.27	-.34	.16

SOURCE: U.S. Bureau of the Census, "Women by Number of Children Ever Born," Subject Report PC(2), 3A, 1960 Census of Population (Washington: Government Printing Office, 1964), Table 39.
[a]Excludes: Husband unemployed, not in civilian labor force, no income in 1959, or occ. not reported.

ple of classification in this table—apart from the socioeconomic variables themselves—is wife's age at marriage.

These data reveal unmistakably significant interactions. For wives marrying at young ages differential fertility on the classic pattern is clearly in evidence: fertility is inversely related to husband's occupational status, his educational attainment, and his income. For women marrying at age 22 and over, however, this is no longer true. Indeed, a distinct positive relationship with income emerges in this group, exactly reversing the finding for women marrying young. Late age at marriage, of course, reduces fertility considerably, but this effect by itself does not account for the interaction of socioeconomic characteristics with age at marriage. The latter requires an explanation on grounds other than the simple diminution of the period of exposure to the risk of childbearing.

If one cared to make the argument, one could hypothesize that youthful age at marriage is selective of persons disinclined to postpone gratification or to plan their lives over long periods ahead. Those marrying late, on the contrary, seem to behave quite "rationally," especially in terms of adjusting fertility to income. A final interesting feature of these data is that the effect described seems somewhat more pronounced for the younger of the two groups of cohorts. Although the inference is risky, we might venture the guess that the age difference represents the emergence of a relatively new phenomenon. Unfortunately, the insight provided by these census data became available too late to affect the design and analysis of the OCG fertility data. We may speculate just a little, however, in the hope of suggesting useful clues for the next investigation along these lines.

Apparently social mobility in the generic sense is not a very important source of differential fertility. Socioeconomic differentials in the population at large are becoming attenuated, yet it is possible to isolate groups wherein vestiges of the classic pattern of "inverted birth rates" still prevail, to wit, couples with farm background and women marrying at early ages. If other such sectors can be identified it would seem strategic to pursue the mobility hypothesis by way of a comparison of these with the sectors wherein differentials have become extremely slight or have even been reversed. Unfortunately this strategy cannot be recommended for small-scale studies, for all the evidence in the present investigation shows that the effects we are seeking are small on the whole and easily masked by sampling and other errors.

AN ALTERNATIVE PERSPECTIVE

Instead of a summary of the detailed analysis in this chapter, we offer, in conclusion, an alternative way of thinking about the results that leads to a compact presentation and that some readers may find more informative.

The viewpoint governing the discussion in the chapter to this point should be clear. It has been concerned with the question of what possible demographic consequences follow from the volume of mobility observed in an economically advanced society, insofar as fertility is concerned. We have placed the analysis in the historical context of a classic concern with the problem of differential fertility, within which some writers were led to expect that investigations of social mobility would shed important light on the genesis of class variations in fertility. On this point of view one is constrained to inspect the results not merely for statistically significant departures from the model proposed as an alternative to the mobility hypothesis, but for departures large enough to be of some demographic consequence. Such departures were not found. We have concluded that occupational mobility, in general, is not a very productive variable for purposes of demographic analysis.

On the other hand, a specific type of spatial and social mobility—

the movement off farms—may indeed be of some considerable demographic importance. This movement is accompanied not only by a reduction in the over-all level of fertility, but also, in the generations after it occurs, by a drastic alteration of the pattern of differential fertility. It is this kind of mobility effect that one might have expected to observe as a general consequence of mobility, but little or no evidence of such a consequence is to be found in the OCG data. At the same time we are constrained to note that the OCG results may well fail to reflect the situation that held at the time differential fertility first began to be studied and the mobility hypothesis was formulated. For all we know to the contrary, the mobility hypothesis may indeed have been descriptive of the actual state of affairs at the turn of the century, although it is difficult to see how it will ever be possible to test this supposition. But in the contemporary United States, insofar as we may trust the evidence from cohorts with atypically low general levels of fertility, the demographic consequence of mobility is simply that mobile couples have children at rates intermediate between those prevailing in their respective strata of origin and destination.

If we shift from this demographic-historical frame of reference however, it can be argued that the foregoing results take on a somewhat different meaning. An investigator concerned with theoretical generalizations about the consequences of mobility may have little interest in the demographic effects of mobility as such. For him demographic data are only illustrative of one kind of possible consequence of mobility. If the interest is in generalizing across a variety of dependent variables, the critical question is no longer whether mobility has pronounced demographic effects, but merely whether any consistent mobility effects (of whatever magnitude) can be observed. If so, then the demographic data lend encouragement to the quest for other consequences of mobility in ranges of phenomena that may respond in a more obvious way to the discrepancy between class of origin and class of destination.

As we have seen above, it is difficult to detect any highly consistent departures from the additive model when the data are arrayed in great detail. It is possible, however, that many of the inconsistencies are merely sampling errors that would cancel out in more highly aggregated data. On this supposition, Tables 11.14 to 11.17 have been prepared. These are simply alternative arrangements of the data already presented. The four tables are grouped into two pairs. The first table in each pair (11.14 and 11.16) shows the actual or observed mean fertility for highly condensed mobility categories. Table 11.14 includes

TABLE 11.14.   CHILDREN EVER BORN PER WIFE, BY OCC. CLASSES OF ORIGIN AND DESTINATION, FOR MARRIED COUPLES, SPOUSE PRESENT, WIFE 42 TO 61 YEARS OLD

Occ. Class of Origin	Occ. Class of Destination		
	White-collar	Manual	Farm
DESTINATION: HUSBAND'S OCC. IN 1962			
Husband's father's occ.			
White-collar	1.89	2.18	2.50
Manual	2.14	2.52	2.54
Farm	2.22	2.83	3.26
Wife's father's occ.			
White-collar	2.00	2.34	2.60
Manual	2.01	2.48	2.63
Farm	2.29	2.77	3.41
Husband's first job			
White-collar	1.91	2.09	1.85
Manual	2.09	2.57	3.20
Farm	2.93	2.93	3.32
DESTINATION: HUSBAND'S FIRST JOB			
Wife's father's occ.			
White-collar	1.90	2.26	2.74
Manual	1.93	2.38	2.83
Farm	2.12	2.66	3.24

information for the four types of mobility when the data on census major occupation groups are condensed into the three broad occupational classes—white-collar, blue-collar, and farm. Table 11.16 displays a summary by direction of mobility, where mobility refers to a change of one 10-point interval or more on the occupational status scale. Thus the categories in Table 11.16 are simply condensations of those in Table 11.11.

The second table in each of these pairs (Tables 11.15 and 11.17) shows the ratio of the observed fertility by mobility category to the fertility expected on the model specifying merely additive effects of origin and destination. Here, as in other analyses where the data have been aggregated, the grouping was done after the calculated number of children ever born was obtained from a model with the full occupational detail initially available. Had the observed data been aggregated before the values for the additive model were calculated the results might have been slightly different.

For the purpose at hand—an examination of the consistency of mobility effects—we may pass over the observed means in Tables 11.14 and 11.16, and examine immediately the departures from the additive model in the other two tables. Here a departure is signified by a ratio differing from unity. A ratio greater than 1.00 means that observed

TABLE 11.15. RATIO OF ACTUAL NUMBER OF CHILDREN EVER BORN TO NUMBER EXPECTED ON THE MODEL OF ADDITIVE EFFECTS OF ORIGIN AND DESTINATION, BY OCC. CLASSES, FOR MARRIED COUPLES, SPOUSE PRESENT, WIFE 42 TO 61 YEARS OLD

Occ. Class of Origin	Occ. Class of Destination			
	White-collar	Manual	Farm	Summary
DESTINATION: HUSBAND'S OCC. IN 1962				
Husband's father's occ.				
White-collar	1.032	.974	.944	. . .
Manual	1.030	1.011	.877	. . .
Farm	.912	.994	1.003	. . .
All mobile[a]	. . .	. . .	. . .	.985
All nonmobile[b]	. . .	. . .	. . .	1.015
Wife's father's occ.				
White-collar	1.037	.979	.923	. . .
Manual	1.008	1.006	.906	. . .
Farm	.962	.971	1.036	. . .
All mobile[a]	. . .	. . .	. . .	.978
All nonmobile[b]	. . .	. . .	. . .	1.020
Husband's first job				
White-collar	1.036	.967	.762	. . .
Manual	.957	1.021	1.141	. . .
Farm	1.068	.955	.992	. . .
All mobile[a]	. . .	. . .	. . .	.973
All nonmobile[b]	. . .	. . .	. . .	1.021
DESTINATION: HUSBAND'S FIRST JOB				
Wife's father's occ.				
White-collar	1.029	.985	.955	. . .
Manual	1.012	1.008	.966	. . .
Farm	.965	1.003	1.005	. . .
All mobile[a]	. . .	. . .	. . .	.990
All nonmobile[b]	. . .	. . .	. . .	1.010

[a]Sum of off-diagonal cells.
[b]Sum of diagonal cells.

TABLE 11.16. CHILDREN EVER BORN PER WIFE, BY MOBILITY CATEGORIES DEFINED BY STEPS ON THE SOCIOECONOMIC SCALE, FOR MARRIED COUPLES, SPOUSE PRESENT, WIFE 42 - 61 YRS. OLD

Type of Mobility		Direction of Mobility		
Origin	Destination	Upward	Stable	Downward
Husband's Father's Occ.	Husband's 1962 Occ.	2.32	2.62	2.47
Husband's Father's Occ.	Husband's First Job	2.15	2.69	2.47
Husband's First Job	Husband's 1962 Occ.	2.37	2.59	2.38
Wife's Father's Occ.	Husband's Father's Occ.	2.20	2.75	2.32
Wife's Father's Occ.	Husband's First Job	2.12	2.70	2.50
Wife's Father's Occ.	Husband's 1962 Occ.	2.25	2.70	2.55

fertility exceeds that expected on the additive model; a ratio less than 1.00 means that it falls short of expected fertility.

Table 11.15 shows that, with one exception among the four types of mobility, the ratios on the diagonal are greater than 1.00. Thus, with some consistency, nonmobile couples—referring, in this connection, to those not moving from one of the three broad occupation

TABLE 11.17. RATIO OF ACTUAL NUMBER OF CHILDREN EVER BORN TO NUMBER EXPECTED ON THE MODEL OF ADDITIVE EFFECTS OF ORIGIN AND DESTINATION, BY MOBILITY CATEGORIES DEFINED BY STEPS ON THE SOCIOECONOMIC SCALE, FOR MARRIED COUPLES, SPOUSE PRESENT, WIFE 42 TO 61 YEARS OLD

| Type of Mobility | | Direction of Mobility | | |
Origin	Destination	Upward	Stable	Downward
Husband's father's occ.	Husband's 1962 occ.	1.003	1.005	.984
Husband's father's occ.	Husband's first job	.972	1.032	.995
Husband's first job	Husband's 1962 occ.	.999	1.016	.986
Wife's father's occ.	Husband's father's occ.	.976	1.031	.988
Wife's father's occ.	Husband's first job	.969	1.028	1.003
Wife's father's occ.	Husband's 1962 occ.	.983	1.020	1.006

classes to another—have higher fertility than expected on the additive model. It is then virtually a tautology that in most of the off-diagonal cells the ratios are below unity. In each panel of the table, however, there is at least one category of mobile couples with fertility greater than is implied by the additive model.

An even more drastic condensation appears in the last column of Table 11.15, where there is a comparison between all mobile and all nonmobile couples. Ratios for nonmobile couples vary, over the four types of mobility, from 1.01 to 1.02, or from 1 to 2 per cent in excess of the fertility expected on the additive model. The same discrepancy is shown by the four ratios falling below unity for the mobile couples.

In Table 11.17 we find the same sort of consistency for nonmobile couples. For all six types of mobility, their fertility exceeds that expected on the additive model, by an amount varying from 5 per cent to a little more than 3 per cent. For five of the six types of mobility, upwardly mobile couples have fertility falling short of that expected on the additive model, and the same is true for four of the six types of mobility in regard to the downwardly mobile. (The designation of direction of mobility for the combination of wife's father's occupation with husband's father's occupation is, of course, arbitrary; but the decision on this point does not affect the finding.) For all six types of mobility, even those where one category of mobile couples shows a ratio over 1.00, the ratio for stable couples is higher than the ratios for couples moving in either direction.

In sum, these data reveal that mobility in either direction has a slight but rather consistent depressing effect on fertility. If we examine the more detailed data presented earlier with this conclusion derived from the condensed data in mind we can detect the same pattern, though there it is not entirely consistent. When occupations are

grouped into a 5 x 5 matrix, whether intragenerational or intergenerational mobility is considered, fertility exceeds expectations in 4 of
5 diagonal cells and falls short of expectations in 13 of 20 off-diagonal
cells (last panel in Tables 11.3, 11.7, and 11.8, ignoring "not stated").
When the nonmobile couples are compared to the mobile ones with
either the same origins or the same destinations the fertility of the
former exceeds that of the latter in terms of departures from the model
in four of five cases, whatever type of mobility is examined (last panel
of Table 11.5 and both panels of Table 11.9). When farm background
is taken into consideration, the data again reveal that the fertility of
the nonmobile, in terms of these departures, exceeds that of the
mobile in most cases (last column, Table 11.6, and both columns,
Table 11.10). When mobility is defined on the basis of a change in
occupational status, the pattern is not consistent (Table 11.11), but
long-distance mobility from first or from father's to 1962 occupational
status, so defined, does depress fertility, as the previous analysis of
these data has shown. Only significant or exceptional social mobility,
like that involving a change in class position or long distances, has an
independent effect on fertility.

This conclusion does not contradict the earlier one; it merely introduces a new perspective. By and large the fertility of mobile couples,
which is intermediate between that prevailing in their origin and
that prevailing in their destination stratum, can be explained by the
additive influence of these two social strata. Substantial social mobility, however, exerts a further influence, independent of those of
social origin and occupational destination, effecting some reduction in birth rates, which is appreciable in the case of some types
of long-distance mobility. Although this depressing effect of mobility
as such is too small to account for much of the variance in fertility, it
reflects a significant impact of the experience of mobility on family
life. Even this mobility effect, however, does not confirm the mobility
hypothesis as originally conceived. The theory from which this hypothesis derives seeks to explain the inverse relationship between
upward mobility and fertility, and it assumes, by implication, that
downward mobility and fertility are directly related. If many children
are an impediment to successful careers, or if an orientation toward
occupational success is incompatible with an interest in having a
large family, it follows not only that men with few children have better
chances of upward mobility but also that men with many children
are more likely to be downwardly mobile. This inference is contra-
dicted by the finding that pronounced downward as well as upward

mobility inhibits fertility somewhat. (It should be noted that Berent's British data conform to the additive model without revealing such a mobility effect.[18])

Whereas upward and downward mobility are in many ways opposites, the one being a rewarding experience for which men strenuously compete and the other being a punishing experience that men seek to avoid, they also have something in common. Mobility in either direction entails disruptions of established social ties. To be sure, the diffuse class boundaries in the United States facilitate social associations among men with different social backgrounds, yet here as well as elsewhere economic circumstances and class status influence social interaction, and a major change in economic conditions tends to bring about corresponding changes in interpersonal contacts and social relations. Mobility, according to these conjectures, weakens the social integration of individuals in a network of social bonds that furnish stable social support.

The interpretation suggested is that the slightly lower fertility of mobile couples is a manifestation of the attenuation of supportive bonds of social integration that results from a basic change in socio-economic status. One question this speculation raises is whether more direct manifestations of the disturbances purportedly produced by lack of social support are also associated with mobility. Two pertinent pieces of evidence are that social mobility in either direction seems to increase nervousness[19] and the likelihood of mental illness.[20] The studies reaching these conclusions, however, were not designed to distinguish additive from interaction effects of mobility in the way that has been suggested in this chapter. A more recent investigation tested the hypothesis that "occupational mobility creates abnormal strain which is manifested in greater hostility towards Negroes than would be expected from additive effects alone."[21] The results were negative. Despite the strong *a priori* reasons for suspecting the operation of interactive mobility effects, such were not in evidence.

A second question is whether the interpretation of the mobility effect in terms of disruptive social relations is compatible with the other findings presented in this chapter. The influence of mobility itself on fertility is greatly overshadowed by that of a number of related

[18] Berent, *loc. cit.*, and Duncan, "Methodological Issues . . . ," *loc. cit.*

[19] Eugene Litwak, "Conflicting Values and Decision Making," Ph.D. dissertation, Columbia University, 1956.

[20] A. B. Hollingshead *et al.*, "Social Mobility and Mental Illness," *American Sociological Review*, 19(1954), 577-584.

[21] Robert W. Hodge and Donald J. Treiman, "Occupational Mobility and Attitudes Toward Negroes," *American Sociological Review*, 31(1966), 93.

factors. White-collar status and origin depress birth rates more than does mobility *per se*. So do late age at marriage and urbanization, whether the historical trend toward urbanization or differences between families with urban and farm background are considered, and these factors, moreover, reduce the class differential in fertility. Can a set of theoretical principles be discovered that helps explain these more pronounced influences on fertility and that is also consistent with the interpretation advanced concerning the influence of mobility on it? In the next chapter a theoretical explanation will be suggested that meets this requirement, centering on the hypothesis that both fertility itself and class differences in it are reduced by the *Gesellschafts* character that distinguishes modern urbanized society in general and its white-collar component in particular.

CHAPTER 12

Occupational Structure and Stratification System

In this concluding chapter we summarize the main findings of our research and discuss some of their broader implications for social stratification. First, conditions that affect a man's chances of occupational success in the United States are reviewed, starting with an analysis of the factors that govern the process of occupational mobility directly, and proceeding to an examination of other factors that modify this process. Next, attention is centered on the relationship between family life and occupational life—how a man's ascribed status in his family of orientation influences his achieved status in the occupational structure, and what significance his career has for his family of procreation. After this overview of some antecedents and consequences of individual achievement, the focus turns to the analysis of the occupational structure itself, the patterns of movements characterizing it, and the historical trends that can be inferred. Reflecting on the research results in a more speculative mood, we attempt to distinguish between structural and historical causes of social mobility in contemporary industrialized society. Finally, our findings on mobility rates in the United States are compared with those from other countries in order to draw some implications about the significance of mobility and economic progress for social stratification and political stability in a democracy.

CONDITIONS OF OCCUPATIONAL SUCCESS

A question often asked is, "What determines an individual's chances of achieving upward mobility?" This question can easily be answered, but the answer is not very meaningful. The main factor that determines a man's chances of upward mobility is the level on which he

401

starts. The lower the level from which a person starts, the greater is the probability that he will be upwardly mobile, simply because many more occupational destinations entail upward mobility for men with low origins than for those with high ones.[1] The trivial nature of the answer indicates that the question poses the issue poorly. To study what affects occupational mobility we must first decompose this concept into its constituent elements by examining how origins influence later achievements, and then proceed to investigate how several antecedent conditions interact in their effect on achievements. Regression and path analysis have been used to clarify the process of occupational mobility in this manner. All occupational categories for origins as well as destinations were transformed for this purpose into a status score based on the average income and education in each detailed occupation.

Whereas intergenerational mobility and intragenerational mobility are conventionally treated as two separate problems, we have investigated the two simultaneously because the influence of social origin (father's position) and that of career origin (first job) on occupational achievements are, of course, not independent. Given the crucial significance of education for careers in modern society, moreover, the variable of years of schooling has been included in the basic model of the process of stratification. This model dissects the process of occupational mobility by tracing the interdependence among four determinants of occupational achievement, two of which refer to a man's social background (father's education and father's occupation), and two of which refer to his own training and early experience that prepare him for his subsequent career (education and first job).

A man's social origins exert a considerable influence on his chances of occupational success, but his own training and early experience exert a more pronounced influence on his success chances. The zero-order correlations with occupational status are .32 for father's education, .40 for father's occupation, .60 for education, and .54 for first job. Inasmuch as social origins, education, and career origins are not independent, however, their influences on ultimate occupational achievements are not cumulative. Thus the entire influence of father's education on son's occupational status is mediated by father's occupa-

[1] Thus the rates of intergenerational occupational mobility are highest for the men with the lowest social origins and decrease regularly with increasing social origins (father's occupation), ranging from a mean of +25 points of upward mobility for men whose father's occupational status was less than 5 to a mean of −35 for those whose father's status was 90 or more. The extremes of education, which is undoubtedly more discriminating than any other variable, only produce a range between −2 and +28.

tion and son's education. Father's occupational status, on the other hand, not only influences son's career achievements by affecting his education and first job, but it also has a delayed effect on achievements that persists when differences in schooling and early career experience are statistically controlled. Although most of the influence of social origins on occupational achievements is mediated by education and early experience, social origins have a continuing impact on careers that is independent of the two variables pertaining to career preparation. Education exerts the strongest direct effect on occupational achievements (the path coefficient is .39), with the level on which a man starts his career being second ($p = .28$).

Social origin, education, and career beginning account for somewhat less than half the variance in occupational achievement. One may interpret this result, depending on one's expectations and values, either by emphasizing that these three attributes of young men have nearly as much impact on their subsequent careers as all other factors combined, or by stressing that occupational success in our society depends not even so much on the socioeconomic and educational differences measured as on other factors. In any case, as a man gets older, the significance of his past career for his subsequent career becomes increasingly pronounced, and the influences of his social origin and his education as well as those of other factors not directly measured become less and less important. Making inferences about career stages from comparisons of age cohorts, we have estimated that the influence of his past career on a man's occupational status increases from a .30 path coefficient around age 30 to .89 when he is about 60, and the net influence of social origins decreases from .18 to nil, that of education decreases from .48 to .06, and that of all other factors decreases from .82 to .40.

The significance of other conditions, such as ethnic background, for occupational success is not independent of that of social and career origins and of education. It is well known that low social origins are associated with a variety of factors that have adverse effects on occupational chances. Disproportionate numbers of poor people are members of minorities who are discriminated against, have many children among whom their limited resources must be divided, and live in areas where educational and occupational opportunities are severely restricted, as illustrated by the Negro sharecropper in the South. Children who grow up in the lower strata tend to have not only poorer but also less educated parents, receive less education themselves, and must start work early in undesirable jobs. The assumption often made is that these multiple handicaps of men raised in lower strata have cumulative effects on their careers, creating a vicious circle through which poverty is perpetuated from generation to generation. Indeed the· analysis has shown that low social origins are an impediment to occupational success (though most of the differences in occupational achievements are not a result of differences in origins but of other factors independent of origins). Yet these results by themselves do not reveal a vicious circle.

The concept of the vicious cycle of poverty implies not merely that growing up in lower strata affects occupational chances adversely but, more specifically, that the various conditions associated with low social origins reinforce each other and have cumulative adverse effects on occupational chances. The fact that several related factors have disadvantageous consequences for occupational achievements, however, does not necessarily indicate that each one adds a further impediment to those produced by the others. On the contrary, it frequently means that their combined effects are in large part redundant and not cumulative. Thus a man's career is adversely affected if his father had little education, if his father's occupational status was low, and if he himself has little education. But these three influences are not cumulative, as the preceding analysis showed. Father's low education only depresses occupational chances because it is associated with father's low occupational status and with son's low education. Once these two intervening factors that mediate the influence of father's education have been taken into account, father's education exerts no further influence on occupational achievements. The influence of father's occupational status on son's career, in turn, is in large part mediated by education, though not entirely. Given such minimum cumulation, it hardly seems justified to speak of a vicious cycle for the population at large, particularly in view of the fact that most of the differences in occupational achievements are not the result of differences in social origins. There are underprivileged groups in our society, however, who suffer serious occupational disadvantages as the result of cumulative handicaps, and whose situation may properly be described as resulting from a vicious cycle. The cases of three minorities—Negroes, Southerners, and sons of immigrants—illustrate the difference between background handicaps that are cumulative and those that are not.

A Negro's chances of occupational success in the United States are far inferior to those of a Caucasian. Whereas this hardly comes as a surprise to anyone familiar with the American scene, it is noteworthy that Negroes are handicapped at every step in their attempts to achieve economic success, and these cumulative disadvantages are what produces the great inequalities of opportunities under which the Negro American suffers. Disproportionate numbers of Negroes live in the South, where occupational opportunities are not so good as in the North. Within each region, moreover, Negroes are seriously disadvantaged. They have lower social origins than whites, and they receive less education. Even when Negroes and whites with the same amount of education are compared, Negroes enter the job market on lower levels. Furthermore, if all these differences are statistically controlled and we ask how Negroes would fare if they had the same origins, education, and career beginnings as whites, the chances of occupational achievement of Negroes are still considerably inferior to those of whites. Within the same occupation, finally, the income of Negroes is lower than that of whites. The multiple handicaps associated with being an American Negro are cumulative in their deleterious consequences for a man's career.

Whereas the uneducated Negro is the subject of the prejudiced stereotype that serves to justify discrimination, the better educated Negro, who is often explicitly exempt from the stereotype, seems to be the one who suffers most from discrimination. Education does not produce the same career advantages for Negroes as for whites. The difference in occupational status between Negroes and whites is twice as great for men who have graduated from high school or gone to college as for those who have completed no more than eight years of schooling. In short the careers of well-educated Negroes lag even further behind those of comparable whites than do the careers of poorly educated Negroes. This difference probably reflects in part discrimination in employment and in part discrimination in education, as the inferior educational facilities communities provide for Negroes make it likely that Negroes acquire less knowledge and fewer skills in the same number of years of schooling than whites. In any case, the same investment of time and resources in education does not yield Negroes as much return in their careers as it does whites. Negroes, as an underprivileged group, must make greater sacrifices to remain in school, but they have less incentive than whites to make these sacrifices, which may well be a major reason why Negroes often exhibit little motivation to continue in school and advance their education. Here we see how cumulative disadvantages create a vicious circle. Since acquiring an education is not very profitable for Negroes they are inclined to drop out of school relatively early. The consequent low level of education of most Negroes reinforces the stereotype of the uneducated Negro that helps to justify occupational discrimination against the entire group, thus further depressing the returns Negroes get for the educational investments they do make, which again lessens their incentives to make such investments.

The situation of southern whites provides an interesting contrast with that of Negroes. The chances of occupational success of Southerners are inferior to those of Northerners, for both whites and Negroes, whether the Southerners remain in the South or migrate north to pursue careers there. Southerners have lower social origins than Northerners, they are less educated, and they start their careers on lower levels. Although the differences between Southerners and Northerners are not so great as those between whites and Negroes, there are parallel differences in respect to every variable under consideration. However, the handicaps of Southerners do not have cumulative effects on their occupational chances, whereas those of Negroes do. When social origins, education, and career beginnings are controlled the occupational level of southern whites is, on the average, no longer any different from that of northern whites. In other words, the inferior background and education of southern whites fully account for their limited occupational chances, and there is no evidence of discrimination against Southerners once these initial differences have been taken into consideration; whereas the chances of Negroes remain inferior to those of whites under controls, which probably is the result of discrimination. Moreover the occupational chances of southern Negroes remain inferior to those of northern Negroes under controls, in contrast to the case of southern whites, which undoubtedly reflects the more severe discrimination against Negroes in the South. Southerners have many competitive disadvantages in the struggle for occupational success, just as Negroes do, but the handicaps of southern whites do not produce cumulative impediments for their careers, while those of Negroes do. It may well be that ethnic discrimination is at the root of such cumulative adverse effects on careers and that without discrimination there is no vicious cycle of poverty.

The case of a third minority—sons of immigrants—differs from that of Southerners as well as that of Negroes. The background of all three minorities creates hardships in their occupational lives. The initial handicaps do not fully account for the inferior occupational chances of Negroes but do account for the inferior chances of southern whites. However in both cases the initial handicaps are accompanied by inferior subsequent achievements, whereas the occupational achievements of the second generation, despite its initial handicaps, are not inferior to those of northern whites of native parentage. That is, sons of immigrants have lower social origins and less education than the majority group of northern whites with native parents, yet their occupational achievements are on the average as high as those of the majority group, not only if initial differences are controlled but also without such controls. Although these results seem to indicate that white ethnic minorities do not suffer discrimination in the American labor market, a possible alternative interpretation is that some white ethnic groups are disadvantaged in their careers but the effects of these disadvantages are neutralized, and hence obscured in the data, by the overachievement of selected members of the white minority groups. There is some evidence in support of this interpretation. Thus second-generation men of northern or western European descent have slightly more successful careers than those with less prestigeful origins (primarily southern and eastern Europe). Besides the data on education show that the second generation has initial disadvantages, but those men among them who overcome these disadvantages are exceptionally successful.

Minority group handicaps are challenges for as well as impediments to achievement. They create obstacles to success and simultaneously provide a screening test of the capacity to meet difficulties, with the result that those members of the minority who have conquered their initial handicaps and passed the screening test are a select group with high potential for continuing achievement. The background handicaps of the second generation are evident in the finding that fewer of them than of the majority group complete eight years of schooling, go on to high school, and remain in high school until graduation. In order to graduate from high school sons of immigrants had to meet more serious challenges than sons of native parents. High-school graduation, consequently, is a particularly effective screening test for the second generation, which is manifest in exceptional rates of proceeding to higher educational levels once the initial handicaps are overcome. The proportion of high-school graduates who go on to college is larger among the second generation than among the majority group, and so is the proportion of college entrants who graduate and the proportion of college graduates who proceed to professional or graduate school. Men who had to overcome competitive disadvantages progress to higher levels subsequently than those never confronted by such difficulties, partly because having to pass through this screen selects men with high initiative or ability, and partly because success in meeting challenges steels men in further competitive struggles. For hardships to be such a spur to achievement, however, requires that those members of minorities who have conquered their initial handicaps are then permitted to enjoy the fruits of their success and that persisting disadvantages and discrimination do not rob them of these hard-won benefits. At least, this conclusion is suggested by the findings that Negroes, whose occupational chances remain inferior when education and background are controlled, do not have exceptionally high probabilities of continuing their education on advanced levels, whereas white minorities, whose occupational rewards for given educational investment are not inferior, do have such high rates.

The significance of processes of selection for contemporary occupational life is most evident in migration. Migrants achieve generally higher occupational status than nonmigrants, whether reference is to a man's leaving the region of his birth or to his moving after age 16 from the community where he was raised. To be sure, there are a few exceptions to the prevailing superiority of migrants, notably in the farm sector. For example, Southerners and, particularly, Negroes, though least qualified for urban careers, are most likely to leave farms. Nevertheless even migrants off farms are on the average superior in occupational achievements to the men who stay on farms, though not to the men in the communities to which they have come; and the achievements of urban migrants are superior to those of the non-migrants in their place of destination as well as in their place of origin. Since the predominant stream of migration is from less to more urban places, where occupational opportunities are better, the greater achievements of migrants may be a result of the improvement in opportunity structure migration usually produces. Indeed migrants from all types of places achieve higher occupational status if they move to an urban community than if they migrate to a rural area. Contrary to expectations, however, the place in which a migrant grew up exerts a more pronounced and more consistent influence on his occupational chances than the place in which he now works. Regardless of the size of the place in which a migrant works, the more urbanized the community was where he grew up, the higher is the occupational status he attains. The superior education and early experiences more urbanized communities with their diversified facilities offer give men raised there a competitive advantage.

The question arises whether migration itself is associated with superior occupational achievements, quite independent of the type of community to which or from which a migrant moved. To answer this question, migrants from one to another large city are compared with nonmigrants in large cities, and parallel comparisons between migrants within the same community type and nonmigrants are made for small cities, rural communities, and farms. In both large and small cities such migrants are considerably superior in occupational status to nonmigrants. The status difference is smaller in rural communities, and it is reversed in farm areas, with migrants being inferior to non-migrants on farms. Since the major variations in environmental opportunities resulting from degree of urbanization have been controlled in these comparisons, the findings suggest that urban migration is a process of selection of men predisposed toward occupational success, though this is less true for rural migration and not at all for farm migration. If this conclusion is correct, it would follow that urban migrants, but not rural ones, should be superior to nonmigrants already before the former actually leave their homes. The data confirm this inference. The social origins, education, and first jobs of urban migrants are superior to those of nonmigrants, whereas rural migrants reveal no such early superiorities. When the differences in these potentials for occupational success are statistically controlled, urban migrants continue to exhibit superior occupational achievements. The implication is that urban migration selects men with high potential for occupational success, and their actual migration raises their chances in fact to realize this potential.

Migration plays an important role for occupational mobility in urbanized society. The dominant stream of migration from rural to urban areas, which improves the opportunities of migrants, and the process of selective migration, which makes migrants particularly qualified for occupational success, combine to produce the superior occupational achievements of migrants. The communication facilities in modern society that make it easy to migrate enable men with initiative and ability but living in areas with restricted opportunities to translate their potential into actual achievements by migrating. To be sure, the poor preparation for urban careers men reared in rural areas tend to receive limits their occupational chances when they migrate to cities. As a result of this very fact, however, rural migration to metropolitan areas promotes not only the occupational mobility of the migrants themselves but also that of the urban natives.

Rural migrants to large cities achieve higher occupational status than the men who remain in rural areas but not so high status as the city natives. They are attracted to the metropolis because of the higher achievements the better opportunities make possible there, and their achievements fall short of those of city-raised men because of their poorer occupational preparation. The influx of poorly qualified rural migrants into the lower ranges of the metropolitan occupational hierarchy permits more of the better qualified city natives than would otherwise be possible to move into relatively higher occupational positions. Thus the role in the metropolitan structure once occupied by immigrants from Europe has been assumed today by migrants from rural areas. The metropolitan natives are advantaged by the inflow of rural migrants, and so are these migrants; even the men who remain in rural areas probably benefit some from the outflow of others, which lessens the competitive struggle for jobs. The rural migration to big cities in the United States has a structural effect on occupational mobility, for it furthers the chances of upward mobility of the natives who never migrated as well as of the migrants themselves.

FAMILY AND OCCUPATIONAL LIFE

Family life has important bearing on occupational life. Broken families spell lower occupational achievements for both the children and the husband, though it is not clear whether the husband's less successful career is a consequence of the marriage break-up or helps to precipitate it. The future occupational chances of children are not only affected by their parents' stable marriage but also by the number of siblings they have, their position among their siblings, and the educational encouragement the family provides.

Many siblings are a considerable occupational handicap. Men from large families are less likely to achieve high status in their careers than those from small families of the same socioeconomic stratum. The most likely reason is that parents of many children must divide their time and resources and cannot expend as much as parents of few children on the training and education or on the guidance and support of any one child. When educational attainments as well as social origins are held constant, the differences in occupational achievements between men from large and those from small families virtually disappear. Although family size affects occupational achievements primarily by affecting education, which in turn affects achievements, and not otherwise, this makes the ultimate depressing effect of large families on career chances no less real.

It is often assumed that oldest sons achieve higher status than younger sons. This assumption must be revised in the light of our findings. To be sure, eldest sons who are also the first-born child in a family have more successful careers than sons in intermediate positions. First-born sons who have older sisters, however, are not superior in occupational achievement to other sons in intermediate sibling positions. Moreover the occupational achievements of sons who are the youngest child in a family are just as high as those of sons who are the oldest child. In brief men in the two extreme sibling positions have more successful careers than those in intermediate positions. This difference is due to the better education oldest and youngest children receive, and it largely disappears when social origins and education are controlled. Parents appear to devote disproportionate resources to the training of their oldest child, who may also be particularly close to the parents and identified with adult values, and that of their youngest child, who benefits from their no longer having to economize for the sake of younger children. The consequent superior education of these first-born and last-born children enables them to surpass middle children in career achievements.

The relations among siblings in various positions also appear to influence achievements. An increase in the size of the family reduces the advantages of the oldest child and enhances that of the youngest one. In technical terms, number of siblings and sibling position interact in their effects on achievements. The adverse influence of a large family on future success is most pronounced for oldest children, less pronounced for middle children, and least pronounced for youngest children. These differences are manifest in educational attainments as well as occupational achievements, whether or not social origins are controlled, though not in achievements when both education and origins are controlled. The interpretation suggested for this finding is that the role relations and normative expectations in the family encourage older siblings to assume some responsibility for younger ones and assist them in their progress. The assumption that the future interests of older children are to some extent set aside in favor of those of their younger siblings could account for the asymmetry observed. The lower a child's position in the birth order, the more does the balance of receiving help from older and giving help to younger siblings turn in his favor, and the less disadvantageous it is, therefore, to have many siblings. To view it from a slightly different perspective, it is more of a handicap to have many younger than to have many older siblings, because older children are expected to make some sacrifices for their younger brothers.

The data on family size support the previous conclusion that men who successfully have overcome obstacles to their advancement are more likely to progress to still higher levels of attainment than those who had never to confront such problems. The disadvantage of men from large families is evident in their conditional probabilities of continuing education from one level to the next. At every step of the educational ladder up to college, the proportion of men who continue is not so high for sons from large families as for those from small ones. Among college graduates, consequently, large-family men are a more highly selected group than small-family men, and this finds expression in the greater tendency of men from large families to proceed to postgraduate levels of university education. Middle children, similarly, are less likely than youngest ones to continue their education at every level up to college, and they are more likely to go beyond college provided that they come from small families though not if they come from large ones, possibly because the compounded disadvantages of middle position and large family are too severe to be overcome by considerable numbers, just as the serious multiple disadvantages of the Negro are. In any case, the process of overcoming special difficulties, whether produced by many siblings or immigrant parents or, presumably, other handicaps that are not crushing, is selective of men with high potential for success, with the result that those members of the disadvantaged groups who have conquered their initial handicaps have better prospects of future success than other men.

The educational attainments of sons, and hence their occupational chances, may be assumed to be influenced by variations in the educational climate of their parental families, specifically, the extent to which conditions in the family stimulate an interest in learning and achievement. The family's educational climate depends undoubtedly in large part on the education of the father, which does, indeed, exert a considerable influence on his son's education. Within each educational origin level, however, the educational stimulation and encouragement children receive from their parents are not the same. Differences in family's educational climate within each educational class can be inferred from the educational attainments of the oldest brother when the father's education is held constant. Intraclass variations in the educational climates of families, so defined, have a pronounced impact on the educational attainment of sons. Even with race and some other conditions as well as father's education held constant, men with the most educated oldest brothers have, on the average, nearly four years more of schooling than those with the least educated oldest brothers. The introduction of a hypothetical variable representing this factor into the formal model of stratification reveals how this interpretation compares with alternative ones in terms of the plausibility of the assumptions made and the precise predictions advanced. The differences within educational classes in the degree to which family conditions stimulate the educational striving of children seem to have a profound impact on their progress in school.

One mechanism through which a favorable family climate apparently elevates the educational level of sons is by motivating them, or possibly the parents, to take full advantage of available resources to further educational attainments. Intraclass variations in family climate affect the education of sons more in small families than in large ones. Controlling father's education and other relevant conditions, the educational advantage of men from small over those from large families is zero if the oldest brother only went to elementary school and increases with oldest brother's advancing education. More resources are available for each child's education in small than in large families, but unless the family climate makes education an important goal there is no inclination to utilize the more abundant resources of the small family to remain longer in school. In brief the more favorable the family climate is to education, the greater is the tendency of men to divert available resources from other uses to attaining a higher education.

Occupational life has important connections with a man's family of procreation as well as his family of orientation. The phenomenon of differential fertility by occupational class is widely known. Higher occupational classes have fewer children than lower ones, though the relationship is not entirely linear because the lower rather than the top white-collar strata have the smallest number of children. The influence of occupational position on fertility extends over two generations. Classification by the occupation of either husband's father or wife's father reveals parallel differences in fertility, as does classification by husband's first job, except that in these cases the dip in the curve for lower white-collar strata is not evident. By and large, then, the higher a family's present social standing or social origins, the smaller is the number of children in it, though a decrease in this differential has accompanied the long-term downward trend in fertility.

These class differences in fertility have been interpreted by some as the result of the association between low fertility and upward mobility. The assumption is that a low birth rate is a prerequisite for upward mobility, inasmuch as a large family is an impediment for career success. Given this upward movement of families with few children, lower strata are depleted of small families and higher strata have an overabundance of them, and this is responsible for the lower fertility that can be observed in higher strata. It should be noted that this interpretation, which may be called the mobility hypothesis in its strong form, has been advanced in the absence of systematic empirical information on the relationship between fertility and mobility. The mobility hypothesis in its weak form merely asserts that fertility and mobility are inversely related, without assuming that this inverse relationship accounts for the observable class differences in fertility.

The strong hypothesis, according to which the lower birth rate of higher strata is due to the presence of upwardly mobile families with few children there, implies that the fertility of nonmobile couples does not differ by social class. The OCG data clearly show that the fertility of nonmobile couples in different occupational strata is not the same but varies parallel to that for all couples, whether mobility—or its absence—from first, father's, or father-in-law's occupation is considered. On the contrary, class differences in fertility are more pronounced for nonmobile families than for all families, undoubtedly because the influences of present and origin status reinforce rather than counteract one another in the case of the nonmobiles. In its strong form the mobility hypothesis must be unequivocally rejected. The association between mobility and fertility does not account for existing class differences in fertility. The question arises whether the underlying assumption that upward mobility is associated with a low birth rate is correct, which is all the hypothesis in its weak form claims.

Upwardly mobile couples tend to have fewer children than others with the same origins. Whereas this finding is in accord with the weak hypothesis, it does not suffice to confirm it, for it does not necessarily reflect the significance of mobility as such. Upwardly mobile couples tend to have more children than others in their class of destination, and the fertility of downwardly mobile couples is also intermediate between that typical for their origin and that typical for their destination. As a matter of fact, the fertility of each origin stratum varies similarly by destination, and the fertility of each destination stratum varies similarly by origin. This pattern suggests that the additive effects of occupational origin and present occupation may account for fertility, with the experience of mobility itself playing no role. To test this inference a model incorporating the two additive effects was constructed, departures from which disclose the uncontaminated influence of mobility in its own right. The model accounts for most differences in fertility in the tables, but there are statistically significant departures, though they are usually very small. Upward occupational mobility appears to depress fertility slightly, and so does downward mobility. In sum the experience of mobility in either direction has a minor depressing effect on fertility, which is greatly overshadowed by the cumulative effects of present occupational status and origin status on fertility.

A number of conditions that reduce fertility simultaneously reduce class differentials in fertility. Thus men in towns and cities whose fathers were farmers, as well as men themselves living on farms, have higher rates of fertility than those two generations removed from the farm. Differences in fertility by occupational status are also more pronounced for men with farm backgrounds than for the second generation of urban dwellers, as fertility declines more sharply with rising status for men with farm background than for urban natives. Similarly the long-term historical trend has been toward lower fertility and lesser differences in it among social strata, as noted. The expansion of urbanization in modern society may well be responsible for this historical trend. An extreme instance of such a double effect on both fertility and its class differential is provided by age at marriage. Couples who married young have more children than those married when the bride was older than 21. If the couple married early, husband's occupational status, education, and income are inversely related to fertility. If the couple married late, however, the birth rate is not related to either occupational status or education, and its relationship to income is reversed. In contrast to the otherwise observable tendency of lower socioeconomic strata to have more children than higher ones, couples who married late have more children if they are well off than if they are poor.

A clue for a possible interpretation of the observed patterns of fertility is provided by the significance of urbanization for them, whether reference is to the growing urbanization of society at large or the increasing urbanization of individuals as they become further removed in time from farm life. A distinctive characteristic of urbanized social structures is that *Gesellschafts* relations prevail over *Gemeinschafts* relations, to use Toennies' famous terminology.[2] *Gemeinschaft* implies that men are imbedded in a matrix of close social ties most of which have existed since birth. In such a context human relations are conceived as part of the natural order, and they are valued for their own sake. Men do not judge their relations with fellow men by some external universalistic standard, but the established social bonds themselves define their particularistic significance. With slight exaggeration we may say that men look upon others as either friend or foe; there is hardly any middle ground. *Gesellschafts* relations differ decidedly from either extreme, involving social contacts that are neither of intrinsic significance nor hostile but simply means for a variety of ends. Urbanized society with its advanced division of labor requires its members in the course of their work and everyday life to enter into relatively superficial relations in segmental roles with many others. Few objectives of individuals in contemporary society can be accomplished without engaging in social interaction with others for this purpose. In these social relations, exemplified by those between buyer and seller or supervisor and subordinate, the

2 Ferdinand Toennies, *Community and Association,* London: Routledge & Kegan Paul, 1955.

objective sought is the external standard for evaluating their significance. As most social contacts of modern man are entered into as means for further ends, an instrumental orientation to social intercourse becomes pervasive and intrudes even on intimate human relations. Family life is not exempt from this tendency. Whereas the traditional view has been that getting married and having children are natural processes outside the realm of rational deliberation, men today are not merely permitted but normatively expected to base their decisions to get married and have children on rational calculation, as the disapproval of teen-age marriages and the high birth rate of the very poor illustrate.

The interpretation suggested is that the deliberate approach to human relations guided by rational calculation, which is embodied in the concept of *Gesellschaft,* is a major factor depressing fertility. Since the tasks of most white-collar workers entail dealing with people and achieving goals by influencing others, whereas blue-collar as well as farm workers primarily work on things, white-collar workers would be expected to be especially imbued with a calculating viewpoint toward social relations. Urbanization, which tears people out of the network of permanent social bonds in the small community and leads to social contacts among erstwhile strangers thrown together in close proximity, is assumed to foster more deliberate attitudes in social intercourse. Accordingly the trend toward increasing urbanization in the society at large and the degree of urbanization of its individual members both should be reflected in a more pronounced *Gesellschafts* orientation. The willingness to postpone marriage is a particularly straightforward expression of the inclination to permit rational deliberation to influence decisions about the most intimate human relations. All these conditions lower fertility rates. Class differentials in fertility, too, can be accounted for by the explanatory hypothesis advanced.

The paradox of class differences in birth rates is that the couples who can least afford it have most children. Calling this a paradox, however, itself reveals our calculating orientation toward family life, since it implicitly assumes that having children is not simply a natural process but ought to result from deliberate decisions based on rational economic considerations. Only people with a profound *Gesellschafts* orientation plan the size of their families in such a deliberate manner. Postponement of marriage manifests a calculating orientation toward family life rather directly, and couples who marry late not only have fewer children than others but also are rationally influenced by their financial resources in deciding how many children to have, as indicated by the positive association between income and fertility for them, in contrast to the negative association for other couples. There is reason to think that the social life of white-collar workers is most extensively guided by *Gesellschafts* principles, and the more affluent higher strata among them have more children than the less affluent lower ones, as rational deliberation would dictate. Thus a major consequence of a *Gesellschafts* orientation, late marriage, as well as a major determinant of it, white-collar work, finds expression in rational planning of family size. Less extreme forms of the calculating orientation toward human relations, like those produced by urbanization, merely attenuate the usual class differences in fertility without reversing them. The usually observable class differential in birth rate results, according to the interpretation, from the less deliberate and more spontaneous orientation toward family life of the lower social strata. The slight depressing effect of mobility regardless of direction on fertility, finally, may be due to the disruptions in social relations often engendered by mobility, inasmuch as men removed from a matrix of established social ties are prone to become more calculating in social intercourse.[3]

What are the implications of differential fertility for society? It has been argued that the lower birth rates of the higher strata, as well as the lower birth rates of the more advanced societies compared to the less industrialized ones, are a deplorable waste of human resources and may spell the doom of civilized societies. Sorokin, who is not an extreme spokesman for this viewpoint, concludes his discussion of the topic in these words: "If we desire the continuation of our civilization, differential fertility and a generally low birth rate are scarcely favorable conditions for this purpose."[4] This argument assumes that the sons of families in higher strata are better qualified for leading positions than men who have moved up from lower strata. There is no need to enter into a discussion of the significance of heredity here, since it can readily be granted that men raised in better educated and more affluent families are more likely than others to have superior qualifications, if only by reason of the advantage their environment creates for their development.

[3] In short disruptions of social integration depress fertility, just as they promote suicide. Note that there are many parallels between low fertility and high suicide rates, both being associated with the historical trend, urbanism, economic depressions, and, inversely, with Catholicism and being Negro. Emile Durkheim formulated the germ of his theory of suicide in a paper analyzing the relationship between fertility and suicide; "Suicide et Natalité," *Revue Philosophique de la France et de l'Etranger*, **26**(1888), 446-463.

[4] Pitirim A. Sorokin, *Social Mobility*, New York: Harper, 1927, p. 504.

To say that the sons of the elite are superior in ability to the entire group of sons of other strata, however, does not imply that they are superior to those sons of other strata who succeed in moving up into the elite. The population of nonelite sons constitutes a large pool of human resources that is sifted in the process of selection entailed in upward mobility, which makes it likely that the ones who do achieve elite status are more outstanding than the initially superior but unselected elite sons, just as the more selected large-family college graduates are more successful in pursuing higher degrees than the initially advantaged small-family college graduates. Moreover Sorokin himself notes that "a greater versatility and plasticity of human behavior is a natural result of social mobility,"[5] and he points out that this encourages intellectual endeavors and creativity. These qualities would give the upwardly mobile a further advantage over those who have inherited elite status. Given the existing family structure it is hardly conceivable that men in the elite would not attempt to assure that their sons remain in this top stratum, and their resources and power often enable them to do so. Differential fertility makes it possible, without any change in the institution of the family, for the elite to be invigorated by fresh blood and for sons from lower strata to have opportunities to move into the elite. Unless we assume that the nonelite sons with the highest potential are inferior to the elite sons with the lowest qualifications, the process of selection inherent in upward mobility can be expected to have the result that the most successful men from lower strata bring not only new perspectives but also superior qualifications to the elite.

OCCUPATIONAL STRUCTURE AND HISTORICAL TRENDS

The movements of individuals from various origins to different occupational destinations, conditioned by the factors that influence chances of achievement, find expression in the occupational structure of the society. The occupational structure can be studied in its own right, and so can its development over time. Any structure consists of relations among parts, and two crucial questions are how the parts are distinguished and what the criterion for defining relation is. In our analysis of the occupational structure the parts are the ten major occupational groups or, more usually, a subdivision of them into 17 occupational strata, and the criterion of relation is the flow of manpower from occupational origins to occupational destinations.

As a starting point let us distinguish the 10 major occupational

5 *Ibid.*, p. 508; see also pp. 509-15.

groups on the basis of their growth or decline since the beginning of this century and the patterns of mobility associated with this change in size. It should be noted that the aggregate trend in an occupation, which is most strongly influenced by differences between successive age cohorts, cannot be inferred from the patterns of intergenerational mobility, because the generation of fathers does not represent a distinctive age cohort but overlaps many (and similar considerations apply to first jobs with respect to intragenerational mobility). The expansion of an occupation may be associated with the intergenerational inflow of men into it, the intragenerational inflow of men into it, or both, and the contraction of an occupation may be associated with the intergenerational outflow of men from it, the intragenerational outflow of men from it, or both. This schema yields six types of occupational groups.

The first type is an occupation that has expanded in the last half-century as increasing numbers of sons have moved into it, despite the fact that intragenerational mobility exhibits a net outflow, that is, in the course of their lifetime careers more men moved out of than into this occupation. The prototype of such an occupation expanded by intergenerational inflow notwithstanding intragenerational outflow is clerical work, and two other cases are salesmen and operatives. The second kind is an occupation that has increased in size because disproportionate numbers of men from other pursuits moved into it in the course of their careers, although the number of sons starting this career line falls short of the number of fathers who pursued it. Many of the occupations in the three groups that manifest this type—managers, proprietors, and officials (combined into one group), craftsmen, and service workers—require some resources, experience, or apprenticeship. Third, one occupational group has grown rapidly as the result of both intergenerational and intragenerational mobility into it, namely, professional, technical, and kindred workers. Fourth, farming is an occupation that has declined since decreasing numbers of sons choose it as their career, despite the fact that there is a net inflow of men who had started to work elsewhere—typically in farm labor—into it. The fifth type is an occupation that has declined as disproportionate numbers who started to work in it later left for other careers, although the number of men starting to work in this occupation exceeds the number of fathers in it. Labor and farm labor represent this type. A final possibility is an occupation whose decline is produced by both intergenerational and intragenerational outflow, but there is no empirical case representing this type. In sum only the two farm occupations and nonfarm labor have decreased in size during this century, whereas the seven other major groups have expanded by various processes and in varying degree.

Turning now to the patterns of mobility themselves, and using 17 occupational strata for this purpose, two basic features can be observed in every matrix, whether intergenerational or intragenerational mobility is considered, and whatever the specific measure employed. There is much upward mobility in the United States, but most of it involves relatively short social distances. Men are much more likely to experience upward than downward mobility, inasmuch as the rapidly expanding salaried professions with low fertility and the contracting farm occupations with high fertility create a vacuum in the form of occupational demand near the top and a pressure of manpower supply at the bottom that have repercussions throughout the occupational structure. An important reason why the growth of high-status professions and the decline of low-status farming have repercussions for the mobility of intermediate strata is that very few men originating in a bottom stratum themselves move all the way to the top, because most upward mobility involves short social distances of two or three steps in the hierarchy.

The socioeconomic rank of occupations, indicated by the education they require and the income they yield, influences mobility among them profoundly, as the preponderance of short-distance movements shows. The similarity between any pair of occupational origins in respect to their destinations, and between any pair of occupational destinations in respect to their origins, can be used as a measure of social distance that is entirely independent of the rank order based on education and income. The major underlying dimension of social distance defined by this similarity measure is the socioeconomic status of occupations, which confirms the assumption that socioeconomic differences are an important determinant of the patterns of mobility among occupations. A second dimension, which is only evident in the similarities of social origins with respect to destination, may refer to whether work is governed by universalistic principles or particularistic skills. Such differences in the organization of work seem to influence the orientation toward occupational life fathers transmit to their sons and hence the career lines sons are likely to follow.

Two class boundaries are manifest in the intergenerational as well as the intragenerational mobility matrix, which divide white-collar from blue-collar and blue-collar from farm occupations. These boundaries restrict downward mobility between virtually any two categories below the level expected on the assumption of independence, although they permit upward mobility in excess of this level. Occupations just below a class boundary, such as skilled crafts, have unexpectedly low recruitment from higher strata, because occupations just above a boundary, such as retail sales, provide opportunities for the unsuccessful from higher strata who are anxious to avoid losing white-collar respectability to find relatively unskilled jobs at low pay within the higher social class. The class boundaries also find expression in excessive social distances between occupations on either side, as shown by the dissimilarity measure discussed above. If the boundaries between the three major social classes restrict occupational mobility, we would also expect them to restrict various forms of social intercourse. As far as intermarriage is concerned, we have data to test this inference.

There is some homogamy by social origins, and it does reflect the class boundaries, as hypothesized. The prediction is that intermarriage exceeds expectations (on the assumption of independence) if the occupations of husband's and wife's father are in the same broad occupational class (white-collar, blue-collar, or farm) but falls short of expectations if the occupations of the two fathers are in different classes. The data essentially confirm this prediction, the major exceptions being that children of craftsmen and of service workers marry children of some of the white-collar strata more frequently than expected. Assortative mating with respect to the education of the spouses themselves, however, is much more pronounced than assortative mating by their occupational origins. These findings suggest that similarities in education and other personal characteristics directly influence marriage, and that origin homogamy is an indirect product of these influences. Although origin homogamy is only reduced and does not entirely disappear when educational homogamy is controlled, this result is not incompatible with the conclusion that similarities in the spouses themselves, which may be related to their social background, are what directly affects selective mating. Because education and other personal characteristics are influenced by social origins, however, mate selection on the basis of these characteristics simultaneously assures some origin homogamy, and parents take this into account when they live in the right neighborhoods and send their children to proper schools in terms of their style of life.

The flow of manpower is not evenly distributed among occupations. Some occupational groups may be considered to be distributive of manpower, inasmuch as they recruit much manpower from different origins and supply disproportionate numbers of sons to different occupational destinations. Other occupations are relatively self-contained, and neither recruit nor supply very much manpower. The occupations located just above one of the two class boundaries—the lowest white-collar and the lowest blue-collar groups—have high rates of both inflow, especially from lower strata, and outflow, especially to higher strata, thus serving as channels for upward mobility. The three self-employed occupational groups—free professionals, proprietors, and farmers—are the most self-contained, implying that proprietorship discourages the inflow of men into as well as their outflow from an occupation. Since self-employment restricts mobility, its decline over time may well have contributed to the high rates of mobility today.

To study the degree of dispersion in the flow of manpower, two different measures were developed. The second was initially intended simply as a refined substitute for the first, but analysis revealed that the two refer to distinct aspects of dispersion that have different properties. The admittedly crude measure is indicative of the width of the recruitment base or of the supply section of an occupation, from how many different origins it recruits more than its share of men or to how many different destinations it supplies disproportionate numbers of men. The refined measure, on the other hand, signifies whether the men recruited into an occupation from the outside or supplied by it to different ones are concentrated in a few other occupations or randomly distributed over all of them.

The width of the recruitment base of an occupation is inversely related to the width of its supply sector in the intergenerational flow of men. Occupational groups that attract more than their proportionate share of men from many different origins send more than their proportionate share to only a few different destinations. This finding has been interpreted with the aid of another, namely, that recruitment from a wide base is directly related to the growth an occupational group has experienced in recent decades. For an occupation to expand in response to an increased demand for its services it must recruit more men than it has in the past. The assumption is that a growing demand can broaden recruitment and effect expansion only by raising income or improving other employment conditions. This increment in rewards does not, of course, obliterate the basic differences in rewards between occupations associated with variations in skill requirements and status. But the heightened incentives presumably attract some men from various backgrounds who otherwise would have gone into different career lines, enabling the occupation to recruit more than its share of manpower from many other origins. The superior economic conditions that outsiders find attractive undoubtedly are also attractive to the occupational group's own sons and, therefore, discourage some of these sons who would otherwise have moved into a variety of other occupations from doing so. This interpretation, though it cannot be tested with our data, would explain the negative correlation between an occupation's recruitment base and its supply sector.

There is a positive correlation between the dispersion in recruitment and the dispersion in supply—that is, between the degree to which the origins of the men recruited into an occupation are dispersed rather than concentrated and the degree to which the destinations of the men supplied by it to others are dispersed rather than concentrated. Moreover intragenerational movements reveal the same direct association between dispersion in inflow and in outflow as intergenerational movements. All these manifestations of the degree of dispersion in the flow of manpower have similar nonmonotonic relations to the status rank order of occupations. The higher blue-collar strata, which constitute the intermediate ranks in the hierarchy, exhibit most dispersion of movement of all kinds. The white-collar strata nearer the top as well as the lower blue-collar and farm strata nearer the bottom have less dispersed patterns of occupational mobility, whatever aspect of mobility is considered. These differences reflect in part the prevalence of short-distance mobility, which restricts the range of likely origins or destinations for those occupational groups located near the top or near the bottom of the hierarchy. The higher degree of dispersion in the social mobility of the intermediate blue-collar workers, however, is also a sign of the poorer chances of upward mobility of these strata.

An important issue is whether the working class has poorer chances of upward mobility than the middle class. It is not easy to answer such a question, as indicated earlier, because even standardized measures of mobility are not free from the pervasive influence of ceiling effects, which makes any direct comparison of the mobility of occupations differently ranked of dubious value. An indirect approach makes it possible, however, to give at least a partial answer to this question. The problem must be reformulated first. Taking advantage of the fact that we have information on father's, first, and 1962 occupation, we ask how men who *enter* careers on different levels compare with respect to the net *inter*generational mobility they experience from father's occupation to their own in 1962. Abstracting from the many compensating moves in opposite direction, the index of net mobility shows how the 1962 occupational distribution of the members of a group entering careers on a certain level differs from the occupational distribution of their fathers. Although information on the direction of mobility is not included in the index, inferences about it can be derived from the analysis.

The reformulated question is whether men who start their careers in manual work are less likely than others to achieve an occupational status that differs from that of their fathers. The answer the data give to this question is yes. Men who start their careers on high white-collar levels as well as those starting to work on farms experience more net mobility from social origins to 1962 occupational destinations than do men entering the labor force as blue-collar workers. The source of the high rates of net mobility of the white-collar and the farm strata is not the same, however, Men who start their working lives in higher white-collar jobs have already experienced much mobility from their social origins, most of which must have been upward mobility, given the elevated destinations. Men who first work on farms have as yet experienced little mobility but experience much subsequently in their careers, most of which also must be upward mobility, given the low positions of the origins. Men who begin their working lives in the working class, by contrast, seem to have a less fortunate fate and end up in occupational positions that differ little from those of their fathers.

Shifting attention to an examination of historical trends, the conservative conclusion is that we find no indication of increasing rigidity in the American occupational structure. Three methods have been used to estimate recent trends in mobility. First, the OCG data were compared with those from national surveys conducted 5, 10, and 15 years earlier, after making needed adjustments in one of these sets of data, though we do not claim that this fully removes the hazards of comparing surveys carried out by different investigators using different procedures. The findings reveal a small increase in occupational mobility, primarily owing to higher rates of upward mobility. Second, to make indirect inferences from the OCG data, supplemented by other sources, the transition matrix for each younger cohort was applied to the origin distribution of the cohort 10 years older, and the destination distribution so derived was compared with that observed. The results suggest that upward mobility has somewhat increased. Third, the correlations between the status of father's occupation and of first job were computed for four age cohorts, 25 to 34, 35 to 44, 45 to 54, and 55 to 64. These data show that the influence of social origins on career beginnings has not changed at all in the last 40 years. None of these comparisons reveals any decrease in social mobility, and two of them imply that there may have been a slight increase in it.

A few other trends deserve brief mention. There is some indication, though the evidence is by no means conclusive, that the influence of educational attainments on occupational achievements has increased in recent decades. Migration apparently has become more pervasive and more selective of men with high potential for success than was the case in the past, making occupational chances less dependent on the accident of a man's birth place. These trends signify an extension of universalistic principles in contemporary occupational life—as does another phenomenon.

Discrimination against Negroes seems to have subsided somewhat, enabling them to begin to narrow the gap between themselves and whites, though only on lower levels of attainment and not on higher ones. The OCG data indicate that the differences between Negroes and whites in average education and in first jobs have decreased, particularly in the North. But resort to census data on education for more refined analysis discloses a different picture. To be sure the gap between the two groups in the proportion who completed eight years of schooling has narrowed since the early part of this century, in both the North and the South. However the differences between Negroes and whites in the likelihood of graduating from high school and in the likelihood of graduating from college have widened, in the North as well as in the South, and so has the difference in income. It would be misleading to interpret these findings as the result of an intensification of discrimination, for which there is no evidence. Yet even if Negroes were not at all discriminated against today, and this surely is still far from the true state of affairs, they would not thereby be enabled to overcome the consequences of centuries of slavery and subjugation and in one big leap jump to the level of the whites. Equitable treatment in terms of universalistic standards is not sufficient for a seriously underprivileged and deprived group to catch up with the rest or, for that matter, to keep abreast of their progress. It requires a helping hand.

CAUSES OF SOCIAL MOBILITY IN CONTEMPORARY SOCIETY

"The land where the streets are paved with gold"—that is how Europeans traditionally have thought of America, meaning the United States. The allegory had some basis in fact. The expanding continent with its open frontier combined with the impact of the industrial revolution, which could be fully exploited in the absence of an aristocracy with a feudal heritage, to create unheard-of opportunities for economic advancement. After the closing of the frontier itself vast open spaces and a rapidly expanding industrial economy absorbed still larger numbers of immigrants and continued to supply much opportunity for social mobility.

The high rates of upward mobility in the United States have been attributed to these and other special historical circumstances, for example by Sibley: "Technological progress, immigration, and differential fertility contributed to a great excess of upward over downward circulation in American Society."[6] The substitution of manual work by machines resulting from technological developments greatly reduced the need for men to perform physical labor and made it possible for a larger proportion of the labor force to be engaged in white-collar work, thus fostering upward mobility. As millions of disadvantaged immigrants moved in disproportionate numbers into the lower ranks of the occupational hierarchy, they freed many sons of men in these lower strata to move up to higher occupational levels. The relatively low birth rates of the white-collar class, finally, opened up additional opportunities for upward mobility.

Two of these three historical conditions that gave a strong impetus to upward mobility in this country, however, no longer exist to the extent that they did in the early part of this century. The once huge stream of immigrants to the United States has declined to a mere rivulet. Differential fertility also has become less pronounced, as we have seen, with the birth rates of the higher white-collar strata now exceeding those of the lower ones. Although technological progress has continued, its further development has not always served to replace more men by machines but often to simplify tasks for the sake of efficiency, thereby lowering rather than raising the skill level of the labor force, as exemplified by assembly-line production, which substitutes semiskilled operatives for skilled craftsmen. In brief upward mobility no longer benefits from large numbers of immigrants to this country; there is less class differential in fertility to promote it; and the influence of technological advances on it has become equivocal.

The rates of upward mobility in the United States today are still high, however, notwithstanding the changes in the historical circumstances that have been held responsible for the high mobility rates in the past. To be sure we have no way of knowing whether the opportunities for upward mobility in the last century were not much superior to those now, although the data do show that the chances of upward mobility have by no means declined in recent years. Be that as it may, the special historical conditions in the nineteenth century that ceased to exist early in the twentieth cannot explain the high rates of social mobility observable in the middle of the twentieth century. The interpretation to be advanced is that basic structural

[6] Elbridge Sibley, "Some Demographic Clues to Stratification," *American Sociological Review*, 7(1942), p. 322.

features of contemporary industrial society are the source of its high rates of occupational mobility, and that the three historical causes of mobility discussed were merely special cases of these generic structural causes, though these special historical conditions may have produced particularly high chances of mobility in nineteenth-century America.

Superior opportunities for occupational achievements attract migrants from other places in which conditions are not so favorable. The poorer environment in which the migrants were raised makes their qualifications inferior to those of the natives, enabling the natives to move to higher positions as the newcomers fill lower ones in the hierarchy. Whereas immigrants from Europe, who used to play this role, have ceased to arrive in large numbers in American metropolitan centers, in-migrants from rural areas have taken their place. Although chances are that the stream of migrants from farms to urban centers will dwindle in the future as the farm population becomes an increasingly smaller proportion of the total population, this would not alter the general principle, only its specific manifestation. Occupational opportunities will unquestionably continue to vary substantially in different places, and they will continue to change as new industries develop in some urban centers and technological advances make the industrial activities in another obsolete. These variations give men incentives to migrate from areas with lesser to areas with better opportunities, and the flow of migrants from disadvantaged environments acts as a catalyst for occupational mobility.

The class differential in fertility has been declining, and prospects are that it will decline further. Thus the inverse relationship between education and birth rate is less pronounced for younger women than for older ones, and it is less pronounced for those who do not have a farm background than for those who do, from which we can infer that this inverse association will further diminish as decreasing proportions of the population have a farm background. Nevertheless there is reason to believe, on theoretical grounds, that some differential fertility is an ingrained characteristic of industrialized and urbanized society and will persist. We have speculated above that an important determinant of lower differential fertility as well as lower fertility rates is the calculating orientation toward human relations typical of *Gesellschafts* structures. Whereas *Gemeinschaft* implies that men derive their major gratification from the intimate social bonds in which their whole existence is rooted, *Gesellschaft* involves a predominant orientation toward achievement and success without which men cannot find satisfaction. The ceaseless and unsatiable striving for success that sometimes results has often been satirized in modern fiction. These extremes only highlight the supreme value achievement assumes generally. Not everybody can be equally successful in the competitive struggle for superior status, however, regardless of the affluence of a society and the equality of opportunity in it.

Men who attain positions of superior prestige and power in the occupational hierarchy receive supportive and gratifying social acknowledgment of their prowess, but those who fail to attain superior status must find other sources of social support and gratification. The very importance of success makes failure to achieve it a threatening experience against which men seek to defend themselves lest it debilitate them, often by denying institutional values. Unsuccessful men may reject the political values of their society and organize an opposition against its government. Alternatively they may reject the prevailing *Gesellschafts* orientation and seek satisfaction and support from their families. Having many children not only expresses the rejection of a calculating approach in the most intimate sexual relation but also supplies a man with a group whose ascribed status as children requires them to submit to his authority. Whereas successful achievers have their status as adult men supported by their superior occupational roles and authority, the unsuccessful find a substitute in the authority they exercise in their role as fathers over a number of children. The significance parental authority has for lower strata is manifest in the tendency of these strata to treat their children in more authoritarian fashion than do higher strata, as students of child rearing have found.[7] If these speculations have any validity, it follows that differential achievement in societies strongly oriented toward achievement will continue to be mirrored in differential fertility.[8]

Technological advances have sometimes led to serious economic depressions, which worsened chances of upward mobility and seriously disrupted careers in general, and they have sometimes effected routinization of formerly skilled tasks, which can only have an adverse effect on mobility. In the long run, however, technological progress has undoubtedly improved chances of upward mobility and will do so in the future. Technical improvements in production and farming have made possible the tremendous expansion of the labor force in tertiary industries—those other than agriculture or manufacturing—

---

[7] See, for example, Robert R. Sears, Eleanor E. Maccoby and Harry Levin, *Patterns of Child Rearing*, Evanston: Row, Peterson, 1957, pp. 426-447.

[8] We had expected, in accordance with these notions, that downward mobility raises fertility, but the data disconfirm this prediction, which weakens the interpretation suggested.

and, particularly, in professional and semiprofessional services since the turn of the century. For example, the number of professional, technical, and kindred workers was less than one-tenth the number working on farms in 1900; today the first group outnumbers the second nearly two to one. This great expansion of the occupational group at the top of the hierarchy,[9] in combination with the simultaneous contraction of the bottom strata, has been a major generator of upward mobility. The elimination of routine jobs by automation, though it may well immediately set back the careers of some men, should ultimately open up additional avenues of upward mobility. The general principle is that as long as some jobs are more routine and less rewarding than others—and the time is hardly foreseeable when this will not be the case—incentives exist to apply scientific and engineering talents to the task of developing mechanical procedures for doing them or finding some other substitute for human labor. The recurrent elimination of the least-skilled occupations is a continual source of upward mobility in advanced industrial societies.

The basic assumption underlying these conjectures is that a fundamental trend toward expanding universalism characterizes industrial society. Objective criteria of evaluation that are universally accepted increasingly pervade all spheres of life and displace particularistic standards of diverse ingroups, intuitive judgments, and humanistic values not susceptible to empirical verification.[10] The growing emphasis on rationality and efficiency inherent in this spread of universalism finds expression in rapid technological progress and increasing division of labor and differentiation generally, as standards of efficiency are applied to the performance of tasks and the allocation of manpower for them.[11] The strong interdependence among men and groups engendered by the extensive division of labor becomes the source of their organic solidarity, to use Durkheim's term, inasmuch as social differentiation weakens the particularistic ingroup values that unite men in common bonds of mechanical solidarity.[12] The attenua-

[9] When the professional group is divided into the self-employed and the salaried, the latter are seen to account for the great expansion of this occupational group, whereas self-employed professionals have expanded very little.

[10] The last point is particularly stressed in Pitirim A. Sorokin, *Social and Cultural Dynamics*, 4 volumes, New York: American Book, 1937–41, *passim*.

[11] Talcott Parsons' theory of social change, modifying Weber's principle of progressive rationalization, focuses on progressive differentiation; *The Social System*, Glencoe: Free Press, 1951, pp. 480-535. For the concepts of universalism and particularism, see *ibid.*, pp. 58-67, 101-112.

[12] Emile Durkheim, *On the Division of Labor in Society*, New York: Macmillan, 1933.

tion of particularistic ties of ingroup solidarity, in turn, frees men to apply universalistic considerations of efficiency and achievement to ever-widening areas of their lives.

Heightened universalism has profound implications for the stratification system. The achieved status of a man, what he has accomplished in terms of some objective criteria, becomes more important than his ascribed status, who he is in the sense of what family he comes from. This does not mean that family background no longer influences careers. What it does imply is that superior status cannot any more be directly inherited but must be legitimated by actual achievements that are socially acknowledged. Education assumes increasing significance for social status in general and for the transmission of social standing from fathers to sons in particular. Superior family origins increase a son's chances of attaining superior occupational status in the United States in large part because they help him to obtain a better education, whereas in less industrialized societies the influence of family origin on status does not seem to be primarily mediated by education.[13] Universalism also discourages discrimination against ethnic minorities, though it does not furnish incentives for giving them the assistance they may need to overcome the handicaps produced by long periods of deprivation and suppression. At the same time, universalism fosters a concern with materialistic values at the expense of spiritual ones; an interest in achievement and efficiency rather than religious devotion, philosophical contemplation, or artistic creation; a preoccupation with the outward signs of success and little patience for probing the deeper meanings of life. The crass materialism and invidious striving for status in today's world that have often been deplored are an integral part of the universalistic system that has also helped produce many things we cherish, including technological progress, a high standard of living, and greater equality of opportunity.

The three structural causes of upward mobility in industrialized society discussed above have their roots in the predominance of universalism. A pervasive concern with efficiency is an essential incentive for devoting much energy to accelerating technological progress, and such progress helps raise standards of living and promote upward mobility from obsolete lower occupational positions to expanding higher ones. The weakening of particularistic ties to kin and

---

[13] Even in Sweden, where the levels of industrialization and education are high but not so high as in the United States, "differential access to educational facilities as such does not go very far in explaining . . . the correlation between parental and filial status." Gösta Carlsson, *Social Mobility and Class Structure,* Lund: Gleerup, 1958, p. 135.

neighbor that would keep a man in the community where he was raised encourages migration to places with better opportunities for achievement, and this migration stimulates occupational mobility. The counterforces set in motion by the dominant significance of occupational achievement among those who cannot achieve superior status in their careers may constrain them to have larger families from whom they can obtain, in their role as fathers, the status support and gratification denied them in their occupational roles. The resulting differential fertility gives another impetus to upward mobility. According to these speculations—and this is all they are, of course—the structural conditions in our industrialized society governed by universalistic principles, and not merely the special historical circumstances in which they find expression at one time or another, are the causes of its high rate of occupational mobility.

The great potential of society's human resources can be more fully exploited in a fluid class structure with a high degree of mobility than in a rigid social system. Class lines that restrict mobility and prevent men born into the lower strata from even discovering what their capacities might be constitute a far more serious waste of human talent than the often deplored lower birth rates of the higher strata. In previous periods the knowledge and skills society was able to utilize were severely limited, which made this waste of talent regrettable from the standpoint of individuals but unavoidable from the perspective of the social order. Indeed Simmel has suggested that the major reason for the inevitable discrepancy between personal qualifications and social positions "is that there are always more people qualified for superordinate positions than there are such positions."[14] This is much less true in today's highly industrialized society than it was in earlier times, for technological progress has created a need for advanced knowledge and skills on the part of a large proportion of the labor force, not merely a small professional elite. Under these conditions society cannot any longer afford the waste of human resources a rigid class structure entails. Universalistic principles have penetrated deep into the fabric of modern society and given rise to high rates of occupational mobility in response to this need. The improvements in opportunities for social mobility resulting from the wider application of universalistic standards permit greater utilization of society's human potential, and they have important implications for the stability of democracy.

[14] Georg Simmel, *The Sociology of Georg Simmel*, Glencoe: Free Press, 1950, p. 300.

OPPORTUNITY AND DEMOCRACY

Lipset and Bendix found in their secondary analysis of mobility surveys from nine different countries that the rates of occupational mobility in all those industrial societies are high, with surprisingly little difference between them.[15] Contrary to the belief that America is a land of superior opportunities, the comparison revealed that the rates of upward mobility in several countries are higher than those in the United States, and so are the combined rates of upward and downward mobility. The authors' conclusion that generic conditions in industrialized societies—not any distinguishing features of the United States—are responsible for the high rates of occupational mobility observerable conforms to the conclusion we have reached. Nevertheless the specific point that opportunities for upward mobility in the United States are not as good as those in several European countries or in Japan (the only other non-European country included) may be questioned on several grounds. The prevailing impression that chances of social mobility are superior in the United States should not be dismissed out of hand, particularly in view of the doubtful reliability of some of the data with which Lipset and Bendix had to work. The outstandingly high degree of industrialization and level of education in American society as well as the less pronounced and less formalized distinctions in social status here compared to Europe or Japan would lead one to expect more social mobility in this country. Last but not least, whereas Lipset and Bendix only examine movements from the blue-collar into the white-collar class and vice versa, a meaningful study of national differences in opportunities must take into account differential chances of achieving elite status in one of the top strata. Industrialization may have the result that many sons of craftsmen become clerks, but such movements would hardly constitute evidence of great opportunities.[16]

As far as mobility between the blue-collar and the white-collar class is concerned, the conclusion of Lipset and Bendix is essentially confirmed by the OCG data, which are more reliable than the American data that were available to them. The combined rate of mobility in either direction between the manual and the nonmanual class is 34 per

[15] Seymour M. Lipset and Reinhard Bendix, *Social Mobility in Industrial Society*, Berkeley: Univer. of California Press, 1960, pp. 17-28.

[16] See Lewis A. Coser, Letter to the Editor, *Commentary*, **19**(1955), 86-87. Although Lipset and Bendix do point out that mobility into the professions is probably higher in the United States than elsewhere (*op. cit.*, p. 38), their theoretical analysis tends to ignore this point and centers on the lack of differences in opportunity for mobility between the United States and other countries.

cent for the OCG sample, slightly higher than that reported for any other country, the second-highest rate being Germany's 31 per cent. With respect to upward mobility of working-class sons into white-collar occupations, the rate in the United States, 37 per cent according to the OCG sample, is exceeded by that in two of the nine countries, France's 39 per cent and Switzerland's 45 per cent. It should be noted, however, that the Swiss data, which are not based on a representative sample, were judged to be unreliable by Miller.[17] To sum up, there is indeed little difference among various industrialized nations in the rate of occupational mobility between the blue-collar and the white-collar class, though the United States has higher rates than most countries, corresponding to its advanced level of industrialization and education.

To investigate national differences in opportunities for upward mobility into a top stratum, the comparative data assembled by Miller are used.[18] Miller's own secondary analysis of these data centers on the proportion of sons from a given social class who move up into the top stratum. But since both the occupational composition and the proportionate size of the elite strata in different countries vary widely, the direct comparison of the proportion of men moving into the elite, ignoring differences in its size and composition, may easily be misleading. For this reason we have decided to use, in addition to the proportions, the mobility ratios that standardize for size, despite the reservations we have about employing mobility ratios in comparative analysis, as discussed in Chapter 3. The data presented in Table 12.1 are derived from the raw frequencies in Miller's tables, except that the original source was used for Sweden because Miller does not present this table, and that Lopreato's recent study of mobility in Italy has been substituted for the one used by Miller, which he considered to be of questionable reliability.[19] Only countries for which national samples are available are included, and the OCG data are substituted for the American ones used by Miller. The broader of his two criteria for elite (Elite I and II) is employed, and the two professional strata in the United States are considered to comprise the Ameri-

[17] S. M. Miller, "Comparative Social Mobility," *Current Sociology*, 9(1960), 37. It should also be noted that if the OCG data are compared with those of other countries presented by Miller (p. 30) instead of with those presented by Lipset and Bendix, the proportion of American working-class sons who move up into white-collar strata is greater than that in any other country. These differences show that all such international comparisons must be interpreted with a great deal of caution.

[18] *Ibid.*, pp. 1-89.

[19] Carlsson, *op. cit.*, p. 93; and Joseph Lopreato, "Social Mobility in Italy," *American Journal of Sociology*, 71(1965), 311-314.

TABLE 12.1. OUTFLOW FROM SPECIFIED ORIGINS INTO ELITE[a] DESTINATIONS: INTERNATIONAL COMPARISONS

Country	Per Cent of All Men in Elite (1)	Working Class into Elite		Manual Class into Elite		Middle–Class into Elite	
		Per Cent (2)	Mobility Ratio (3)	Per Cent (4)	Mobility Ratio (5)	Per Cent (6)	Mobility Ratio (7)
Denmark	3.30	...	...	1.07	.32	4.58	1.39
France I (Bresard)	8.53	4.16	.49	3.52	.41	12.50	1.46
France II (Desabie)	6.12	1.99	.33	1.56	.25	10.48	1.71
Great Britain	7.49	...	...	2.23	.30	8.64	1.15
Italy	2.77	.48	.17	.35	.13	5.76	2.08
Japan	11.74	...	...	6.95	.59	15.12	1.29
Netherlands	11.08	...	...	6.61	.60	11.55	1.04
Puerto Rico	13.79	11.42	.83	8.60	.62	23.17	1.68
Sweden	6.66	4.43	.67	3.50	.53	18.09	2.72
USA (OCG)	11.60	10.41	.90	9.91	.85	20.90	1.80
West Germany	4.58	1.55	.34	1.46	.32	8.28	1.81

SOURCE: S. M. Miller, op. cit., pp. 69–80, except for Sweden (Carlsson, op. cit., p. 93), Italy (Lopreato, op. cit., p. 314), and the U.S.A. (OCG).

[a] "Elite" here is equivalent to Miller's "Elite I and II" for data taken from Miller and Carlsson, to Lopreato's "Ruling Class" for Italy, and to "Professional, Technical and Kindred" for the United States.

can elite. (The considerable gap in social distance between the two professional groups and all other occupational strata makes their designation as elite not entirely unjustified.) Following Miller's procedure, we examine movement into the elite from the working class (blue-collar), from the manual class (blue-collar and farm laborers, who could not always be separated from other manual workers), and from the middle class (white-collar excluding the elite).

Upward mobility from the working class into the top occupational stratum of the society is higher in the United States than in other countries. The proportion of American sons originating in the working class who move into the elite is exceeded only by that in Puerto Rico (column 2), and when differences in the size of the elite, which includes business owners as well as professionals for Puerto Rico, are taken into account, the mobility ratio for the United States is higher than that for any other country (column 3). Farm laborers must be combined with the various blue-collar workers into a manual class to permit comparisons with all countries. The chances of manual sons to experience upward mobility into the elite are greater in the United States than in any other country, whether raw proportions (column 4) or mobility ratios (column 5) are considered. The countries with the next best chances of mobility from manual origins into top-ranking positions are Puerto Rico, Japan, and the Netherlands. The likelihood that the middle class, consisting of the white-collar strata below the elite, sees its sons moving up into the elite is greater in the United States than in most countries, though not in all. The proportion of

American men originating in the middle class who move into the elite is only exceeded by that in Puerto Rico (column 6), but when the size of the elite is taken into account, the mobility ratio reveals Sweden to be in the first place, with Italy, West Germany, and the United States following in that order (column 7). It should be noted that the mobility ratio for the middle class is not entirely independent of that for the manual class in the same country, so that a high manual ratio tends to depress the middle-class ratio. What is of special significance for an understanding of the opportunities of the poor is the relative size of the mobility ratio for manual sons.

The relative opportunities of underprivileged Americans with manual origins to move up into the top stratum are particularly good compared to those in other societies. Nearly 10 per cent of manual sons achieve elite status in the United States, a higher proportion than in any other country. Lest it be suspected that this result is misleading because it only reflects the large size of the American elite —close to 12 per cent of the population—the mobility ratios have been compared, despite the reservation we have about this measure. Doing so merely accentuates the earlier result. The proportion of manual sons who achieve elite status is six-sevenths of that of all men occupying such status in the United States (.85), whereas this proportion is in no other country as great as two-thirds of that of the total (Puerto Rico being in second place with .62). In respect to mobility from the middle class into the elite, however, the ratio for the United States, though high, is not outstanding. It is the underprivileged class of manual sons that has exceptional chances for mobility into the elite in this country. There is a grain of truth in the Horatio Alger myth. The high level of popular education in the United States, perhaps reinforced by the lesser emphasis on formal distinctions of social status, has provided the disadvantaged lower strata with outstanding opportunities for long-distance upward mobility.[20]

[20] Correlations between father's and son's occupational status, however, do not reveal a similar superiority of American opportunity. Thus, Kaare Svalastoga ("Social Mobility: The Western European Model," *Acta Sociologica,* **9**, 1965, 176) concludes his regression analysis of data from nine European nations by stating "that it would not be very far off the mark in any industrialized European country to predict a father-son mobility equal to $r = .4$," which is the same correlation exhibited by the OCG data for the United States. The apparent contradiction may well be a result of the fact that the amount of mobility, even when presumably standardized, is not the same thing as the degree to which son's status depends on father's. The exceptionally large amount of occupational mobility in the United States, a result of the structural changes that have occurred with rapid industrialization, has inclined people to ignore the degree to which social origins influence occupational achievements here as well as in other societies.

The stimulating theory Lipset and Bendix present on the relationships between mobility, egalitarian values, and stable democracy is in need of a few revisions in the light of these findings as well as some other considerations.[21] They start by challenging the assumption of various observers of the political scene, such as Tocqueville, that the high chances of occupational mobility in the United States are the fundamental source of the political stability of American democracy. Since high rates of mobility characterize all industrial societies and opportunities in this country are no better than those elsewhere, according to Lipset and Bendix, the absence of extremist political parties and recurring political upheavals in the United States cannot be explained by the better chances of workers in cities and on farms "to attain positions of prominence and privilege."[22] They suggest instead that the egalitarian American ideology, which has no real counterpart in nations with a feudal past, is responsible for the stability of American democracy. The egalitarian ideology does not nullify the great differences in wealth and power that exist in this country, but it alters their significance and thereby robs them of their sting. The profound belief in the essential equality of all men combines with the often-noted materialism of American society to make people view differences in status as mere differences in accumulated resources and rewards rather than as inherent distinctions between persons born into families of varying ranks in the social order. There is no hereditary aristocracy that commands deference as a matter of birthright in the United States, and attempts to establish its equivalent, like those of the Daughters of the American Revolution, are not taken seriously by the rest of the population. The emphasis on equality and opportunity in the American ideology makes status distinctions less important, despite the great actual differences in rank and authority. By contrast, "in a society in which prevailing views emphasize class differences, even a high degree of mobility may not suffice to undermine these views."[23]

The first question this thesis raises is what perpetuates the firm American belief in equality and opportunity, which differs from the common beliefs in other countries, if, as presumed, there is neither more equality of rank and privilege nor more opportunity for mobility here than elsewhere. Although ideologies often distort reality, one does not have to be an orthodox Marxist to accept the proposition that ideologies and social values are rooted in existential conditions of the

[21] Lipset and Bendix, *op. cit.*, pp. 76-113.

[22] *Ibid.*, p. 76.

[23] *Ibid.*, p. 81. The criticisms raised below apply also to the fuller discussion of the significance of American egalitarian values in Seymour M. Lipset, *The First New Nation*, New York: Basic Books, 1963.

social structure. To be sure social values, in turn, influence the structure of social relations in the society. The ideological conviction of Americans that superior class position reflects primarily not an ingrained superiority of persons but only superior possessions and privileges that anybody with adequate abilities or sufficient luck can attain in fact reduces the significance that status distinctions *per se* have in social life. This perceptive observation of Lipset and Bendix, however, begs the question of why Americans continue to believe that class differences merely indicate differences in material advantages and rewards that are accessible to all, whereas men in other societies do not, if the actual chances of men from lower strata to achieve superior class positions are no better in the United States than in other industrial nations. These inconsistencies are resolved by the finding that the opportunities of men originating in lower social strata to move into top positions in the occupational hierarchy are greater in the United States than in other countries. The superior opportunity for upward mobility in American society is what sustains the egalitarian ideology, which expresses this opportunity in exaggerated form, and which has profound implications for the status structure.

The crass materialism of Americans has often been deplored, but the dominant emphasis on material values plays a crucial role, in conjunction with the egalitarian ideology, in reducing the patterns of deference and social subordination that otherwise accompany class differences in rank, income, and power. The elevation of material possessions into the most important distinguishing feature of differential status diminishes the significance of ascribed criteria of status and enhances the significance of achieved, which implies achievable, criteria of status. This makes it easier to translate economic improvements into advancements in accepted social status. The great value material possessions assume, moreover, provides incentives for devoting much energy to producing them. Hence the materialistic orientation prevalent in American society is probably not not unrelated to the high standard of living it has achieved, as Lipset and Bendix point out. "Every indicator of economic productivity and consumption patterns clearly demonstrates that the United States is much wealthier than any other country in the world today. In the present context this is significant because the *distribution* of consumers' goods has tended to become more equitable as the size of national income has increased."[24] The outstandingly high standard of living in this country enables most families in the lower occupational strata to enjoy a variety of consumer goods that are luxuries reserved for the rich in poorer

[24] *Ibid.,* p. 108 (italics in original).

countries. Although most Americans, despite the relatively great chances of upward mobility, do not achieve high occupational positions, of course, the high and rising standard of living makes it possible for most to experience some improvement in their economic welfare, to which the high valuation of material possessions lends added significance.

The joint effect of the materialistic orientation and the high standard of living it helps to produce is to further lessen the import of status distinctions in the United States. In a society in which material goods are highly valued but the standard of living is low, great differences in valued material possessions would intensify status distinctions. In a society in which the standard of living is high but an antimaterialistic orientation denigrates sheer material possessions, the wide distribution of material goods would have little influence on the distinctions in status resting on other grounds. It is the combination of a high standard of living and a materialistic orientation that reduces class differences, because it makes the widely available consumer goods important symbols of social status. Conspicuous consumption under these conditions extends to the lower social strata of society and reflects their endeavors to achieve social recognition by displaying the generally valued material symbols of status. The condemnation of such unrefined display by groups whose higher status rests on more secure foundations seems to be an attempt to deny men recognition as equals on the basis of material possessions alone. These defensive reactions of established elites to the ostentatious exhibition of material symbols of status, including the disapproval of materialism itself, reveal the threat to inherent status superiority that is posed by a system in which material achievements are a prime basis of status. Any appreciable economic achievement in such a materialistic system gives a man a right to claim higher status, which discourages the crystallization of lasting status differences between families that can be inherited.[25]

Impermanent status superiority does not command deference and compliance as a matter of inherent right. It constrains others to defer to a man and comply with his wishes only to the extent to which his resources obligate them to do so. He must pay them to do his bidding, as exemplified by the employer and his representative, or he must furnish them with services that command their respect and make it in

[25] The differences in style of life between social classes, which Warner emphasizes, promote status crystallization, counteract the materialistic orientation, and make the American stratification system less different from European ones than it otherwise might be. See W. Lloyd Warner and Paul S. Lunt, *The Social Life of a Modern Community*, New York: Yale Univer. Press, 1941.

their interest to follow his guidance, as exemplified by the professional expert. Lasting status distinctions tend to become surrounded with social norms that make deferential behavior and obedience to superiors a moral obligation of inferiors. Men in lower social strata are expected to be humble and deferential in social intercourse with their "betters." With the notable exception of race relations in the South, the expectations governing the social interaction between lower and higher strata in the United States are less discriminating, though subtle ways of deferring to men of acknowledged stature occur here too. Americans do not humbly express deference to a man of superior status, but they typically defer to his wishes if he uses his resources to make doing so to their advantage. This reflects once more the materialism of Americans and, simultaneously, the lesser import distinctions of social status *per se* assume for them. Although the differences in wealth and power in the United States are no less than those in other countries, the associated differences in social status in its own right are less pronounced and less lasting. The same attenuation of status distinctions may be anticipated in other industrial societies with the spread of universalism and the consequent improvements in occupational opportunities.

The stability of American democracy is undoubtedly related to the superior chances of upward mobility in this country, its high standard of living, and the low degree of status deference between social strata. For these conditions make it unlikely that large numbers of underprivileged men experience oppression, despair of all hope, and become so disaffected with the existing system of differential rewards as well as with political institutions that they join extremist political movements committed to violent rebellion. Thus a comparative study by Fox and Miller suggests that high rates of both upward and downward mobility distinguish stable democracies from other nations.[26] But Carlsson poses an intriguing paradox about the bearing of mobility on inequality. "Though a high rate of mobility may have the effect previously discussed of diminishing some of the gaps between classes, it may also tend to conserve the system and ultimately even create inequality."[27] He envisages a fictitious society in which high rates of mobility would assure the allocation of men to differential occupational positions on the basis of ability alone. Under these conditions, inequality would be pronounced, groups whose inferior ability

26 Thomas G. Fox and S. M. Miller, "Economic, Political and Social Determinants of Mobility," *Acta Sociologica*, 9(1965), 76-93.

27 Gösta Carlsson, "Sorokin's Theory of Social Mobility," in Philip J. Allen (ed.), *Pitirim A. Sorokin in Review*, Durham: Duke Univer. Press, 1963, p. 137.

has been demonstrated by their failure to progress to higher levels of education would have no chance to improve their position, and these "groups at the bottom of the scale would no longer have the consolation that society distributes its rewards unfairly, for what can be fairer than giving everyone a chance to prove his native ability and go ahead as far as it permits him?"[28] Carlsson actually raises three issues here, regarding the implications of mobility unhampered by ascribed status for fairness, inequality, and stability of the system.

The implicit assumption that we, with our universalistic orientation, readily make is that fairness demands that differential rewards be distributed on the basis of differences in abilities, whether native or acquired. From a wider perspective devoid of such universalistic bias this assumption must be questioned. Giving special privileges to men with socially valued abilities, which are the only abilities that are highly rewarded, is, in principle, no fairer than giving special privileges to any other group, though it may well serve important social functions by supplying men with incentives for nurturing these abilities and choosing occupations in which they can be applied.[29] Turning to the second point, it is not unreasonable to expect that high rates of mobility intensify the differential distribution of social rewards. Men who see little opportunity for improvement in their own economic status or, at least, that of their children, have greater inducements than those anticipating advancements in status to organize a union to raise wages or to vote for a party that advocates higher taxes for the wealthy, though many other factors unquestionably play a part. It follows from these unproved but plausible considerations that high rates of mobility permit extant differences in rewards to persist and even to grow. Inasmuch as high chances of mobility make men less dissatisfied with the system of social differentiation in their society and less inclined to organize in opposition to it, they help to perpetuate this stratification system, and they simultaneously stabilize the political institutions that support it, as already noted.

High rates of occupational mobility, therefore, do not assure unquestionable fairness in the allocation of rewards, may reinforce the unequal distribution of privileges, and may protect the system of social stratification against change. It would be by no means warranted, however, to infer that high chances of mobility make the stratification system more rigorous and magnify the social constraints it imposes.

[28] *Ibid.*, p. 138.
[29] See Kingsley Davis and Wilbert E. Moore, "Some Principles of Stratification," *American Sociological Review*, **10**(1945), 242-249. We take exception, however, to some of the assumptions made in this theory.

Although high rates of vertical mobility may preserve the status differences observable between *some* individuals, they undermine the status differences between the *same* families that are inherited from one generation to another. The consequent impermanence of status differences, even if they are no less pronounced, weakens the hold they have on people's conduct. In contrast to status differences persisting over many generations and becoming part of the established tradition, impermanent class differences do not confer the claim to deference and compliance on superiors as a matter of inherent right invested in ascribed status by social conventions. There is a fundamental difference between a stratification system that perpetuates established status distinctions between particular families over generations and one that perpetuates a structure of differentiated positions but not their inheritance.[30] Industrial societies, and the United States in particular, approach the latter type, but no society exhibits either extreme in pure form, for there is a minimum of mobility in the most rigid systems and some occupational inheritance in the most fluid social structures.

FUNCTIONS OF MOBILITY RESEARCH

Some conjectures about stratification theory informed by our research findings have been advanced in the last sections. As the comparative data from a variety of societies needed for refining the theory of stratification are not available in our study, it has been supplemented with data from mobility surveys of other countries. We have not hesitated to let our imagination roam in theorizing about social stratification, but the empirical findings provided a solid springboard for our speculations. Unfortunately information on occupational mobility is available only for a few countries, and some of it is of dubitable reliability. One function of the systematic empirical investigation of occupational mobility in the United States presented in this book is to provide, once similar studies from many nations become available, an adequate foundation for testing and refining stratification theory.

More limited theories pertaining to occupational differentiation, as distinguished from an over-all theory of stratification, could be directly explored and, occasionally, tested in our research. For instance, the hypothesis advanced by Lipset and Bendix that rural migrants to urban centers have taken the place formerly occupied by immigrants from Europe, and thus serve as catalysts of social mobility,

30 See Walter Buckley, "Social Stratification and the Functional Theory of Differentiation," *American Sociological Review*, 23(1958), 369-375.

is supported by our data. A generalization suggested by the OCG findings is that spatial as well as social movements tend to entail processes of selection, which promote chances of success and the allocation of men to positions on the basis of universalistic criteria. Migration is such a process of selection. Another example is that men who have overcome initial handicaps, like the sons of immigrants and the boys from large families who attain a high level of education, are more likely than others to achieve success subsequently. The experience of having succeeded in meeting a challenge may help them in later competitive struggles, but their superior attainments are undoubtedly in large part due to the fact that they are more highly selected groups than men who never had to conquer the same initial handicaps. These illustrations suffice to indicate that another function of our research is to suggest theoretical generalizations about occupational achievement and mobility.

The OCG inquiry provides a wealth of information on the American occupational structure, conditions that affect success in careers, and the consequences of occupational achievement for fertility. The size and representativeness of the sample, in conjunction with the rigorous methods of data collection and analysis, make this extensive body of material a highly reliable description of important aspects of occupational life in the United States. The availability of this material, partly by providing national standards with which studies of local communities and special groups can be compared, should prove useful to students of class differences and related problems.

A final function of the research is the practical one of providing policy makers and interested parties with knowledge essential for effective action programs to better social conditions. Thus the findings imply that helping children from large families to obtain a better education would suffice to remove the occupational disadvantages they now tend to experience, but that the compounded handicaps of Negroes cannot be relieved in such a straightforward manner and would have to be attacked on many different levels. Information of this kind cannot resolve conflicts over policy, but it can clear the air by settling some questions of fact—though of course not all—and thereby laying bare the value premises underlying the presumably disinterested policy disagreements.

APPENDIX A

Bibliography of Official Government Publications Relating to the Population Covered in OCG

1. REPORTS BASED ON OCG AND MARCH 1962 CPS

U. S. Bureau of the Census, "Lifetime Occupational Mobility of Adult Males: March 1962," *Current Population Reports,* Series P-23, No. 11, May 12, 1964.

———, "Educational Change in a Generation: March 1962," *Current Population Reports,* Series P-20, No. 132, September 22, 1964.

2. REPORTS BASED ON MARCH 1962 CPS

U. S. Department of Labor, *Monthly Report on the Labor Force: March 1962,* April 1962.

U. S. Bureau of Labor Statistics, "Marital and Family Characteristics of Workers, March 1962," *Special Labor Force Report,* No. 26, January 1963.

———, "Educational Attainment of Workers, March 1962," *Special Labor Force Report,* No. 30, May 1963.

U. S. Bureau of the Census, "Households and Families, by Type: 1962," *Current Population Reports,* Series P-20, No. 119, September 19, 1962.

———, "Educational Attainment: March 1962," *Current Population Reports,* Series P-20, No. 121, February 7, 1963.

———, "Income of Families and Persons in the United States: 1961," *Current Population Reports,* Series P-60, No. 39, February 28, 1963.

———, "Marital Status and Family Status: March 1962," *Current Population Reports,* Series P-20, No. 122, March 22, 1963.

443

———, "Household and Family Characteristics: March 1962," *Current Population Reports,* Series P-20, No. 125, September 12, 1963.

———, "Continuing Increase in the Average Number of Children Ever Born: 1940 to 1964," *Current Population Reports,* Series P-20, No. 136, April 16, 1965.

3. SELECTED REPORTS FOR DATES PROXIMATE TO MARCH 1962

U. S. Bureau of Labor Statistics, "Multiple Jobholders in May 1962," *Special Labor Force Report,* No. 29, May 1963.

———, "Labor Force and Employment, 1960-62," *Special Labor Force Report,* No. 31, May 1963.

———, "Employment of High-School Graduates and Dropouts in 1962," *Special Labor Force Report,* No. 32, July 1963.

———, "Economic Status of Nonwhite Workers, 1955-62," *Special Labor Force Report,* No. 33, July 1963.

———, "Employment of School-Age Youth, October 1962," *Special Labor Force Report,* No. 34, August 1963.

———, "Job Mobility in 1961," *Special Labor Force Report,* No. 35, August 1963.

———, "Job Tenure of American Workers, January 1963," *Special Labor Force Report,* No. 36, October 1963.

———, "Work Experience of the Population in 1962," *Special Labor Force Report,* No. 38, January 1964.

———, "Geographic Mobility and Employment Status, March 1962—March 1963," *Special Labor Force Report,* No. 44, August 1964 .

U. S. Bureau of the Census, "Estimates of the Population of the United States, by Age, Color, and Sex: July 1, 1950 to 1962," *Current Population Reports,* Series P-25, No. 265, May 21, 1963.

———, "Mobility of the Population of the United States: April 1961 to April 1962," *Current Population Reports,* Series P-20, No. 127, January 15, 1964.

———, and U. S. Department of Agriculture, Economic Research Service, "Estimates of the Farm Population of the United States: April 1962," *Farm Population,* Series Census-ERS (P-27), No. 33, March 14, 1963.

4. REPORTS ON SURVEY METHODS

U. S. Bureau of the Census, *The Current Population Survey: A Report on Methodology,* Technical Paper No. 7, 1963.

U. S. Bureau of Labor Statistics and Bureau of the Census, "Concepts and Methods Used in Household Statistics on Employment and Unemployment from the Current Population Survey," *BLS Report,* No. 279 and *Current Population Reports,* Series P-23, No. 13, June 1964.

APPENDIX B

Questionnaire for OCG Survey

OFFICE OF
THE DIRECTOR
FORM CPS-516
(12-15-61)

U. S. DEPARTMENT OF COMMERCE
BUREAU OF THE CENSUS
WASHINGTON 25, D. C.

March 19, 1962

Dear Mr._____ :

We appreciate your cooperation in connection with our regular Current Population Survey program. Now we would like to ask you to answer a few additional questions about your earlier background and on the occupation of your father. If you are married, there are also a few questions about your wife and her father's occupation. This information is needed to help in forecasting the kinds of changes that are likely to occur in the future and to help develop programs to meet changing conditions.

Please complete this form and mail it within the next three days in the enclosed envelope, which requires no postage. All information provided will be held in strict confidence and only statistical totals will ever be published.

Sincerely yours,

Richard M. Scammon
Director
Bureau of the Census

Control and line number		
		BUDGET BUREAU NO. 41-4155 *APPROVAL EXPIRES JUNE 30, 1962*

445

QUESTIONNAIRE FOR OCCUPATIONAL CHANGES IN A GENERATION

1. **Where were you born?** *(Name of State, foreign country, U.S. possession, etc.)*

2. **In what country was your father born?**

   United States ☐

   or

   _____
   (Name of foreign country; or Puerto Rico, Guam, etc.)

3. **In what country was your mother born?**

   United States ☐

   or

   _____
   (Name of foreign country; or Puerto Rico, Guam, etc.)

4. **Number of brothers and sisters**

   (Count those born alive but no longer living, as well as those alive now. Also include stepbrothers and sisters and children adopted by your parents.)

   a. How many sisters did you have? .... _____

       or ☐ None

   b. How many of these sisters were older than you (born earlier)? .... _____

   c. How many brothers did you have? .... _____

       or ☐ None

   d. How many of these brothers were older than you (born earlier)? .... _____

   e. Did any of your older brothers live to age 25?

   ☐ Yes   ☐ No
   (Answer Question 5)   *(Skip to Question 6)*

7. **Which of the following types of school did you attend before you were 16 years old?**

   (If you attended more than one kind, please check all that you did attend.)

   Public .... ☐ 1

   Parochial .... ☐ 2

   Other private .... ☐ 3

8. **Please think about the first full-time job you had after you left school. (Do not count part-time jobs or jobs during school vacation. Do not count military service.)**

   a. How old were you when you began this job? _____

   b. What kind of work were you doing?

   _____

   (For example: Elementary school teacher, paint sprayer, repaired radio sets, grocery checker, civil engineer, farmer, farm hand)

   c. What kind of business or industry was this?

   _____

   (For example: County junior high school, auto assembly plant, radio service, retail supermarket, road construction, farm)

5. If "Yes" in 4e, please indicate the highest grade of school the oldest brother completed.

(Check one box: if you are not sure, please make a guess.)

Never attended school .... ☐

Grades 1 to 12 ......
| 1 ☐ | 2 ☐ | 3 ☐ | 4 ☐ | 5 ☐ | 6 ☐ |
| 7 ☐ | 8 ☐ | 9 ☐ | 10 ☐ | 11 ☐ | 12 ☐ |

College (Academic years)
| 1 ☐ | 2 ☐ | 3 ☐ | 4 ☐ | 5 or more ☐ |

---

6. Where were you living when you were 16 years old?

a. The same community (city, town, or rural area) as at the present time? .... ☐ 1

b. Different community *(Check one):*

in a large city
(100,000 population or more)? ...... ☐ 2

in a suburb near a large city? ...... ☐ 3

in a middle-sized city or small town
(under 100,000 population) but
not in a suburb of a large city? ...... ☐ 4

open country (but not on a farm)? ...... ☐ 5

on a farm? ...... ☐ 6

---

d. Were you -- *(Check one)*

an employee of a PRIVATE company,
business, or individual for wages,
salary, or commissions? .... ☐ 1

a GOVERNMENT employee (Federal,
State, County, or local government)? .... ☐ 2

self-employed in OWN business, professional practice, or farm? .... ☐ 3

working WITHOUT PAY in a family
business or farm? .... ☐ 4

working FOR PAY in a family business
or farm? .... ☐ 5

---

9. Were you living with both your parents most of the time up to age 16?

☐ Yes ☐ No

(Skip to Question 10) *(Answer Question 9a)*

a. If "No" above, who was the head
of your family? *(Check one)*

Father ...... ☐ 1

Mother ...... ☐ 2

Other male ...... ☐ 3

Other female ...... ☐ 4

447

10. Now we would like to find out what kind of work your father did when you were about 16 years old. If you were not living with your father, please answer for person checked in Question 9a.

a. What kind of work was he doing?

(For example: Elementary school teacher, paint sprayer, repaired radio sets, grocery checker, civil engineer, farmer, farm hand)

b. What kind of business or industry was this?

(For example: County junior high school, auto assembly plant, radio service, retail supermarket, road construction, farm)

c. Was he --   (Check one)

an employee of a PRIVATE company, business, or individual for wages, salary, or commissions? .... ☐ 1

a GOVERNMENT employee (Federal, State, County or local government)? .... ☐ 2

self-employed in his OWN business, professional practice, or farm? .... ☐ 3

working WITHOUT PAY in his family's business or farm? .... ☐ 4

---

12. Are you now married?

(If "Yes," please answer Questions 13 and 14 below concerning your wife. If you are not sure of the answer, please ask her for the information.)

☐ Yes --

☐ No -- (Omit the next two questions)

13. a. How many brothers did your wife have? ....

or ☐ None _____

b. How many sisters did your wife have? ....

or ☐ None _____

14. Now we would like to find out what kind of work your wife's father did when she was about 16 years old. If she was not living with her father, please check here ...... ☐ and answer for the person who was the head of her family at that time.

a. What kind of work was he doing?

(For example: Elementary school teacher, paint sprayer, repaired radio sets, grocery checker, civil engineer, farmer, farm hand)

b. What kind of business or industry was this?

(For example: County junior high school, auto assembly plant, radio service, retail supermarket, road construction, farm)

c. Was he -- (Check one)

an employee of a PRIVATE company, business, or individual for wages, salary, or commissions? .... ☐ 1

a GOVERNMENT employee (Federal, State, County, or local government)? .... ☐ 2

self-employed in his OWN business, professional practice, or farm? .... ☐ 3

working WITHOUT PAY in his family's business or farm? .... ☐ 4

11. What is the highest grade of school your father (or person checked in Question 9a) completed? *(Check one box. If you are not sure, please make a guess)*

Never attended school ..... ☐

Grades 1 to 12 ....
1 ☐ 2 ☐ 3 ☐ 4 ☐ 5 ☐ 6 ☐
7 ☐ 8 ☐ 9 ☐ 10 ☐ 11 ☐ 12 ☐

College (Academic years) .. 1 ☐ 2 ☐ 3 ☐ 4 ☐ 5 or more ☐

Please use this space to clarify any problems the questions caused.

_____

_____

_____

_____

_____

_____

449

APPENDIX C

Notes on Coverage of OCG Tabulations and Comparability with Other Sources

Tabulations of OCG data are in the form of frequencies (in thousands) that represent estimates of the corresponding numbers in the "civilian non-institutional population" residing in the United States. As in many CPS tabulations, the civilian noninstitutional population includes members of the Armed Forces living off post or with their families on post. It excludes other members of the Armed Forces stationed in the United States, members of the Armed Forces stationed abroad, and inmates of institutions.

The OCG population estimates, like all CPS estimates, are produced by inflating sample totals "to independent estimates of the civilian population of the United States by age, sex, and color," which are in turn derived by demographic accounting procedures. It should be noted that these independent estimates are considered to be very reliable. They use the most recent decennial census as a benchmark, and after a decade has passed the error of closure between current estimates and the new census is quite small.

One of the great strengths of the OCG inquiry, therefore, as compared with previously published studies of occupational mobility, is that its conclusions automatically translate into statements about the entire covered portion of the U. S. population. For the same reason, moreover, it is possible to make meaningful comparisons between OCG data and other national figures, provided careful attention is paid to the coverage of the respective sets of statistics and to procedural variations likely to affect comparability.

These notes go into some detail about the coverage of the OCG data, because this appears to be a significant consideration in making interpretations of the findings. In approximate terms, the OCG tabulations represent a population of 45 million males 20 to 64 years of age residing in the United States in March 1962, or about 96 per cent of the total of 47 million males, in-

451

TABLE C.1. POPULATION ESTIMATES FOR THE UNITED STATES RELATING TO COVERAGE OF OCG–CPS DATA, FOR MALES 20 TO 64 YEARS OLD, BY AGE, 1962 (FREQUENCIES IN THOUSANDS)

| Age (Years) | Estimates for July 1, 1962 | | | | Estimates for March 1962 | | | Approximate Per Cent Coverage by OCG[b] (8) |
	Civilian Resident Population of the U.S. (1)	Armed Forces Stationed Abroad (2)	Armed Forces Stationed in U.S. (3)	Inmates of Institutions (4)	Armed Forces Covered in CPS[a] (5)	Civilian Noninstitutional Population (6)	Covered in OCG Data, (5) + (6) (7)	
20 to 24	4,955	280	710	81	211	4,804	5,015	85.4
25 to 34	10,326	213	579	148	435	10,179	10,614	95.5
35 to 44	11,590	111	311	155	225	11,384	11,609	97.1
45 to 54	10,311	21	69	155	54	10,108	10,162	98.2
55 to 64	7,770	...	5	146	4	7,580	7,584	98.1
Total, 20 to 64	44,952	625	1,674	685	929	44,055	44,984	95.6

SOURCE: Cols. (1) to (3) from Bureau of the Census, "Estimates of the Population of the United States, by Age, Color, and Sex: July 1, 1950 to 1962," Current Population Reports, Series P-25, Population Estimates, No. 265, May 21, 1963; cols. (4) to (7) from unpublished estimates of the Bureau of the Census used as control figures for March 1962 CPS.

[a]Includes only those living off post or with families on post.

[b]Col. (7) divided by sum of cols. (2), (3), (4), (6). This calculation assumes no change in size or age distribution of the Armed Forces between March and July of 1962. According to Current Population Reports, P-25, No. 253, August 16, 1962, the total strength of the Armed Forces was 2,885,000 on March 1, 1962, and 2,855,000 on July 1, 1962, representing a decrease of about 1 per cent. Note that males aged 20 to 64 comprised about 80 per cent of the total personnel of the Armed Forces in March.

cluding all Armed Forces, those stationed abroad as well as in the United States, and inmates of institutions (see Table C.1.). If we simply point out that the OCG findings on occupational mobility do not apply to career military men or to inmates of institutions, it seems safe to discuss the results as though they applied to the whole population in the designated age range.

There is one exception to this advice, however, that must be carefully noted. Only 85 per cent of the U. S. male population 20 to 24 years of age is covered by OCG tables, owing primarily to the concentration in this age group of men temporarily in military service. Many of the older men in the study, of course, had seen such service. The young men are not exceptional from that standpoint. The OCG survey does, however, catch them at a stage in the life cycle when the interruption of careers by military service is sufficiently frequent that it becomes dangerous to generalize for the cohort as a whole from data available on that portion eligible for OCG coverage.

The detailed statistics supporting these summary statements on coverage are given in Table C.1, which show not only that military service claims larger proportions of younger men but also that the proportion of those in the service who are covered in the CPS increases with age.

Although it is unlikely that many readers will go to the trouble of doing so, it would be possible for them to discover slight discrepancies between the population estimates in Table C.1 and those published in Table 2 of the March 1962 *Monthly Report on the Labor Force,* issued by the Bureau of Labor Statistics in April 1962. The reason for these discrepancies is

TABLE C.2.   YEARS OF SCHOOL COMPLETED, FOR MALES 20 TO 64 YEARS OLD IN MARCH 1962, AS SHOWN IN OCG TABULATIONS AND IN PUBLISHED CPS TABULATIONS

Years of School Completed	Number in Thousands		(B) minus (A)	Per Cent Distribution	
	(A) OCG	(B) CPS[a]		OCG	CPS
No school	562	541	− 21	1.3	1.2
Elementary					
1 to 4 years	1,901	1,979	78	4.2	4.3
5 to 7 years	4,317	4,596	279	9.6	10.1
8 years	6,128	6,300	172	13.6	13.8
High School					
1 to 3 years	8,478	8,642	164	18.9	18.9
4 years	12,788	13,021	233	28.4	28.5
College					
1 to 3 years	5,277	5,119	−158	11.7	11.2
4 years	3,256	3,251	− 5	7.2	7.1
5+ years	2,276	2,220	− 56	5.1	4.9
Total	44,984	45,669[b]	685	100.0	100.0

[a]Bureau of the Census, Current Population Reports, Series P-20, No. 121, "Educational Attainment: March 1962" (February 7, 1963).
[b]Includes 685 inmates of institutions.

that in early 1962 it was still necessary to inflate CPS sample totals to U. S. population estimates compiled on the basis of the 1950 census benchmark. By the time the OCG data were tabulated, however—and the same thing holds for publications by the Bureau of the Census derived from the March 1962 CPS—it was possible to substitute revised population estimates based on the 1960 benchmark.

Another kind of minor discrepancy that could attract attention is illustrated in Table C.2, which compares published tabulations from the CPS with OCG data ostensibly on nearly the same population. There is, first of all, a difference in coverage, inasmuch as these CPS data include the institutional population whereas the OCG tables do not. If this were the only cause for the discrepancy, however, all the differences in frequencies should be positive. The other cause relates to the fact that OCG data are derived from only 83.7 per cent of the eligible sample, those returning OCG questionnaires that could be matched to CPS records. After the initial return of these questionnaires a subsample of nonrespondents was subjected to intensive follow-up, so that it was possible to form unbiased estimates of the characteristics of initial nonrespondents and hence of the whole eligible sample. Nevertheless the estimates incorporating differential sample inflation weights for initial nonrespondents could not be expected to show precisely the same distributions as estimates based on the full sample.

As the per cent distributions in the last two columns of Table C.2 indicate, the education distributions in the two sources are very similar and for most purposes interchangeable.

A final example of comparability between OCG and other CPS data con-

TABLE C.3.   CIVILIAN NONINSTITUTIONAL MALE POPULATION 20 TO 64 YEARS OLD, BY MARITAL STATUS, MARCH 1962, ESTIMATED FROM ALTERNATIVE SOURCES (FREQUENCIES IN THOUSANDS)

Marital Status	Civilian[a] Population March 1962 CPS (1)	Institutional Population April 1960 Census (2)	Estimated Civilian[a] Noninstitutional Population March 1962 (3)	Civilian[a] Noninstitutional Population CPS–OCG March 1962 (4)
Total	45,669	685	44,984	44,984
Married, spouse present	35,575	...	35,575	35,574
Husband in first marriage	30,906	...	30,906	31,075
Husband previously married	4,669	...	4,669	4,499
Widowed	660	27	633	558
Divorced	1,132	77	1,055	1,027
Married, spouse absent	1,570	224	1,346	1,085
Separated	896	46	850	NA
Other	674	178	496	NA
Never married (single)	6,732	357	6,375	6,739

SOURCES: (1) Bureau of the Census, "Marital Status and Family Status: March 1962," Current Population Reports, Series P-20, No. 122 (22 March 1963), Table 1; (2) Bureau of the Census, "Inmates of Institutions," 1960 Census of Population, Final Report PC(2)-8A (Washington: Government Printing Office, 1963), Table 17; (3) Column 1 minus column 2; (4) Unpublished OCG tabulations by Bureau of the Census.

[a] Includes members of the Armed Forces living off post or with families on posts in the United States.

cerns statistics on marital status. The frequencies in the OCG tables differ slightly from published data derived from the March 1962 CPS (see Table C.3) for two reasons. First, the published tables include 685,000 inmates of institutions, who were excluded from the OCG tabulations. Second, although the OCG sample (comprising about five-sixths of the eligible persons in the CPS sample) was so weighted as to yield a correct total population estimate and to eliminate most of the bias of nonresponse, some bias remains in the data. The calculations summarized in Table C.3 suggest that the OCG tables, relative to the full CPS data for March 1962, overstate the number of single men and understate the numbers whose marriages were disrupted by separation, divorce, or death of the spouse. There is no way, however, to estimate what bias (if any) may pertain to the OCG data on socioeconomic characteristics of men by marital status.

APPENDIX D

Chicago Pretest Matching Study

The Chicago pretest covered 570 males 20 to 64 years old in the Chicago metropolitan area who were included in selected rotation groups of the CPS sample for the survey month. Altogether, 485 returned OCG questionnaires or were contacted in a follow-up by an interviewer. (Only a subsample of rotation groups were followed up.) Of these, about 70 per cent gave an answer to the question, "What was your address when you were 16?" such that it seemed feasible to locate the address in the records of an earlier census. (This question was not asked in the main study, but only in the pretest.) Of the cases that were submitted for matching only about 40 per cent were completed successfully. Some major reasons for failure to match were: address outside of the United States; address located, but family was not listed at that address in the census record; family was located, but father was not a member of the household; and address could not be found. Records of the census of 1920, 1930, or 1940—whichever was nearest the respondent's sixteenth birthday— were searched. This means that a period of up to five years may have separated the respondent's sixteenth birthday and the date of the census. Hence a low proportion of matches is not surprising. According to recent data, about 20 per cent of the U. S. population changes its address each year, about 50 per cent every five years. If geographic mobility is occupationally selective (which it is), then the matched cases need not be a representative sample of all cases. In summary, the case base for the matching analysis was derived as follows:

> 570 males in target sample for pretest
> 485 OCG questionnaires completed
> 342 names searched in census
>   29 matched to 1920 census
>   46 matched to 1930 census
>   62 matched to 1940 census
> —
> 137 total names matched and father identified.

For the 137 matched names, three-digit occupation and industry codes were assigned to the questionnaire response and to the occupation reported in the census. On this detailed level of coding the agreement between the two sources is not high; here are the relevant frequencies:

> 60 same occupation and same industry (three-digit codes)
> 15 same occupation but different industry
> 16 different occupation but same industry
> 46 different occupation and different industry
> ———
> 137 total

Thus for only 44 per cent of the cases was there complete agreement between the two sources. There was partial agreement for an additional 23 per cent.

This result, of course, is relative to the system of occupational classification. It is perhaps unduly discouraging for the reason that none of the analyses contemplated for this study will make use of the full detail of occupation and industry. We must consider, therefore, some alternative classifications that are more nearly relevant to the study design, and also point out some reasons why disagreements between the two sources are not so serious as may appear on first examination.

One portion of the study makes use of major occupation groups. Hence the summary of agreements and disagreements between the two matched sources in Table D.1 is pertinent. We may note first that 51, or 37 per cent, of the cases lie off the diagonal of the table; this is the percentage of dis-

TABLE D.1.   FATHER'S OCC. AS REPORTED ON QUESTIONNAIRE COMPARED WITH OCC. IN CENSUS RECORD, FOR MALES IN CHICAGO PRETEST WHO WERE LOCATED IN CENSUSES OF 1920, 1930, OR 1940

	Census											
Questionnaire	(1)	(2)	(3)	(4)	(5)	(6)	(7)	(8)	(9)	(10)	(11)	Total
(1) Prof., tech.	6		2		1			1				10
(2) MOP, exc. farm		4	4			1					1[a]	10
(3) Sales			3								2	5
(4) Clerical				5							1	6
(5) Crafts		2	1		32	1	1	4	1		1	43
(6) Operatives		1		1	3	11	1	5			1	23
(7) Service							9					9
(8) Laborer					2	2		7			2	13
(9) Farmer					1				8			9
(10) Farm labor								1	1	1		3
(11) NA				1	1	1	2	1				6
Total	6	7	10	7	40	16	13	19	10	1	8	137

[a]"Retired" in census record.

agreement based on major occupation groups. The base for this percentage, however, includes six questionnaires that failed to state father's occupation and eight census records in which occupation was not given (there were no cases of NA in both sources). If we are interested in estimating the accuracy of the questionnaire report on father's occupation, when that occupation actually is reported, it may be well to omit the NA's from consideration (not to neglect, but simply to treat separately, the problem of NA bias). On the basis of 123 cases with father's occupation reported in both sources, the proportion of disagreements between the two is 37/123 = 30 per cent.

At this point, we may consider whether 30 per cent is a "high" or a "low" percentage of discrepancies. In the first place, although complete accuracy would be desirable, it is more realistic to ask how this figure compares with the reliability of other survey data. Perhaps the most relevant information comes from the 1950 post-enumeration study (PES) of the Bureau of the Census. The PES was an intensive operation with relatively highly trained enumerators; it was taken shortly after the 1950 census in an effort to assess the amount of error present in the data supplied by the regular census enumerators. According to the report on the study,[1] 17.1 per cent of the employed males classified in both the census and the PES were in a different major occupation group in the census from that reported in the PES. Note that this is an estimate of the extent of unreliability in reports on the *same* labor force experience at a current, or very recent, date.

A second consideration is that our questionnaire–census match could well show discrepancies due to occupational mobility of the father over a period ranging up to as long as five years. As noted above, if the family were geographically mobile during the relevant period, a match was not likely to be made. But many of the fathers may have changed jobs and occupations without shifting residences. How much occupational mobility there may have been at the various times to which the data refer cannot be known with any precision. We may, however, cite a figure that is at least suggestive. The Bureau of the Census reported[2] that of males who were employed in both August 1945 and August 1946 (excluding those in the Armed Forces), 12.4 per cent were in a different major occupation group on the second date from that stated for the first. Admittedly, this was a period of great instability, as the nation shifted from a war to a postwar economy (that, presumably, was the reason for taking the survey, which remains unique in the work of the Bureau of the Census to date). Nevertheless, the time period involved is only one year.

Surely it is only a coincidence that adding the PES estimate of unreliability (17.1 per cent disagreement with the census) to the CPS estimate of one-year occupational mobility (12.4 per cent) yields a total, 29.5 per cent, which hardly differs from the 30 per cent disagreement between our pretest questionnaires and the census records to which our respondents were matched. Yet such a calculation, despite its conceptual looseness, does suggest that the order of

[1] Bureau of the Census, Technical Paper No. 4, "The Post-Enumeration Survey: 1950," Washington, 1960, Table N.

[2] Bureau of the Census, "Industrial and Occupational Shifts of Employed Workers: August, 1945 to August, 1946," *Current Population Reports*, Series P-50, No. 1, July, 1947.

magnitude of the unreliability in the questionnaire reports of father's occupation is not hopelessly greater than that in other commonly used survey data.

The figure previously given on disagreement at the three-digit occupation code level may be combined with the data in Table D.1 and the summary thereof in Table D.2 to indicate the levels at which discrepancies occurred; the total of 62 discrepancies breaks down as follows:

- 11 different three-digit occupations within same major occupation group
- 26 different major occupation groups within same broad occupation category
- 11 different broad occupation categories
- 14 NA in one source
- 62 total

The broad categories just referred to may be of particular interest to some readers, given the prevailing interest in mobility across the white-collar–manual boundary. Table D.2 reveals that only five fathers reported as manual workers in the questionnaire were in white-collar occupations according to census records and that the obverse discrepancy occurred three times. All three discrepancies involving fathers reported as farm workers had to do with their being reported as manual workers in the alternate source. Assuming, as we have argued above, that at least some of the discrepancies represent actual mobility on the part of the fathers, we may conclude that the classification of fathers as white-collar or manual workers is made with reasonably high reliability.

TABLE D.2.   SUMMARY BY BROAD OCCUPATION CATEGORIES

Questionnaire	Census				
	(1)-(4)	(5)-(8)	(9)-(10)	(11)	Total
(1)-(4) White-collar	24	3	0	4	31
(5)-(8) Manual	5	78	1	4	88
(9)-(10) Farm	0	2	10	0	12
(11) NA	1	5	0	0	6
Total	30	88	11	8	137

There are only one or two other points in Table D.1 that may be suggestive. Note the appreciable number of fathers returned as MOP's (managers, officials, and proprietors) on the questionnaire who were counted as sales workers in the census. Actual mobility may well account for such discrepancies, but a reporting error in this direction would not be surprising either. There is another cluster of cases in which the father was recorded as a laborer in the census but reported as a craftsman or operative by his son in the questionnaire. A similar observation applies; both actual parental mobility and respondent recall error probably are involved.

A related question is that of the reliability of reports on father's occupation from the standpoint of the socioeconomic status score (SES). A considerable number of the tabulations on occupational mobility and fertility employ this score as an independent variable. The properties of the score have been fully stated in the source publication[3] and need not be recapitulated here. The point to emphasize is that occupations may be quite different in job description and yet have the same or similar SES scores. Hence a response or coding error that puts the father in the "wrong" major group or detailed occupation is of consequence for this part of the analysis only if it simultaneously results in his being assigned a very erroneous occupational score.

A scatter diagram of the status scores derived from questionnaire reports on those derived from census records was prepared for 115 matched cases in which father's occupation was reported in' both sources and in which the father was not a farmer in both. The latter omission was made because a considerable part of the analysis will concern men of nonfarm origins. Since farm fathers seem to be reliably reported the omission will, if anything, reduce the apparent reliability.

Before mentioning the finding in regard to reliability, some effort can be made to assess the representativeness of the matched cases. We have, first, a group of 110 *un*matched questionnaires wherein father's occupation was reported, omitting farm fathers and respondents whose address at age 16 was in a foreign country. A second comparison group consists of 1,207 males reporting "father's longest job" in the 1951 Chicago portion of the Six City Survey of Labor Mobility. This sample was studied in an earlier paper,[4] although the data given here do not appear in the same form in that paper. Means and standard deviations of the occupational status of reported father's occupations are given in the summary below:

	N	Mean	S. D.
Males 25 to 64 years old, nonfarm origin,			
1951 Chicago Labor Mobility Survey	1,207	32.3	22.2
Chicago pretest, OCG Study, males 20 to			
64 years old, nonfarm origin, 1961			
Unmatched questionnaires	110	28.6	23.5
Matched questionnaires	115	—	—
Questionnaire report	—	31.9	22.0
Census record	—	29.8	21.7

There is, of course, a 10-year lapse between the two studies, as well as a slight difference in the age range of respondents; the Labor Mobility data (for "father's longest job"), moreover, are for the city of Chicago, the OCG pretest data (on father's occupation when the respondent was age 16) for the Chicago metropolitan area. Hence comparability is by no means precise. The

3 Albert J. Reiss, Jr. *et al., Occupations and Social Status,* New York: Free Press, 1961.

4 Otis Dudley Duncan and Robert W. Hodge, "Education and Occupational Mobility," *American Journal of Sociology,* **68**(1963).

similarity of the statistics from the two studies, however, suggests that the smaller and somewhat selected OCG samples are representing approximately the same universe of fathers' occupations as did the Labor Mobility Survey. There seems to be reasonable similarity, too, between the unmatched and matched questionnaires as concerns the central tendency and dispersion of status score distributions. Finally, the questionnaire and census records are not far apart in these respects, although the upward bias in the mean for the questionnaire reports is perhaps in the direction we would expect for a retrospective question.

The critical question here, of course, is not whether the questionnaire gives about the same average and spread of scores as does an independent source, but how high the correlation between the sources is on a case-by-case basis. The scatter diagram reveals a heavy concentration of frequencies on the diagonal $Y = X$, that is, of cases with the same or closely similar occupational SES scores: in 65 cases the father's SES is the same in the two sources, and in an additional eight cases the two sources differ by less than five SES points. There is, however, considerable scattering off the diagonal in both directions, some with questionnaire-derived scores markedly higher than those derived from census reports, and some deviating almost as much in the opposite direction. The Pearsonian correlation between the two series is .74. The reader may recall the old rule of thumb that reliability coefficients should be at least .90, and this order of reliability apparently is attained in survey work. Thus the census–PES match, which was mentioned earlier, was studied by assigning to each *major* occupation group the mean occupational status score for the group, and correlating the census with the PES reports for matched cases. This correlation is .878. Hence, our correlation of .74 between pretest questionnaire and census may seem disappointingly low. Yet, as has been mentioned before, some of the failure of the two sources to correspond may be a result of actual mobility of fathers between the time to which the census record pertains and the time for which the respondent was asked to report. It is difficult to say how much the correlation might be lowered by this factor. In the Duncan-Hodge study mentioned above the interannual correlation between status scores of the 1950 and 1940 occupations of respondents was .77 for men 45 to 54 years old at the later date and only .55 for men aged 35 to 44. Evidently a 10-year period gives ample time for men old enough to have 16-year-old sons to change their occupational rank considerably. The interannual correlation would doubtlessly be higher for a shorter period, and was perhaps higher in the earlier time periods that are relevant for some of the fathers reported on in the OCG study. Any substantial allowance for actual mobility on the part of the fathers, however, would be compatible with the assumption that the reliability of the questionnaire reports is considerably greater than is suggested by the questionnaire–census correlation of .74.

APPENDIX E

Census Checks on Retrospective Data

Many items in the OCG questionnaire call for retrospective data, and it is a matter of some importance to ascertain whether such data are reported with reasonable accuracy. Checking each report against an independent source is perhaps the most trustworthy means of reaching a judgment in this question. This approach could be taken only on a small scale, in connection with the pretest (see Appendix D). When individual reports cannot be checked it may still be possible to detect major biases in retrospective data by checking their aggregate distributions against independent sources. This type of check is available for several of the questionnaire items.

FATHER'S EDUCATIONAL ATTAINMENT

The OCG questionnaire item on the number of school years completed was designed to be comparable in concept—though it was slightly different in form of presentation—with the same item used in the 1940, 1950, and 1960 censuses. In OCG the respondent reported his father's educational attainment; in the censuses males living in the United States reported their own attainment. If we could identify in the census the men who were fathers of men who were, say, 25 to 34 years old in 1962, the distributions of educational attainment in the two sources should, ideally, be the same (neglecting the problem of differential fertility).

There is no way to make such a comparison completely rigorous. Certain of the reasons will be obvious to the reader. Some fathers were no longer alive, or were not residents of the United States at the date of the census. The census data on educational attainment do not segregate fathers of men who were to be of a specified age in March 1962 from contemporaries of the fathers. The OCG reports, moreover, are somewhat selective, in that some 11 per cent of respondents failed to state father's education, and some of the reports (as a result of the instruction to respondents) pertain to a person other than the father who was the head of the family in which the respondent grew up. For these reasons a comparison between OCG reports and independent estimates derived from census data can only be roughly indicative of the accuracy of the former. Let us, nevertheless, see what a set of estimates prepared with reasonable care may show. The steps in preparing them are listed seriatim.

(1) *Distribute respondents by year of birth.* This was done on the basis of single-year-of-age distributions of males in the 1960 census. Consider the group of male respondents 25 to 34 years old in March 1962 as an example. It was assumed that all these men were born during the years 1927 to 1936. The number of males reported as age 23 in 1960 was divided by the total number of registered births in 1936, to provide an adjustment to use in the next step; the number of males age 24 was divided by the 1935 births; and so on. It will be seen that this procedure automatically takes into account the sex ratio at birth and annual variation in completeness of birth registration.

(2) *Distribute birth cohorts of respondents by age of father.* Annual vital statistics publications provide a count of births by age of father at the time of the birth. The number in each five-year interval of father's age was adjusted by multiplying the reported births by the ratio obtained in the preceding step. The resulting distribution was broken down into a distribution by single years of father's age, using Sprague multipliers as published by Jaffe,[1] together with some arbitrary adjustments at the two tails of the distribution.

(3) *Distribute respondents by birth year of father.* After the previous step was accomplished for each annual birth cohort of respondents it was necessary to merge the 10 cohorts included in the group of respondents 25 to 34 years old in March 1962 into a single distribution of those respondents by birth year of father. It should be noted that age of father at birth of son does not precisely specify father's birth year. Thus the 27-year-old father of a son born in 1936 may himself have been born in either 1918 or 1919, whereas a 28-year-old father was born in either 1918 or 1917. Each single year of father's age, therefore, was allocated half and half to the two included years of father's birth. At this point fathers of respondents in all 10 cohorts could be aggregated to provide a single distribution of respondents by birth year of father, and fathers' birth years could be so grouped as to correspond with age intervals in the census educational attainment tables. Table E.1 shows the estimated distribution by father's birth year for the two groups of respondents for which this analysis was carried out.

(4) *Estimate educational attainment of "fathers."* A distribution of an aggregate of birth cohorts by birth year of father does not, of course, refer to a sample of fathers, for each father appears in the distribution once for each son born to him. But this is to our advantage in the present case because the OCG respondents were reporting father's education even though they had

---

[1] A. J. Jaffe, *Handbook of Statistical Methods for Demographers,* Washington: Government Printing Office, 1951, Chapter 4.

TABLE E.1. ESTIMATED DISTRIBUTION OF MALES 25 TO 34 AND
35 TO 44 YEARS OLD IN MARCH 1962, BY BIRTH YEAR OF FATHER
(PER MILLION)

Birth Year of Father	25 to 34 (Born 1927–36)	35 to 44 (Born 1917–26)
1855 to 1859	...	817
1860 to 1864	...	3,876
1865 to 1869	774	12,254
1870 to 1874	4,634	33,884
1875 to 1879	13,145	73,903
1880 to 1884	32,954	139,770
1885 to 1889	73,893	208,001
1890 to 1894	134,321	248,643
1895 to 1899	192,740	193,905
1900 to 1904	237,581	76,904
1905 to 1909	210,316	8,035
1910 to 1914	90,050	8
1915 to 1919	9,582	...
1920 to 1924	10	...
Total	1,000,000	1,000,000

one or more brothers eligible to be included in the survey. The assumption made at this point is that "fathers" born during a given five-year period had the same educational attainment as all men born in that period who were enumerated in one of the censuses. Let f_i = proportion of men in an aggregate of birth cohorts whose fathers were born in period i. Let p_{ij} be the probability that a male born in a period i and included in the census will be enumerated in educational attainment category j in the census. The estimation of f_i has just been described, and numerical values are given in Table E.1. Values of p_{ij} were calculated from tables on educational attainment by age in the censuses of 1940, 1950, and 1960. We define the estimated proportion with fathers in the jth educational attainment category as

$$e_j = \sum_i f_i p_{ij}.$$

The numerical values of e_j are shown in Table E.2, together with the distributions of respondents by father's educational attainment as reported in OCG.

The results are distinctly encouraging. The OCG distributions closely resemble those synthesized from independent data. Perhaps the only major bias is an apparent tendency to report as high-school graduates fathers who attended only one to three years of high school. This is especially evident for respondents 35 to 44 years old.

The reader will note the variation between the estimates based on different census years. Because f_i was the same irrespective of the census year, this

TABLE E.2. PER CENT DISTRIBUTION OF MALES 25 TO 34 AND 35 TO 44 YEARS OLD IN MARCH 1962, BY FATHER'S EDUCATIONAL ATTAINMENT, AS REPORTED IN OCG AND AS ESTIMATED FROM CENSUS DATA ON AGE BY EDUCATIONAL ATTAINMENT AND VITAL STATISTICS ON FATHER'S AGE BY YEAR OF BIRTH

Educational Attainment of Father	Males 25 to 34 Years Old			Males 35 to 44 Years Old			
		Estimate, using				Estimate, using	
	OCG	1950 Census	1960 Census	OCG	1940 Census	1950 Census	1960 Census
No school	4.15	2.68	3.74	6.66	4.82	4.65	6.69
Elementary							
1 to 4 years	9.35	10.29	10.21	12.84	12.77	14.21	14.27
5 to 7 years	19.11	18.95	19.99	21.76	20.41	21.37	22.51
8 years	25.74	24.50	24.17	27.76	31.30	26.74	26.00
High school							
1 to 3 years	14.96	15.97	15.96	9.41	12.02	11.91	11.72
4 years	15.40	14.47	12.81	12.49	9.48	10.70	8.72
College							
1 to 3 years	5.68	6.18	6.55	4.27	4.35	4.89	5.28
4 years	2.74	}6.95	{3.48	2.73	}4.84	5.45	{2.79
5 or more years	2.87		{3.01	2.08			{2.02
Total[a]	100.0	100.0	100.0	100.0	100.0	100.0	100.0

[a]Excludes father's educational attainment not reported.

variation is due entirely to intercensal variation in p_{ij}. Real causes of such variation may be subsumed under the categories of differential mortality and differential net immigration by years of school completed. Artifactual causes are intercensal variation in completeness of enumeration and in net errors in reported distributions of educational attainment. Such errors—assuming the other sources to be minor—apparently are sizable. In several instances intercensal variation in e_j covers a range large enough to include the proportion derived from OCG reports.

The conclusion is that OCG data on father's educational attainment are subject to relatively minor biases. The distributions by educational attainment could, of course, be correct despite a high incidence of compensating inaccuracies or "gross" errors in the OCG reports. The present analysis does not enable us to evaluate this possibility.

FATHER'S OCCUPATION

The procedure used for assessing the reported distributions of father's education is not applicable to the data on father's occupation. Education (years of school completed) is virtually a fixed characteristic once adulthood is attained; hence we could estimate educational attainment of fathers from data collected in the census long after those fathers had completed their schooling. Occupation, on the other hand, may change at any time in a man's life. To use census data in evaluating the OCG occupation data, therefore, requires that we find in the census information pertaining specifically to the fathers of a definite group of cohorts represented by OCG respondents.

To this end, special tabulations of OCG data on father's occupation were made for three groups of respondents whose fathers would have been reported (and classified by occupation) in the 1910 and 1940 census fertility data on children under 5 years of age (see source note to Table E.3).

TABLE E.3. FATHER'S OCC., AS REPORTED FOR SELECTED COHORTS OF CHILDREN IN CENSUS FERTILITY TABLES AT AGES 0 TO 4 AND IN OCG FOR AGE 16 (PERCENTAGE DISTRIBUTIONS)

Father's Occ.	Children Born in 1905–09 to Native White Women		Children Born in 1905–09 to Native Negro Women		Children Born in 1935–39 to Native White Women	
	1910 Census	OCG (Males)	1910 Census	OCG (Males)	1940 Census	OCG (Males)
Total[a]	100.0	100.0	100.0	100.0	100.0	100.0
Prof., tech., & kindred	3.2	3.7	1.0	4.2	5.1	7.6
Mgr., off'l, propr. exc. farm	8.6	10.8	0.8	1.9	7.5	12.8
Sales and clerical	7.5	7.0	0.7	1.6	10.5	13.0
Craftsmen, foremen, etc.	14.8	16.8	3.1	7.4	15.0	20.8
Operatives and kindred	9.2	13.1	4.1	5.8	22.4	19.8
Service workers	2.1	3.8	4.1	3.2	3.2	5.4
Laborers, exc. farm	8.6	3.8	17.5	13.5	14.3	5.3
Farmers, farm mgrs.	40.1	38.5	54.3	56.3	17.1	13.8
Farm laborers, foremen	5.9	2.5	14.4	6.1	4.9	1.5

SOURCE: Data on children under five years old are from U. S. Bureau of the Census, Population: Differential Fertility 1940 and 1910, Women by Number of Children under 5 Years Old (Washington: Government Printing Office, 1945), Tables 41, 42, 43. Data are restricted to women married once, husband present.

Data from OCG are from tabulations for white males 52 to 56 years old in 1962, mother born in the U. S.; Negro males 52 to 56 in 1962; and white males 22 to 26 in 1962, mother born in the U. S.

[a]Excludes father's occupation not reported.

The census fertility data show, for example, the number of children under 5 years of age in 1940 by father's occupation. This is to be compared with OCG reports on father's occupation made by males 22 to 26 years old in 1962. Because the census data are confined to children of mothers married once, husband present, there is a minor discrepancy between the two sets of data in coverage of fathers. Both sets are subject to sampling error and to any bias that may have been present in cases for which father's occupation was not reported.

The most serious obstacle to comparability, however, is the fact that the census data pertain to fathers of children 0 to 4 years old, but the OCG questionnaire required respondents to report father's occupation as of the respondent's age 16. Although essentially the same fathers are represented in the two sets of data, a period of some 12 to 16 years separates the two dates to which the occupation reports apply. As will be shown, this is ample time for substantial mobility of fathers to occur.

For this reason the comparisons in Table E.3 can be only roughly indicative. The pattern of discrepancies is much the same in the three comparisons.

Relative to the census distributions the OCG data show excessive proportions of white-collar workers and of craftsmen and deficits of laborers and farm laborers. In the two samples of white respondents there are deficits of farmers. In view of the sample sizes it is unlikely that these discrepancies could have arisen by sampling variation alone in the two comparisons for white respondents. The data for Negroes, however, are based on a very small sample. The OCG-census differences are, on the whole, rather larger for the 1935 to 1939 than for the 1905 to 1909 cohorts of white respondents.

How much these discrepancies should be discounted for intragenerational mobility of fathers is difficult to say. We can, however, exhibit a comparison that demonstrates substantial net mobility of fathers over a 10-year period. Table E.4 shows the distribution by father's occupation in 1950 and in 1960

TABLE E.4. PERSONS BORN BETWEEN 1945 AND 1949 BY FATHER'S OCC. IN 1950 AND 1960.

Father's Occ.	1950	1960	1960 Minus 1950
Number in millions			
Total in cohort	16.2	16.8	...
Not classified by father's occ.	3.7	3.7	...
Classified by father's occ.	12.5[a]	13.1[b]	...
Per cent distribution			
All occupations	100.0	100.0	...
Professional, technical and kindred workers	8.2	9.6	1.4
Managers, officials and proprietors, except farm	9.3	13.0	3.7
Sales, clerical and kindred workers	11.9	11.7	-0.2
Craftsmen, foremen, and kindred workers	19.7	23.6	3.9
Operatives and kindred workers	23.6	22.0	-1.6
Service workers, including private household	3.7	4.6	0.9
Laborers, except farm	8.2	6.3	-1.9
Farmers and farm managers	12.0	7.1	-4.9
Farm laborers and foremen	3.4	2.1	-1.3

[a]Children under 5 years old of women 15 to 49 years old, married once and husband present, husband in experienced civilian labor force and reporting occupation. (Source: 1950 Census of Population, Vol. IV, Part 5, Chapter C, "Fertility," Tables 48 and 49.)

[b]Persons 10 to 14 years old living with employed father (estimated as persons 10 to 13 plus one-half of persons 14 and 15 years old), excluding father's occupation not reported. (Source: 1960 Census of Population, Final Report PC(2)-5A, "School Enrollment," Table 7.)

of a cohort of children 10 to 14 years old on the latter date. There are minor disturbances of comparability between the two sets of figures which should not, however, distort unduly the estimate of net mobility. For every occupation but one (sales and clerical), the direction of net mobility, 1950 to 1960, is the same as the direction of the discrepancy between the OCG distribution in Table E.3 and the 1940 Census distribution for children born in 1935 to 1939. The latter discrepancies are, however, somewhat larger in most instances. The reasonable inference is that by no means all the difference between the OCG distribution and that taken from the 1940 Census is due to response bias in the OCG data. Although some of the difference is a result of upward mobility of fathers, some of it probably does reflect response bias.

In the nature of the case, our conclusion here cannot be as unambiguous as for the comparisons of educational attainment distributions. It is impossible to dispose of the possibility of systematic error in the OCG reports on father's occupation, operating as an over-all upward bias with respect to occupational status. Nevertheless, if we make a realistic allowance for net upward mobility of fathers between the time their sons are 0 to 4 years old and the date at which the sons reach age 16, the comparison between OCG and census distributions is seen seriously to overstate the magnitude of the bias.

APPENDIX F

Effect of Nonresponse on Correlation Results

The problem of NA bias, which was mentioned in Chapter 4, refers to respondents who returned the OCG questionnaire with one or more questions unanswered or with answers that were unclassifiable.

This question differs from either of two others: (1) the CPS respondents who failed to return an OCG questionnaire, and (2) households not responding to the CPS interview itself. As far as the second of these questions is concerned, we can only say that CPS procedures for adjusting for nonresponse exist and the problem has been studied, but "We do not know of an unbiased or even consistent method of making adjustments for nonresponse. The magnitudes of the biases resulting from the adjustment procedures used in CPS are not known."[1] As for question (1), CPS respondents who initially failed to return an OCG questionnaire were sampled, and sampling weights were so determined as to make OCG tabulations essentially unbiased *with respect to CPS estimates,* although OCG and CPS tables for the same items are not necessarily identical.

Leaving these two questions aside, we turn briefly to the problem of *item nonresponse.* Table F.1 shows the proportions of cases tabulated as reporting the item for each of the status variables, for males with nonfarm background, by age. The reader should understand a basic difference between two categories of items. The first category, including respondent's occupational status (Y), respondent's education (U), and wife's education (S), comprises the status variables ascertained within the regular CPS interview. The other category comprises the items on the supplemental OCG questionnaire: occupational status of respondent's first job (W), respondent's father's occupational status (X), father's education (V), and wife's father's occupational

---

[1] U. S. Bureau of the Census, *The Current Population Survey—A Report on Methodology,* Technical Paper No. 7 (Washington: Government Printing Office, 1963), p. 53.

TABLE F.1.   PER CENT OF RESPONDENTS REPORTING STATUS VARIABLES, BY AGE, FOR MALES WITH NONFARM BACKGROUND

Variable, or Combination of Variables[a]	Age (years)				
	20 to 24	25 to 34	35 to 44	45 to 54	55 to 64
All males, number in thousands	4,289	8,438	8,478	6,936	4,737
Per cent reporting:					
Y[b]	78.2	92.6	95.3	94.9	87.7
W	81.0	94.0	95.6	96.5	95.8
U[b]	100.0	100.0	100.0	100.0	100.0
X	91.9	89.9	88.3	87.7	85.6
V	94.6	93.0	87.8	86.3	81.8
Y and W	72.0	88.9	91.8	92.1	84.7
Y and U	78.2	92.6	95.3	94.9	87.7
Y and X	72.3	83.1	84.2	83.8	75.1
Y and V	73.4	86.1	83.4	82.0	71.7
W and U	81.0	94.0	95.6	96.5	95.8
W and X	74.0	85.3	85.3	85.7	83.5
U and X	91.9	89.9	88.3	87.7	85.6
U and V	94.6	93.0	87.8	86.3	81.8
X and V	88.4	85.4	80.7	79.2	73.3
W and V	76.2	88.4	85.0	84.1	79.2
Married males (wife present), number in thousands	1,919	6,783	7,383	5,810	3,882
Per cent reporting:					
U[b]	100.0	100.0	100.0	100.0	100.0
S[b]	100.0	100.0	100.0	100.0	100.0
Y[b]	...[c]	93.7	95.8	96.1	89.9
V	92.1	92.3	88.4	86.2	82.0
Z	90.9	90.6	89.5	89.4	90.9
Y and S	...[c]	93.7	95.8	96.1	89.9
S and Z	91.0	90.6	89.5	89.4	90.9
Y and Z	80.5	84.9	86.1	86.5	81.9
Z and X	86.1	82.8	80.8	79.8	80.2
S and U	100.0	100.0	100.0	100.0	100.0
S and V	92.1	92.3	88.4	86.2	82.0

[a] Y: 1962 occ. status.
  W: Status of first job.
  U: Education.
  X: Father's occ. status.
  V: Father's education.
  S: Wife's education.
  Z: Wife's father's occ. status.
[b] Nonresponse eliminated by computer allocation in CPS processing.
[c] Not available.

status (Z). In the CPS interview, item nonresponse is low, because the trained and closely supervised interviewer is on hand to probe for answers to all questions. In CPS data-processing procedures, moreover, all "unknown" or missing entries are allocated or assigned by a computer routine as part of the mechanical editing process. Hence there are no NA's on the CPS items as far as final tabulations are concerned. The reason why we have NA's tabulated for Y is that occupation is ascertained only for members of the experienced civilian labor force, whereas the OCG tabulations were run for the entire civilian noninstitutional population (including members of the Armed Forces living off post or on military posts in families). Members of the Armed Forces, persons unable to work, retired persons, and individuals attending school without engaging in gainful economic activity are among the categories of persons not in the experienced civilian labor force.

It would have been possible, of course, to confine the OCG tabulations to respondents in the experienced civilian labor force; but this would have reduced the sample size for tabulations of variables that do not depend on labor-force status, for example, respondent's education by father's education.

Our concern with nonresponse, therefore, reduces to the problem of NA bias as it may occur in the four OCG status variables.

The age patterns of nonresponse are no doubt significant. Reporting of W is low for young respondents. Some of them, though currently employed in part-time or temporary jobs, may not yet actually have entered a "first job" of the kind specified on the OCG questionnaire. Even among men 20 to 24 years old, however, more report a first job than are currently employed or experienced workers seeking work. (Compare Y and W.)

By contrast, nonresponse increases with age for both items concerned with the respondent's father—his occupational status (X) and his educational attainment (V). The age gradient is especially sharp for the latter. We can only conjecture as to the reasons for this contrast. If men were simply more likely to know or to remember one item of information about their fathers than another, there should be a difference in the same direction for all age groups between the proportions reporting X and V. If the age gradient were simply due to memory failure, it should be the same for the two items. The observed pattern suggests, however, differentials among cohorts of respondents in access to or retention of information on father's education relative to father's occupation. This pattern would appear if in recent decades educational attainment has gained in salience as an achieved status in comparison with occupation. In this event, young men should differ from older men more widely in their ability to report father's education than in their ability to describe his occupation.

This kind of reasoning, however, does not help to interpret the curious contrast in the nonresponse patterns, by respondent's age, for X (father's occupation) and Z (father-in-law's occupation), the latter being reported only for married men, spouse present. Although nonresponse on X increases with age of respondent, there is little variation by respondent's age in completeness of response on Z. It would appear, too, that females are better informed than males about their fathers' occupations; but this difference may only reflect the difference in population covered by the two questions.

The proportion responding to both items of a pair depends not only on the proportion responding to each of the two items but also on the correlation between response proportions. If 95.6 per cent respond on W and 88.3 per cent on X, as is the case for respondents 35 to 44 years of age

(Table F.1), the maximum proportion that could have answered both items is, of course, 88.3 per cent. The minimum percentage who must have reported both items (computed on the assumption that no one failed to report on both) is 83.9 per cent. If there were no correlation between the two items in terms of tendency to report, then the expected proportion reporting both items would be $(.883)$ $(.956) = .844$, or 84.4 per cent. According to Table F.1, 85.3 per cent of respondents actually reported both W and X. There is, therefore, some correlation between the two response proportions; yet, appreciable numbers not reporting each item did report the other.

The proportions reporting do not as such indicate how serious the NA problem is. Failure to respond does, of course, reduce the sample size. This would be a modest loss, however, providing the nonrespondents were, in effect, a random sample of the population. Actually, our concern, even here, is not so much with NA bias in means and standard deviations—although for some purposes (as in the discussion of Table E.3) such bias could be serious. We are most concerned with the question of whether the estimates of relationship between variables are seriously biased.

It must be admitted at once that there is no way to determine definitely the degree of this type of bias. Yet we can gain some appreciation of the magnitude of an allowance that might reasonably be made for it.

Let us continue with the example of response on items W and X by men 35 to 44 years old. For 85.3 per cent of these men we have reports on both items; 10.4 per cent reported W but not X, 3.1 per cent X but not W; and 1.3 per cent reported neither. Both variables were tabulated against U (respondent's education), for which response was 100 per cent, after the CPS computer allocation, which did not depend at all on either W or X. The (W, U) and (X, U) tables, therefore, may be used to form some estimate of the univariate distributions of NA's on W and X. The NA cases were distributed proportionally to the known cases *within* categories of educational attainment, and these distributions were summed to secure the estimated W-score distribution of the NA's on W and the estimated X-score distribution of the NA's on X. To these estimated or imputed distributions were added the cases that were known on the one variable but unknown on the other. For the 14.7 per cent of cases not included in the (W, X) correlation because one or both items were not reported we can now compute means and standard deviations for both items.

With respect to W, the mean and standard deviation of occupational status scores are 29.5 and 21.5 in the 85.3 per cent of cases that comprise the (W, X) correlation table; corresponding figures (based on partly known, partly imputed distributions) for the remaining 14.7 per cent are 24.7 and 19.9. Combining the known with the imputed data, the estimates for the entire population are 28.8 for the mean and 21.4 for the standard deviation of W.

Similar calculations for X give as the mean and standard deviation respectively: 33.1 and 23.0 for the cases in the (W, X) correlation table; 29.8 and 22.9 for the remaining cases; 32.6 and 23.0 for all cases.

Evidently there is a biased selection for nonresponse on both items; not surprisingly, nonrespondents have somewhat lower statuses than respondents. Yet the bias is not great enough to make the estimates of central tendency and dispersion of W and X, based on cases reporting the two variables, seriously in error.

There remains the question of NA bias in the computed correlation between the two variables. Here we can only indicate what would happen under various assumptions about the unknown correlation between W and X in the 14.7 per cent of the cases not included in the initial calculation. Let us employ this notation: r_1 is the correlation between W and X computed from the 85.3 per cent of all cases reporting both (the correlation used in all calculations in this research); r_2 is the (unknown) correlation between W and X in the remaining 14.7 per cent of the cases; and r (with no subscript) is the (unknown) correlation between W and X for all cases. Now it can be shown that $r = mr_2 + k$, where m and k are constants that can be computed from known or assumed values of r_1 together with the means and standard deviations of W and X. We know r_1 and we have offered plausible estimates of the means and standard deviations. Note that these estimates are based on 95.6 per cent of all cases for W and 88.3 per cent for X reporting the respective items, with imputations based on education being used for the remainder. Given the numerical values in the present example, we determine that $r = .137r_2 + .327$.

Obviously the implied "true" value of r will depend somewhat on what we care to assume about the unknown value of r_2. Look first at the mathematically possible extreme assumptions. If $r_2 = -1.0$, $r = .190$; if $r_2 = 1.0$, $r = .464$. (Actually, r_2 could attain precisely either of these two extreme values only if the distributions permitted. The arithmetically possible extreme is probably not far short of unity, however.) We know, virtually for certain, that the true correlation between W and X, estimated at .377 from the reporting cases, cannot be lower than .190 or higher than .464. We cannot disprove rigorously any claim that it takes on any designated value within this range. Yet, the maximum range is based on wild assumptions. There certainly is no reason to think the correlation between W and X would be likely to approach ± 1 in the cases when one or both variables were not reported. The correlation might, indeed, be different in these than in the reporting cases. Let us assume a really considerable difference. If r_1 is .377, what would happen to r if $r_2 = r_1 \pm 0.2$? If $r_2 = .177$, then $r = .351$; if $r_2 = .577$, then $r = .406$. In other words, we might write $r = .377 \pm .03$ and feel that we had allowed for every "reasonable" possibility of the effect of NA bias on our calculation of the correlation between W and X. Thus it turns out that errors in correlation coefficients owing to NA bias are perhaps of about the same order of magnitude as the sampling errors of these coefficients, given the size of the OCG sample.

It is interesting to note what happens if we assume $r_2 = r_1$. If, in the present example, we set $r_2 = r_1 = .377$, then r is not .377 but the slightly different value, .379. The slight difference is a result of discrepancies in the means and standard deviations between the reporting and the NA cases.

In the specific illustration used here—the correlation between W and X for men 35 to 44 years old—we have considered a case that is fairly typical in terms of NA proportions. The potential NA bias may be somewhat greater or somewhat less for other pairs of variables. Table F.1 makes it plain that calculations for the 20-to-24 age group are especially vulnerable, a fact already mentioned in the text. It hardly seems worthwhile to compute illustrative estimates of possible NA bias for other correlations. We must, of course, exercise special caution in interpreting such correlations as r_{YV} and r_{XV} for respondents 55 to 64 years old.

APPENDIX G

Estimated Standard Errors of Percentages in OCG Data

The accompanying table is reproduced from Bureau of the Census, "Educational Change in a Generation: March 1962," *Current Population Reports,* Series P-20, No. 132 (September 22, 1964), Table G. The table is provided for OCG data on occupation and education; different estimates might be required for other items. The table is constructed in such a way that the relevant base for percentages is not the actual sample size but rather the inflated figure representing estimated number in the population (in thousands).

TABLE G.1. STANDARD ERRORS OF ESTIMATED PERCENTAGES (68 CHANCES OUT OF 100)

	Base of Percentage (Estimated Population, In Thousands)								
Estimated Percentage	50	100	500	1,000	2,500	5,000	10,000	25,000	50,000
1 or 99	2.6	1.9	0.8	0.6	0.4	0.3	0.2	0.1	0.1
2 or 98	3.7	2.6	1.2	0.8	0.5	0.4	0.3	0.2	0.1
5 or 95	5.8	4.1	1.8	1.3	0.8	0.6	0.4	0.3	0.2
10 or 90	7.9	5.6	2.5	1.8	1.1	0.8	0.6	0.4	0.3
15 or 85	9.5	6.7	3.0	2.1	1.3	0.9	0.7	0.4	0.3
20 or 80	10.6	7.5	3.3	2.4	1.5	1.1	0.7	0.5	0.3
25 or 75	11.5	8.1	3.6	2.6	1.6	1.1	0.8	0.5	0.4
35 or 65	12.6	8.9	4.0	2.8	1.8	1.3	0.9	0.6	0.4
50	13.2	9.4	4.2	3.0	1.9	1.3	0.9	0.6	0.4

The table is to be used after the fashion of the following example: An estimated 1,714,000 men 25 to 64 years of age in March 1962 had fathers who were professional, technical and kindred workers. Of these, 38.9 per cent were themselves currently engaged in this type of occupation in March 1962. A rough interpolation in the table suggests that the standard error is about 2.3 percentage points. In the wording suggested by the Bureau of the Census, "chances are 68 out of 100 that a complete census would have disclosed a figure between 36.6 and 41.2 per cent, and 95 chances out of 100 that the figure would have been between 34.3 and 43.5."

APPENDIX H

Summary of Results of Multiple-Classification Analysis

The accompanying tables (H.1 to H.6) show the percentages of sums of squares in the three main dependent variables of the study—occupational status in 1962 (Y), status of first job (W), and educational attainment (U)—accounted for by the several independent variables or combinations of variables studied by means of multiple-classification analysis. Problems in the interpretation of these "explained" sums of squares were illustrated in Chapter 4. In presenting this summary of our calculations we must warn the reader that their meaning is not always self-evident. Results are shown for some combinations for which we cannot necessarily offer a cogent interpretation. The reason is that the calculations were partly exploratory. More-over, a number of results were obtained as a by-product of calculations that were of direct interest. These are shown for whatever interest they may hold, but with no implication that we regard them as affording an adequate basis for conclusions going beyond those stated in the text.

The description of the dependent variables has been given in the text of Chapter 4 and elsewhere. Here we supply the details of the categories involved in the several independent variables. The accompanying frequencies are the U. S. population estimates (in thousands) for the male population 20 to 64 years of age covered in the OCG survey, a total of 44,984,000. Sample frequencies can be estimated by dividing the population estimates by 2.17.

A: *Size of place* (1960 classification of residence in March 1962)

1. Urbanized area of 1,000,000 or more, central city of a
   standard metropolitan statistical area   7,143
2. Urbanized area 1,000,000 or more, not in central city   6,361
3. Urbanized area 250,000 to 999,999, central city of a
   standard metropolitan statistical area   3,903

4. Urbanized area 250,000 to 999,999, not in central city	2,483
5. Urbanized area 50,000 to 249,999, central city of a standard metropolitan statistical area	2,954
6. Urbanized area 50,000 to 249,999, not in central city	1,937
7. Other urban place 2,500 to 49,999, not in urbanized area	6,736
8. Rural nonfarm	9,849
9. Rural farm	3,618

(Note: For several reasons, CPS field procedures do not yield populations by residence strictly comparable to decennial census data; the foregoing figures are not approved by the Bureau of the Census as population estimates by size of place, but are shown to indicate the relative magnitude of size categories in this survey.)

B: Ethnic-migration (color, nativity, parentage, region of birth, and 1962 residence in region of birth or other region)

Native white, native parentage, including state of birth and/or parentage not reported

Born in North or West, or state of birth not reported

1. Living in region of birth, including state of birth not reported	16,513
2. Living in other region	3,759

Born in South

3. Living in South	7,831
4. Living in North or West	2,101

Native white, foreign or mixed parentage

Parent(s) born in Northern or Western Europe or Canada

5. Living in region of birth, including state of birth not reported	2,419
6. Living in other region	574

Parent(s) born elsewhere

7. Living in region of birth, including state of birth not reported	3,797
8. Living in other region	895
9. Foreign-born white	2,515

Nonwhite

Born in South, including state of birth not reported

10. Living in South	2,155
11. Living in North or West	1,672

Born in North or West

12. Living in region of birth	665
13. Living in other region	87

(Note: If both parents foreign-born, classified by country of birth of father.)

C: Family type (with whom respondent was living most of the time up to age 16)

1. Both parents	37,087
2. Father was head of family, mother absent	1,617

3. Mother was head of family, father absent   4,019
4. Other male was head of family   1,403
5. Other female was head of family   530
6. No response   326

D: *Geographic mobility* (type of community where respondent lived at age 16 by 1960 classification of residence in 1962)

Same community at age 16 as in 1962

1. 1962 residence in urbanized area (50,000 or more)   10,224
2. 1962 residence in other urban place (2,500 to 49,999, not in urbanized area)   2,817
3. 1962 residence in rural territory   6,422

Different community at age 16 from residence in 1962

4. Large city or suburb of large city at age 16, urbanized area in 1962   5,567
5. Large city or suburb of large city at age 16, other urban place in 1962   677
6. Middle-sized city or town at age 16, urbanized area in 1962   4,718
7. Middle-sized city or town at age 16, other urban place in 1962   1,649
8. Urban at age 16 (large city, suburb of large city, middle-sized city, or town), rural in 1962   3,224

Rural at age 16 (open country, not on a farm; or farm)

9. Urbanized area in 1962   3,809
10. Other urban in 1962   1,527
11. Rural nonfarm in 1962   2,622
12. Rural farm in 1962   1,013
13. Residence at age 16 not reported   714

(Note: In Chapter 7 an expanded version of this classification is used; it was obtained by subdividing categories 3, 9, 10, and 11 by farm versus nonfarm background of respondent, on the basis of father's occupation—see Appendix I. Sums of squares reported for variable *D,* therefore, are not comparable with those for the expanded geographic mobility classification in Chapter 7.)

E: *Sibling pattern* (number of siblings and sibling position)

1. Only child (no brothers or sisters)   2,921
2. Oldest child, one to three younger siblings   7,073
3. Oldest child, four or more younger siblings (except ten)   3,038
4. Youngest child, one to three older siblings   6,229
5. Youngest child, four or more older siblings (except ten)   3,191

Middle child, two or three siblings, at least one older and one younger

6. No older brother   2,252
7. At least one older brother   3,081

Middle child, four or more siblings (except 10), at least
one older and one younger

8.	No older brother	2,668
9.	At least one older brother	12,638
10.	Exactly ten siblings, or number of siblings not reported	1,894

(Note: Respondents with exactly ten siblings comprise a large majority of category 10; they were inadvertently tabulated with nonrespondents.)

F: Region-color (residence in 1962 by color)

1.	Northeast, white	10,348
2.	Northeast, nonwhite	779
3.	North Central, white	11,943
4.	North Central, nonwhite	955
5.	South, white	10,264
6.	South, nonwhite	2,176
7.	West, white	7,850
8.	West, nonwhite	670

G: Marital status (as of 1962)

1.	Married, spouse present, previously married	4,499
2.	Married, spouse present, not previously married	31,075
3.	Widowed	558
4.	Divorced	1,027
5.	Married, spouse absent (includes separated)	1,085
6.	Never married (single)	6,739

P: Ethnic-education (color and nativity by years of school completed)

Native white, native parentage, including birthplace or parentage not reported

1.	0 to eight years	7,286
2.	High school, one to three years	5,420
3.	High school, four years	8,855
4.	College, one or more years	7,534

Native white, foreign or mixed parentage

5.	0 to eight years	2,316
6.	High school, one to three years	1,702
7.	High school, four years	2,587
8.	College, one or more years	2,190

Foreign-born white

9.	0 to eight years	1,064
10.	High school, one to three years	324
11.	High school, four years	519
12.	College, one or more years	607

Nonwhite

13.	0 to eight years	2,243
14.	High school, one to three years	1,032
15.	High school, four years	827
16.	College, one or more years	477

Q: Brother's education (number of siblings by years of school completed by oldest brother)

1.	No siblings	2,921

One to three siblings

2.	No older brother	12,005
3.	0 to seven school years completed by oldest brother	644
4.	Eight years	817
5.	High school, one to three years	1,055
6.	High school, four years	1,934
7.	College, one to three years	839
8.	College, four years or more	1,180

Four or more siblings (except 10)

9.	No older brother	6,701
10.	0 to seven years	3,192
11.	Eight years	3,548
12.	High school, one to three years	2,731
13.	High school, four years	2,942
14.	College, one to three years	740
15.	College, four years or more	910
16.	Exactly 10 siblings, or number of siblings not reported, or brother's education not reported	2,824

(Note: See note for variable *E*.)

S: Wife's education (years of school completed)

0.	No school	192
1.	One to four years	732
2.	Five to seven years	2,484
3.	Eight years	4,311
4.	High school, one to three years	7,393
5.	High school, four years	14,199
6.	College, one to three years	3,769
7.	College, four years	1,984
8.	College, five years or more	512
9.	Not applicable (all respondents except married, spouse present)	9,409

(Note: Code numbers, except 9, were used as scores in regression and correlation analyses; all categories used in multiple-classification analyses.)

U: *Education* (years of school completed by respondent)

0.	No school	562
1.	One to four years	1,901
2.	Five to seven years	4,317
3.	Eight years	6,128
4.	High school, one to three years	8,478
5.	High school, four years	12,788
6.	College, one to three years	5,277
7.	College, four years	3,256
8.	College, five years or more	2,276

(Note: Code numbers were used as scores in regression and correlation analyses and in treating U as a dependent variable in multiple-classification analysis.)

V: *Father's education* (years of school completed)

0.	No school	2,702
1.	One to four years	4,803
2.	Five to seven years	8,030
3.	Eight years	10,604
4.	High school, one to three years	4,372
5.	High school, four years	5,486
6.	College, one to three years	1,820
7.	College, four years	1,206
8.	College, five years or more	862
9.	Not reported	5,098

(Note: Code numbers were used as scores in regression and correlation analysis, omitting category 9; all categories were used in multiple-classification analysis.)

Y: Occupational Status in 1962
W: Occupational Status of First Job
X: Father's Occupational Status
Z: Wife's Father's Occupational Status

Score interval	Frequency distribution for—			
	Y	W	X	Z
90 and over	580	381	424	317
85-89	473	98	193	209
80-84	1,446	652	500	436
75-79	1,580	412	756	604
70-74	1,319	848	661	489
65-69	2,024	927	855	599
60-64	2,001	795	1,376	1,139
55-59	589	107	775	533
50-54	2,368	1,263	1,737	1,495
45-49	1,528	776	1,106	850
40-44	3,134	3,419	1,973	1,424
35-39	1,709	2,574	1,495	1,211
30-34	2,430	1,926	2,557	1,926
25-29	1,811	1,766	1,087	929
20-24	2,712	2,663	2,095	1,767
15-19	7,031	9,249	6,033	5,145
10-14	3,783	4,087	12,421	9,097
5-9	3,630	8,123	3,313	2,529
0-4	926	2,333	1,901	1,560
NA	3,908	2,585	3,727	12,724

(Note: For Y, NA means not in experienced civilian labor force; for W and X, NA means not reported; for Z, NA means not applicable—respondent is not married, spouse present—or not reported. In correlation and regression analysis, or as dependent variables in multiple classification, the categories were represented by the midpoints, 2, 7, 12, . . . , 87, 92. The NA category was omitted in correlation and regression calculations and scored at the mean in multiple-classification calculations.)

TABLE H.1.   PER CENT OF TOTAL SUM OF SQUARES IN 1962 OCC. STATUS (Y) ACCOUNTED FOR BY DESIGNATED VARIABLES AND COMBINATIONS OF VARIABLES IN MULTIPLE-CLASSIFICATION ANALYSIS, FOR MEN 20 TO 64 YEARS OLD, BY FARM BACKGROUND (SEE TEXT FOR IDENTIFICATION OF VARIABLES)

Variables	Background			Variables	Background		
	All	Nonfarm	Farm		All	Nonfarm	Farm
A: Size of place	7.31	2.96	9.18	B,W,U	42.26	41.85	29.90
B: Ethnic-migration	6.70	6.00	5.80	B,U,X	39.16	38.35	...
C: Family type	0.69	1.54	0.11	B,U,V	37.71	37.41	26.75
D: Geographic				B,X,V	19.94	17.60	...
mobility	9.30	5.13	8.07	B,U	37.44	37.15	26.16
E: Sibling pattern	5.35	4.62	1.13	B,W	30.41	29.11	20.39
F: Region-color	5.96	5.25	4.77	B,X	18.30	15.90	...
G: Marital status	1.25	1.28	1.37	B,V	13.73	12.51	8.59
P: Ethnic-education	32.55	32.10	21.35	C,W,U,X,V	42.09	41.36	28.25[a]
Q: Brother's				C,W,U,X	41.98	41.26	...
education	10.94	9.64	5.17	C,U,X,V	37.79	36.84	24.07[a]
S: Wife's education	16.28	16.23	10.31	C,W,U	41.00	40.48	28.04
U: Education	35.48	34.91	23.99	C,U,X	37.65	36.68	...
V: Father's				C,X,V	17.26	15.07	...
education	9.26	8.41	3.95	C,W	27.77	27.03	17.03
W: First job status	27.40	26.25	17.09	C,U	35.59	35.25	23.82
X: Father's occ.				C,X	15.31	13.19	...
status	15.05	12.83	...	C,V	9.71	9.47	3.94
Z: Wife's father's				D,W,U,X,V	43.09	41.76	32.30[a]
occ.	9.35	8.20	...	D,W,U,X	42.95	41.67	...
A,W,U,X,V	43.51	41.88	32.93[a]	D,U,X,V	39.19	37.54	29.02[a]
A,W,U,X	43.38	41.78	...	D,W,U	42.17	40.79	32.11
A,U,X,V	39.55	37.51	29.89[a]	D,U,X	39.01	37.39	...
A,W,U	42.68	40.91	32.88	D,X,V	20.41	17.25	...
A,U,X	39.40	37.34	...	D,X,W	33.31	31.35	...
A,X,V	20.19	16.42	...	D,U	37.67	35.99	28.86
A,W,X	33.62	31.26	...	D,W	30.34	27.95	22.11
A,U	37.99	35.83	22.92	D,X	18.67	15.66	...
A,W	30.55	27.71	22.62	D,V	15.58	11.94	11.59
A,X	18.30	14.63	...	E,W,U,X,V	42.08	41.37	28.44[a]
A,V	14.71	10.62	12.62	E,W,U,X	41.95	41.27	...
B,W,U,X,V	43.22	42.57	30.17[a]	E,U,X,V	37.79	36.91	...
B,W,U,X	43.09	42.49	...	E,W,U	40.98	40.43	28.47
B,U,X,V	39.26	38.49	...	E,U,X	37.65	36.72	...
B,X,W	33.55	32.00	...	E,X,V	18.18	16.13	...

	Background				Background		
Variables	All	Nonfarm	Farm	Variables	All	Nonfarm	Farm
E,X,W	32.14	30.99	...	W,U,X,V	42.04	41.25	28.22[a]
E,U,V	35.97	35.54	24.29	W,U,X	41.93	41.14	...
E,U	35.70	35.23	24.16	U,X,V	37.71	36.75	24.05[a]
E,W	28.74	27.69	17.30	W,U	40.93	40.26	28.13
E,X	16.72	14.80	...	W,X	31.57	30.16	...
E,V	11.63	10.58	4.47	U,X	37.59	36.54	...
F,W,U,X,V	43.10	42.42	29.70[a]	X,V	17.03	14.71	...
F,W,U,X	43.01	42.34	...	Z,X	19.66	17.38	...
F,U,X,V	39.08	38.20	25.84[a]	A,B,W,U,X	44.59	43.03	...
F,W,U	42.19	41.72	29.49	A,B,W,U	44.08	42.42	34.97
F,U,X	38.95	38.07	...	A,B,W,X	35.45	32.88	...
F,X,V	19.51	17.06	...	A,B,U,X	41.00	39.00	...
F,W	30.05	28.85	20.01	A,B,W	33.18	30.20	26.18
F,U	37.26	36.92	25.60	A,B,U	39.93	37.89	32.41
F,X	17.93	15.43	...	A,B,X	21.35	17.38	14.67[a]
F,V	13.17	12.04	7.69	A,P,W,X	42.62	41.03	32.29[a]
G,W,U,X,V	43.03	42.27	29.09[a]	A,P,X	36.61	34.40	28.24[a]
G,W,U,X	42.95	42.19	...	B,D,E,W,U,X	44.29	43.07	...
G,W,X	32.59	31.20	17.87[a]	B,D,E,W,U	43.77	42.54	34.57
G,W,U	41.95	41.29	28.88	B,D,E,U,X	40.77	39.28	...
G,X,V	18.44	16.06	...	B,D,E,W,X	35.78	33.75	26.23[a]
G,U	36.70	36.16	24.91	B,D,E,U	39.88	38.34	31.81
G,X	16.34	14.03	...	B,D,E,X	23.06	19.96	14.93[a]
G,V	10.72	9.94	5.23	B,E,U,X,V	39.32	38.64	26.98[a]
P,W,X	41.09	40.47	...	B,E,X,V	20.97	18.93	...
P,W	40.18	39.76	27.07	B,E,V	15.72	14.45	9.04
P,X	34.42	33.70	...	B,C,E,U,X	39.28	38.59	26.53[a]
Q,U,X,V	37.97	37.10	24.48[a]	D,E,U,X	39.07	37.53	29.05[a]
Q,X,V	20.03	17.81	...	F,Q,U,X,V	39.32	38.59	26.32[a]
Q,X	19.20	16.98	...	F,Q,X,V	22.14	19.93	...
Q,V	14.61	13.31	7.02	F,Q,X	21.45	19.22	8.68[a]
S,U,V	37.67	37.33	25.42	F,Q,V	17.73	16.37	10.26
S,V	20.27	19.83	11.79				

[a]Independent variables do not include X.

TABLE H.2.   PER CENT OF TOTAL SUM OF SQUARES IN STATUS OF FIRST JOB (W)
ACCOUNTED FOR BY DESIGNATED VARIABLES AND COMBINATIONS OF VARIABLES IN
MULTIPLE-CLASSIFICATION ANALYSIS, FOR MEN 20 TO 64 YEARS OLD, BY FARM
BACKGROUND (SEE TEXT FOR IDENTIFICATION OF VARIABLES)

| Variables | Background | | | Variables | Background | | |
	All	Nonfarm	Farm		All	Nonfarm	Farm
A: Size of place	4.23	1.98	2.13	D, U	34.84	32.45	25.87
B: Ethnic-migration	3.60	2.91	2.03	D, X	18.41	15.64	...
C: Family type	0.34	0.79	0.18	D, V	15.81	12.94	5.59
D: Geographic				E, U, X, V	36.33	34.22	25.42[a]
mobility	8.36	4.74	2.33	E, U, X	36.05	33.82	...
E: Sibling pattern	5.69	4.53	1.97	E, X, V	19.56	16.99	4.83[a]
F: Region-color	3.03	2.30	1.76	E, U	33.25	31.58	25.59
G: Marital status	0.35	0.35	0.49	E, X	17.73	15.06	...
P: Ethnic-education	27.29	25.34	20.37	F, U, X, V	36.52	34.36	26.25[a]
U: Education	32.73	31.18	25.14	F, U, X	36.21	33.96	...
V: Father's education	10.75	9.89	3.58	F, X, V	19.14	16.41	...
X: Father's occ.	16.00	13.21	...	F, U	33.36	31.71	26.01
status				F, X	16.92	14.03	...
A, U, X, V	36.68	34.50	25.87[a]	F, V	12.43	11.18	5.03
A, U, X	36.37	34.09	...	G, X, V	18.53	15.86	...
A, X, V	19.45	16.67	...	G, U	32.77	31.19	25.38
A, U	33.79	31.77	26.07	G, X	16.16	13.38	...
A, X	17.15	14.26	...	G, V	10.96	10.07	3.96
A, V	13.42	11.20	5.41	P, X	30.79	28.21	...
B, U, X, V	36.67	34.61	26.27[a]	U, X	35.86	33.61	...
B, U, X	36.34	34.17	...	A, B, U, X	36.86	34.58	...
B, X, V	19.55	16.96	...	A, B, U	34.49	32.47	26.70
B, X	17.18	14.40	...	A, B, X	18.30	15.30	4.02[a]
B, U	33.44	31.90	25.84	A, P, X	31.28	28.65	21.06[a]
B, V	12.88	11.65	5.04	B, D, E, U, X	37.40	35.16	...
C, U, X, V	36.22	34.14	25.28[a]	B, D, E, U	35.73	33.37	26.89
C, U, X	35.89	33.71	...	B, D, E, X	20.79	18.00	6.20[a]
C, X, V	18.49	15.94	...	D, E, U, X	36.95	34.70	26.07[a]
C, U	32.80	31.34	25.07				
C, X	16.10	13.40	...				
C, V	10.98	10.45	3.67				
D, U, X, V	37.13	34.92	25.99[a]				
D, U, X	36.80	34.54	...				
D, X, V	20.50	17.80	...				

[a]Independent variables exclude X.

TABLE H.3.   PER CENT OF TOTAL SUM OF SQUARES IN EDUCATIONAL ATTAINMENT (U) ACCOUNTED FOR BY DESIGNATED VARIABLES AND COMBINATIONS OF VARIABLES IN MULTIPLE-CLASSIFICATION ANALYSIS, FOR MEN 20 TO 64 YEARS OLD, BY FARM BACKGROUND (SEE TEXT FOR IDENTIFICATION OF VARIABLES)

Variables	Background			Variables	Background		
	All	Nonfarm	Farm		All	Nonfarm	Farm
A: Size of place	4.96	2.44	2.20	D, V	25.69	22.33	17.97
B: Ethnic-migration	9.42	6.31	12.03	E, X, V	30.71	27.98	...
C: Family type	1.11	1.94	1.31	E, X	24.42	22.71	...
D: Geographic				E, V	25.24	22.82	19.53
mobility	9.46	5.97	2.15	F, X, V	30.21	26.50	...
E: Sibling pattern	10.78	9.09	6.03	F, X	23.34	20.23	...
F: Region-color	7.37	4.68	9.30	F, V	24.31	21.16	21.60
G: Marital status	1.37	1.26	1.71	G, X, V	28.62	25.76	...
Q: Brother's				G, X	20.74	18.99	...
education	23.89	19.95	21.23	G, V	21.54	19.67	17.62
S: Wife's education	29.81	27.90	29.65	Q, X, V	36.28	32.37	...
V: Father's education	20.77	18.95	16.55	Q, X	32.55	28.89	...
X: Father's occ.				Q, V	32.20	28.60	28.19
status	19.86	18.17	...	S, V	38.85	36.40	36.25
A, X, V	29.07	26.22	...	X, V	27.94	25.14	...
A, X	21.11	19.39	...	A, B, X	25.36	21.82	13.65[a]
A, V	23.58	20.47	17.94	B, C, E, X	28.45	25.19	17.07[a]
B, X, V	31.08	27.29	...	B, D, E, X	29.85	26.89	18.34[a]
B, X	24.24	20.86	...	B, E, X, V	33.61	29.99	...
B, V	25.62	22.07	22.96	B, E, V	29.42	25.60	25.59
C, X, V	28.22	25.39	...	F, Q, X, V	37.54	33.26	...
C, X	20.24	18.49	...	F, Q, X	34.19	30.05	25.77[a]
C, V	21.33	20.07	17.05	F, Q, V	34.26	29.95	31.62
D, X, V	29.95	27.48	...				
D, X	22.37	21.18	...				

[a]Independent variables exclude X.

TABLE H.4.   PER CENT OF TOTAL SUM OF SQUARES IN 1962 OCC. STATUS (Y) ACCOUNTED FOR BY DESIGNATED VARIABLES AND COMBINATIONS OF VARIABLES IN MULTIPLE-CLASSIFICATION ANALYSIS, FOR MEN 20 TO 64 YEARS OLD WITH NONFARM BACKGROUND, BY AGE (SEE TEXT FOR IDENTIFICATION OF VARIABLES)

Variables	Age (years)				
	20-24	25-34	35-44	45-54	55-64
A: Size of place	2.62	3.24	2.18	3.76	2.69
B: Ethnic-migration	7.24	7.18	5.98	6.32	5.82
C: Family type	2.17	1.40	1.84	1.61	1.72
D: Geographic mobility	3.67	7.16	4.77	5.52	3.45
E: Sibling pattern	6.16	5.10	6.70	3.42	4.95
P: Ethnic-education	19.30	40.06	40.36	33.57	28.84
U: Education	21.11	43.39	42.21	34.66	29.88
V: Father's education	6.56	12.04	12.10	8.15	8.43
W: First job status	27.88	32.64	23.75	26.15	24.40
X: Father's occ. status	7.86	13.19	16.56	15.66	11.86
Z: Wife's father's occ.	2.38	8.31	10.11	9.34	8.75
B, D, E, U, X	27.45	47.14	46.76	40.64	35.11
B, C, E, U, X	26.52	46.79	46.44	39.66	34.36
A, B, U, X	25.90	47.09	46.12	40.30	34.31
A, X	9.47	15.08	18.42	18.38	13.86
C, X	8.54	13.81	17.00	16.21	12.40
D, X	10.08	17.30	19.11	19.06	14.12
E, X	11.30	15.20	19.66	17.02	14.70
P, X	20.44	41.05	42.44	36.32	31.23

TABLE H.5.   PER CENT OF TOTAL SUM OF SQUARES IN STATUS OF FIRST JOB (W)
ACCOUNTED FOR BY DESIGNATED VARIABLES AND COMBINATIONS OF VARIABLES IN
MULTIPLE-CLASSIFICATION ANALYSIS, FOR MEN 20 TO 64 YEARS OLD WITH NONFARM
BACKGROUND, BY AGE (SEE TEXT FOR IDENTIFICATION OF VARIABLES)

Variables	Age (Years)				
	20–24	25–34	35–44	45–54	55–64
A: Size of place	4.27	2.41	2.02	2.23	2.30
B: Ethnic-migration	3.38	3.48	2.99	3.58	4.06
D: Geographic mobility	5.23	5.92	4.56	5.00	5.89
E: Sibling pattern	4.67	6.38	5.00	3.73	3.25
U: Education	19.35	35.61	31.55	32.95	32.16
X: Father's occ. status	10.32	14.26	13.62	15.89	15.76
B,D,E,U,X	25.58	40.16	35.51	38.89	39.43
A,B,U,X	24.47	39.73	34.66	38.97	37.97
E,X	12.60	17.17	15.85	15.99	17.15
D,X	13.25	17.41	16.20	17.49	19.35
A,X	13.05	15.65	14.80	15.71	17.50

TABLE H.6.   PER CENT OF TOTAL SUM OF SQUARES IN EDUCATIONAL ATTAINMENT
(U) ACCOUNTED FOR BY DESIGNATED VARIABLES AND COMBINATIONS OF VARIABLES
IN MULTIPLE-CLASSIFICATION ANALYSIS, FOR MEN 20 TO 64 YEARS OLD WITH NONFARM
BACKGROUND, BY AGE (SEE TEXT FOR IDENTIFICATION OF VARIABLES)

Variables	Age (Years)				
	20–24	25–34	35–44	45–54	55–64
A: Size of place	5.28	3.03	3.82	2.61	2.05
B: Ethnic-migration	9.83	6.50	7.23	6.70	9.05
C: Family type	5.01	1.34	2.37	2.27	2.52
D: Geographic mobility	6.56	9.08	6.80	7.68	6.15
E: Sibling pattern	12.84	24.93	8.62	6.52	7.23
Q: Brother's education	22.70	19.44	18.55	17.66	17.34
S: Wife's education	15.68	25.77	28.11	29.17	37.61
V: Father's education	22.29	19.57	18.51	15.87	15.55
X: Father's occ. status	20.17	18.39	19.35	20.08	17.77
D,X	23.04	18.04	23.08	24.47	21.10
A,X	22.70	14.24	21.65	21.60	19.06
C,X	21.56	13.23	19.97	20.57	18.41
E,X	26.01	16.89	22.54	23.20	21.70

APPENDIX I

Migration Classification

Some explanation of the classification of migration status and size of place of origin and destination, which defines the main independent variable in Chapter 7, is presented here, together with comments about the potential errors to which it is subject.

Migration status is inferred from the respondent's answer to the question, "Where were you living when you were 16 years old?" Those choosing the first alternative, "The same community (city, town, or rural area) as at the present time," are identified as nonmigrants.[1] All others are migrants, and they were further asked to describe the community of their residence at age 16 as:

1. A large city (100,000 population or more)
2. A suburb near a large city
3. A middle-sized city or small town (under 100,000 population) but not in a suburb of a large city
4. Open country (but not on a farm)
5. On a farm

In the tabulations categories 1 and 2 were combined into a single class, "large city." For the sake of conformity with a number of other tabulations, farm residence at age 16 as reported by the respondent was discarded in favor of classification by "farm background," that is, whether the father had a farm occupation or not.

Once a respondent is defined as a migrant, his classification by type of

[1] The identification of the size of community at age 16 by its size in 1962 for nonmigrants poses a problem of growing place size. A city of over 50,000 inhabitants in 1962 was not necessarily a community of over 50,000 ten, twenty, or forty years ago, when the respondent was 16 years old. In comparing "large city" nonmigrants in cities that have grown to large-city status recently to migrants who have moved from one large city to another—a procedure designed to distinguish the effects of origin and destination community size and migrant status—some small error is doubtlessly involved.

491

migration depends on the comparison between his identification of the type of community where he lived at age 16 and the classification of his 1962 residence according to the standard residential categories of the Bureau of the Census. There is, therefore, no element of self-identification in the classification of residence at age 16 for nonmigrants (with the exception of the use of reported father's occupation to identify rural farm origin), whereas there is for migrants.

Categories of 1962 place of residence are not precisely comparable to place at age 16. "Large city" here refers to the "urbanized areas" of the census. These are all places with 50,000 or more inhabitants in 1960 plus the surrounding incorporated places and unincorporated territory settled to a typically urban level of population density. Given the addition of this surrounding suburban and urban fringe area to the core city with its minimum of 50,000 inhabitants, the aggregate population of an urbanized area is unlikely to be much less than 100,000. Although there were 201 individual urban places of 50,000 to 100,000 inhabitants in 1960, only 60 of these were in urbanized areas of less than 100,000 population. (The remaining 141 places were either suburbs of still larger places, or else the urbanized areas of which they were the core included an aggregate of 100,000 persons or more.) Altogether these 60 smaller urbanized areas contained less than 5 per cent of the total population residing in urbanized areas in 1960. Hence the "large city" category for 1962 residence is reasonably comparable to the "large city" plus "suburb near a large city" responses to the question on residence at age 16.

The second largest category for 1962 residence is "small city," equivalent to the census class of urban places other than those included above, that is, places 2,500 to 49,999 inhabitants in 1960. This is a slightly narrower class than the respondent's alternative (3) for place at age 16, which might include places of 50,000 to 100,000 or places under 2,500. Census residential categories discriminate rural nonfarm and rural farm places for 1962 residence.

These four roughly comparable categories of residence for age 16 and 1962, "large city," "small city," "rural nonfarm," and "farm," were employed to classify both migrants within community type and migrants between types of communities. To make these procedures explicit, the following table defines the categories used in Chapter 7 in terms of the self-identification used in the questionnaire (for residence at age 16) and 1962 residence as classified by the Bureau of the Census.

Short Title	Residence at 16	Census Categories 1962 Residence
Nonmigrant		
Large city	"same community"	Urbanized area (50,000+)
Small city	"same community"	Other urban place (2,500-50,000)
Rural nonfarm	"same community" father in nonfarm occupation	Rural
Rural farm	"same community" father in farm occupation	Rural
Migrant within type		
Large city	"large city" (100,000+) or "suburb of a large city"	Urbanized area (50,000+)
Small city	"middle-sized city or small town" (under 100,000)	Other urban place (2,500-50,000)
Rural nonfarm	"open country" or "farm," father in nonfarm occupation	Rural nonfarm
Rural farm	"open country" or "farm," father in farm occupation	Rural farm
Migrant between type		
Large to small city	"large city" (100,000+) or "suburb of a large city"	Other urban place (2,500-50,000)
Small to large city	"middle-sized city or small town" (under 100,000)	Urbanized area (50,000+)
Urban to rural	(all in preceding 2 categories)	Rural
Rural nonfarm to large city	"open country" or "farm," father in nonfarm occupation	Urbanized area (50,000+)
Rural nonfarm to small city	(as above)	Other urban place (2,500-50,000)
Rural farm to large city	"open country" or "farm," father in farm occupation	Urbanized area (50,000+)
Rural farm to small city	(as above)	Other urban place (2,500-50,000)
Rural nonfarm to rural farm	"open country" or "farm," father in nonfarm occupation	Rural farm
Rural farm to rural nonfarm	"open country" or "farm," father in farm occupation	Rural nonfarm

APPENDIX J

Additional Tables

TABLE J2.1. MOBILITY FROM FATHER'S OCC. TO 1962 OCC., FOR MALES 25 TO 64 YEARS OLD IN THE CIVILIAN NON-INSTITUTIONAL POPULATION OF THE UNITED STATES, MARCH 1962 (FREQUENCIES IN THOUSANDS)

Father's Occ.	1	2	3	4	5	6	7	8	9	10	11	12	13	14	15	16	17	No Answer	Total
Professionals																			
1 Self empl.	83	158	49	47	22	20	7	10	9	11	13	8	9	2	11	10	4	23	496
2 Salaried	40	388	157	72	58	93	21	46	54	12	84	63	41	12	7	10	2	58	1218
3 Managers	50	320	275	88	111	108	16	77	75	44	57	36	21	15	12	7	2	100	1414
4 Salesmen, other	32	137	165	101	72	41	27	22	42	15	20	29	13	...	6	8	2	46	778
5 Proprietors	106	390	522	165	455	175	94	100	148	112	146	102	80	14	35	32	11	155	2842
6 Clerical	28	295	141	74	64	111	16	83	89	23	48	58	70	13	22	16	...	106	1257
7 Salesmen, retail	5	92	95	59	77	43	18	39	23	21	59	34	31	1	21	15	...	39	672
Craftsmen																			
8 Manufacturing	22	337	193	54	141	139	39	346	145	99	246	141	105	38	55	10	3	148	2261
9 Other	23	286	236	99	167	195	38	200	313	114	211	236	118	32	71	24	8	199	2570
10 Construction	17	130	138	51	161	153	16	200	158	268	145	119	100	22	84	16	12	142	1932
Operatives																			
11 Manufacturing	30	262	161	82	171	183	44	371	221	96	545	210	156	123	107	24	19	235	3040
12 Other	16	304	134	67	174	165	37	186	246	130	273	330	155	55	110	25	30	198	2635
13 Service	13	151	128	60	103	154	33	138	110	93	201	139	180	46	56	17	4	94	1720
Laborers																			
14 Manufacturing	...	42	37	5	23	31	5	75	42	20	127	66	66	50	41	12	6	55	703
15 Other	6	82	59	41	58	146	29	129	137	95	212	177	135	57	165	15	19	111	1673
16 Farmers	64	439	421	126	677	447	109	580	696	595	1056	890	499	251	557	1696	405	826	10334
17 Farm laborers	2	20	30	6	42	37	13	67	69	61	137	113	78	33	96	60	98	84	1046
No answer	36	232	231	55	210	208	57	212	276	150	394	273	327	87	255	72	53	250	3378
Total	573	4065	3172	1252	2786	2449	619	2881	2853	1959	3974	3024	2184	851	1711	2069	678	2869	39969

TABLE J2.2. MOBILITY FROM FATHER'S OCC. TO FIRST JOB, FOR MALES 25 TO 64 YEARS OLD IN THE CIVILIAN NON-INSTITUTIONAL POPULATION OF THE UNITED STATES, MARCH 1962 (FREQUENCIES IN THOUSANDS)

Father's Occ.	First Job																		No Answer	Total
	1	2	3	4	5	6	7	8	9	10	11	12	13	14	15	16	17		
1 Professionals, Self emp.	52	137	11	22	4	89	22	13	16	...	23	33	10	5	14	6	8	31	496
2 Salaried	15	359	45	26	...	150	73	47	57	19	118	92	41	38	65	6	24	43	1218
3 Managers	27	257	40	50	12	294	83	41	62	24	142	163	25	35	95	7	16	41	1414
4 Salesmen, other	20	132	20	89	8	134	69	11	22	11	70	74	14	9	29	...	18	48	778
5 Proprietors	55	397	111	144	126	355	313	104	109	70	287	268	97	69	169	8	62	98	2842
6 Clerical	5	226	29	21	2	275	54	35	72	12	166	118	39	60	72	9	16	46	1257
7 Salesmen, retail	10	67	17	14	12	130	79	22	20	1	104	54	14	26	54	5	29	14	672
8 Craftsmen, Manufacturing	2	148	19	11	2	325	117	218	82	58	573	201	100	193	109	5	40	58	2261
9 Other	13	158	9	21	8	357	154	99	260	41	386	349	93	100	280	13	111	118	2570
10 Construction	2	110	16	11	...	241	107	80	100	201	329	213	116	60	177	21	111	37	1932
11 Operatives, Manufacturing	8	124	11	29	2	337	120	126	79	51	1091	233	155	261	184	7	92	130	3040
12 Other	7	146	58	8	2	288	120	90	107	43	347	754	92	121	228	10	103	111	2635
13 Service	3	76	24	20	5	238	73	49	103	37	313	222	174	115	144	12	70	42	1720
14 Laborers, Manufacturing	...	27	1	...	...	37	34	8	29	8	163	64	29	156	53	2	54	38	703
15 Other	18	53	3	8	2	157	74	41	52	17	268	214	109	114	367	12	105	59	1673
16 Farmers	24	343	42	40	32	427	234	201	209	186	1006	877	224	418	780	1054	3910	327	10334
17 Farm laborers	2	7	2	2	3	25	12	6	32	10	111	73	30	58	62	16	570	25	1046
No answer	12	140	27	25	14	370	151	97	108	70	470	394	161	177	334	55	365	408	3378
Total	275	2907	485	541	234	4229	1889	1288	1519	859	5967	4396	1523	2015	3216	1248	5704	1674	39969

TABLE J2.3. MOBILITY FROM FIRST JOB TO PRESENT OCC., FOR MALES 25 TO 64 YEARS OLD IN THE CIVILIAN NON-INSTITUTIONAL POPULATION OF THE UNITED STATES, MARCH 1962 (FREQUENCIES IN THOUSANDS)

First Job	1962 Occ.																	No Answer	Total
	1	2	3	4	5	6	7	8	9	10	11	12	13	14	15	16	17		
Professionals																			
1 Self empl.	147	70	5	13	7	4	…	4	2	…	2	…	…	…	7	…	2	12	275
2 Salaried	188	1585	358	82	161	142	11	47	57	12	36	35	28	2	8	28	4	123	2907
3 Managers	6	99	173	21	44	32	11	11	20	14	10	7	6	3	6	3	2	17	485
4 Salesmen, other	3	46	136	128	67	27	15	3	18	7	29	21	15	…	…	2	…	24	541
5 Proprietors	2	16	45	15	85	6	6	4	5	1	10	10	7	2	5	9	…	6	234
6 Clerical	68	551	733	307	227	744	77	194	182	109	237	177	187	41	78	50	9	258	4229
7 Salesmen, retail	39	189	295	139	219	219	96	85	90	54	115	140	58	20	36	19	1	75	1889
Craftsmen																			
8 Manufacturing	11	112	101	32	157	53	9	290	96	55	117	45	48	10	51	29	…	72	1288
9 Other	5	136	101	29	157	63	52	166	323	71	108	83	54	21	26	18	10	96	1519
10 Construction	3	48	29	14	95	27	2	76	113	225	43	37	21	9	27	18	7	65	859
Operatives																			
11 Manufacturing	24	366	317	119	416	367	104	801	400	277	1124	456	280	189	206	122	35	364	5967
12 Other	20	221	268	130	384	189	50	321	476	305	422	661	265	61	187	81	44	311	4396
13 Service	7	108	74	21	95	76	19	52	97	95	202	117	302	38	88	6	7	119	1523
Laborers																			
14 Manufacturing	7	110	79	31	58	125	25	211	107	78	364	177	147	165	126	33	35	137	2015
15 Other	8	176	175	78	216	133	41	196	310	220	339	346	201	78	371	69	30	229	3216
16 Farmers	3	29	32	23	47	38	15	52	74	68	104	63	58	18	45	449	63	67	1248
17 Farm laborers	12	99	135	43	268	156	60	302	362	313	595	529	328	160	382	1101	398	461	5704
No answer	20	104	116	27	83	48	26	66	121	55	117	120	179	34	62	32	31	433	1674
Total	573	4065	3172	1252	2786	2449	619	2881	2853	1959	3974	3024	2184	851	1711	2069	678	2869	39969

TABLE J4.1. OBSERVED PERCENTAGE DISTRIBUTION BY INTERGENERATIONAL MOBILITY (Y-X), FOR MEN IN EACH CATEGORY OF EDUCATIONAL ATTAINMENT

| | Educational Attainment | | | | | | | | | |
| | Elementary | | | | High School | | College | | | Total |
Mobility	0	1-4	5-7	8	1-3	4	1-3	4	5+	
High upward (+26 and over)	2.1	7.7	10.0	15.9	18.4	27.7	31.1	45.7	53.1	24.8
Upward (+6 to +25)	10.1	19.8	24.4	25.7	26.1	25.8	23.1	23.4	22.9	24.7
Stable (-5 to +5)	52.4	44.4	42.9	37.2	31.3	24.5	19.1	13.8	12.3	28.1
Downward (-25 to -6)	33.7	25.7	17.6	17.1	17.2	13.6	15.1	11.7	9.2	15.5
High downward (-26 and under)	1.7	2.3	5.0	4.2	6.9	8.4	11.6	5.4	2.5	6.8
Total	100.0	99.9	99.9	100.1	99.9	100.0	100.0	100.0	100.0	99.9
Population[a] (in thousands)	288	1,413	3,432	5,149	7,197	11,064	4,165	2,861	1,994	37,563

[a]Excludes men not reporting Y and/or X.

TABLE J4.2. EXPECTED PERCENTAGE DISTRIBUTION BY INTERGENERATIONAL MOBILITY (Y-X), ON THE HYPOTHESIS OF INDEPENDENCE WITHIN EDUCATION CATEGORIES FOR MEN IN EACH EDUCATION CATEGORY

| Mobility | Educational Attainment | | | | | | | | | Total |
| | Elementary | | | | High School | | College | | | |
	0	1-4	5-7	8	1-3	4	1-3	4	5+	
High upward (+26 and over)	3.5	9.3	11.2	16.9	21.1	31.8	34.2	46.3	52.9	30.7
Upward (+6 to +25)	14.1	23.4	28.0	29.0	27.5	24.0	20.4	22.4	22.2	21.2
Stable (-5 to +5)	44.5	41.3	35.8	31.0	23.5	17.2	13.4	11.2	10.1	18.5
Downward (-25 to -6)	30.6	22.6	19.1	16.6	17.4	15.6	16.0	13.1	10.6	15.6
High downward (-26 and under)	7.3	3.5	6.0	6.5	10.5	11.4	15.9	7.0	4.1	14.0
Total	100.0	100.1	100.1	100.0	100.0	100.0	99.9	100.0	99.9	100.0
Population[a] (in thousands)	288	1,413	3,432	5,149	7,197	11,064	4,165	2,861	1,994	37,563

[a]Excludes men not reporting Y and/or X.

TABLE J4.3. STANDARDIZED PERCENTAGE DISTRIBUTION BY INTERGENERATIONAL MOBILITY (Y-X), FOR MEN IN EACH CATEGORY OF EDUCATIONAL ATTAINMENT

| | Educational Attainment | | | | | | | | | |
| | Elementary | | | | High School | | College | | | Total |
Mobility	0	1-4	5-7	8	1-3	4	1-3	4	5+	
High upward (+26 and over)	23.4	23.3	23.7	23.8	22.2	20.8	21.7	24.2	25.0	24.8
Upward (+6 to +25)	20.6	21.1	21.2	21.4	23.4	26.4	27.4	25.7	25.4	24.7
Stable (-5 to +5)	36.0	31.3	35.3	34.3	35.9	35.4	33.8	30.8	30.3	28.1
Downward (-25 to -6)	18.6	18.7	14.0	16.0	15.3	13.6	14.6	14.1	14.1	15.5
High downward (-26 and under)	1.2	5.6	5.8	4.5	3.2	3.8	2.5	5.2	5.2	6.8
Total	99.8	100.0	100.0	100.0	100.0	100.0	100.0	100.0	100.0	99.9

NOTE: Obtained by subtracting expected percentage in each cell of Table J4.2 from corresponding observed percentage in Table J4.1 and adding to this difference the observed percentage for all men with the designated degree of mobility, as shown in "Total" column of Table J4.1.

TABLE J5.1.   ALTERNATIVE SOLUTIONS FOR MODEL DEPICTED IN FIGURE 5.2--SYNTHETIC COHORT OF MEN WITH NONFARM BACKGROUND

Correlation or Path	All Sets	Set 1[a]	Set 2[a]	Set 3[a]	Set 4[a]	Set 5[a]
r_{UX}	.418					
p_{WX}	.183	Based on average of correlations for four age groups				
p_{WU}	.478					
p_{1X}	.055					
p_{1W}	.305					
p_{1U}	.465	Based on data for men 25-34 and average r_{UX}				
p_{Wa}	.815					
p_{1b}	.704					
p_{2X}	...	.100	.118	.139	.083	.111
p_{21}	...	.563	.397[b]	.209	.711	.460
p_{2U}	...	.225	.327	.442	.135	.288
p_{3X}	...	-.064	.048	.059	.019	.039
p_{32}	...	1.404	.715[b]	.647	.891	.769
p_{3U}	...	-.274	.118	.156	.017	.087
p_{4X}	...	-.059	-.009	-.014	-.037	-.025
p_{43}	...	1.093	.789[b]	.818	.962	.890
p_{4U}	...	-.048	.112	.097	.021	.059
p_{2c}	...	...	.696	.740	.539	.674
p_{3d}	...	...	.578	.622	.414	.536
p_{4e}	...	...	.504	.487	.278	.401
r_{ca}	...	0.0[b]	.059	.119	-.068	.038
r_{da}	...	0.0[b]	.167	.172	.175	.165
r_{ea}	...	0.0[b]	.119	.111	.093	.098
r_{cb}	...	0.0[b]	-.021	-.043	.024	-.013
r_{db}	...	0.0[b]	-.059	-.061	-.062	-.059
r_{eb}	...	0.0[b]	-.042	-.042	-.034	-.036

Correlation or Path	All Sets	Set 1[a]	Set 2[a]	Set 3[a]	Set 4[a]	Set 5[a]
r_{21}	...	.748	.655	.550[b]	.830[b]	.690[b]
r_{32}	...	1.203[c]	.809	.770[b]	.910[b]	.840[b]
r_{43}	...	1.043[c]	.852	.870[b]	.960[b]	.915[b]
r_{31}	...	...	.563	.480	.758	.602
r_{42}	...	...	.706	.686	.874	.775
r_{41}	...	...	.515	.451	.729	.565

[a]See the discussion in Chapter 5 for a full description of the assumptions of the five solutions.
Set 1: Assumes no intercorrelations among residual factors (R_a, R_b . . . R_e).

Set 2: Assumes path coefficients, p_{21}, p_{32}, and p_{43} of Chicago data (see footnote 11, Chapter 5).

Set 3: Assumes correlation coefficients (r_{21}, etc.) of Chicago data (see footnote 9, Chapter 5).

Set 4: Assumes correlation coefficients of Minneapolis data (see footnote 10, Chapter 5).

Set 5: Average of Sets 3 and 4.

[b]Values assumed to obtain solution.
[c]Impossible values requiring rejection of assumptions.

TABLE J6.1.   GROSS AND NET EFFECTS OF COLOR, NATIVITY, AND EDUCATIONAL ATTAINMENT ON STATUS OF FIRST JOB (W) AND 1962 OCC. (Y), BY FARM BACKGROUND

Background and Educational Attainment	Native White			Non-White	Native White			Nonwhite
	Native Parentage	Foreign or Mixed Parentage	Foreign-Born White		Native Parentage	Foreign or Mixed Parentage	Foreign-Born White	
	Gross Effects on W				Net Effects[a] on W			
All men	(Grand Mean = 25.5)							
None to elementary 8	-10.3	-9.2	-7.5	-11.7	-8.1	-7.4	-6.2	-9.3
High school 1 to 3	-6.1	-3.2	-1.2	-10.6	-5.5	-2.5	-1.4	-8.9
High school 4	-0.6	2.9	1.5	-5.6	-0.9	2.6	1.0	-4.3
College 1 or more	16.7	18.8	21.8	3.8	13.6	16.6	18.6	4.0
Nonfarm background	(Grand Mean = 28.7)							
None to elementary 8	-11.7	-11.1	-8.6	-13.1	-9.8	-9.1	-7.4	-10.9
High school 1 to 3	-7.9	-5.3	-3.3	-12.1	-7.2	-3.9	-2.9	-10.1
High school 4	-1.8	0.8	0.9	-7.0	-1.9	1.3	0.7	-5.2
College 1 or more	14.9	16.4	19.7	1.9	12.2	15.3	17.5	2.1
Farm background	(Grand Mean = 17.7)							
None to elementary 8	-3.9	-3.6	-2.9	-4.9	...	...	...	...
High school 1 to 3	-1.1	-1.0	-1.1	-5.7	...	...	...	...
High school 4	2.0	2.3	0.4	-2.3	...	...	...	...
College 1 or more	18.8	15.3	22.7	8.1	...	...	...	...

[a] Father's occ. status (X) held constant.

[b] Father's occ. (X) and first job (W) held constant for all men and men with nonfarm background; W held constant for men with farm background.

Background and Educational Attainment	Native White				Native White			
	Native Parentage	Foreign or Mixed Parentage	Foreign-Born White	Nonwhite	Native Parentage	Foreign or Mixed Parentage	Foreign-Born White	Non-White
	Gross Effects on Y				Net Effects[b] on Y			
All men	(Grand Mean = 36.3)							
None to elementary 8	-12.7	-8.5	-11.6	-19.5	-8.1	-4.8	-8.2	-14.0
High school 1 to 3	-6.6	-9.2	-2.4	-17.7	-4.3	-7.9	-2.1	-13.1
High school 4	1.5	4.9	3.6	-13.5	1.7	3.6	2.7	-10.5
College 1 or more	20.5	24.3	19.6	4.8	13.4	16.4	10.4	3.0
Nonfarm background	(Grand Mean = 40.1)							
None to elementary 8	-14.7	-13.2	-13.0	-22.1	-10.2	-8.9	-9.6	-16.5
High school 1 to 3	-9.2	-7.9	-3.4	-20.1	-6.3	-5.6	-2.0	-14.8
High school 4	0.1	2.4	0.6	-16.5	0.6	2.5	0.3	-12.7
College 1 or more	18.2	21.4	16.6	4.5	12.1	15.2	9.1	3.8
Farm background	(Grand Mean = 27.3)							
None to elementary 8	-4.6	-5.4	-6.0	-10.5	-3.3	-4.2	-4.8	-9.1
High school 1 to 3	0.0	-3.4	-6.0	-10.8	0.3	-3.3	-5.2	-9.3
High school 4	4.7	4.8	10.2	-6.4	4.3	3.8	10.1	-5.6
College 1 or more	23.5	23.3	26.6	-1.6	17.1	17.8	17.0	-1.1

TABLE J6.2. GROSS AND NET EFFECTS OF ETHNIC-MIGRATION CLASSIFICATION ON OCC.

Dependent Variable and Population	All Classes (Grand Mean)	Native White, Native Parentage			
		Born in North or West, living in--		Born in South, living in--	
		Region of Birth	Other Region	South	North or West
ESTIMATED POPULATION (THOUSANDS)					
All men	44,984	16,513	3,759	7,831	2,101
Nonfarm background	32,879	12,508	3,100	4,633	1,313
Farm background	12,104	4,005	659	3,198	788
OCCUPATIONAL STATUS, 1962 (Y)					
All men					
Gross effects	(36.3)	1.5	8.9	-1.4	-0.5
Net of W, U, X	0.0	-0.1	2.1	1.1	1.3
Nonfarm background					
Gross effects	(40.1)	1.3	7.4	-0.9	-0.5
Net of W, U, X	0.0	0.1	1.6	0.5	0.8
Farm background					
Gross effects	(27.3)	0.5	10.4	2.2	3.6
Net of W, U	0.0	-1.0	4.8	2.4	3.0
STATUS OF FIRST JOB (W)					
All men					
Gross effects	(25.5)	0.8	6.2	-1.7	-2.8
Net of U, X	0.0	-0.6	0.4	0.5	-1.1
Nonfarm background					
Gross effects	(28.7)	0.6	5.4	-1.1	-3.0
Net of U, X	0.0	-0.5	0.5	0.2	-1.8
Farm background					
Gross effects	(17.6)	0.3	4.1	1.3	0.8
Net of U	0.0	-0.7	0.3	1.5	0.7
EDUCATIONAL ATTAINMENT (U)					
All men					
Gross effects	(4.43)	0.29	0.84	-0.37	-0.10
Net of V, X	0.0	0.08	0.38	-0.22	0.01
Nonfarm background					
Gross effects	(4.74)	0.20	0.67	-0.25	-0.07
Net of V, X	0.0	0.02	0.27	-0.24	-0.04
Farm background					
Gross effects	(3.60)	0.45	1.06	-0.16	0.17
Net of V	0.0	0.28	0.85	-0.08	0.18

STATUS IN 1962 (Y), STATUS OF FIRST JOB (W), AND EDUCATIONAL ATTAINMENT (U), BY FARM BACKGROUND

| Native White, Foreign or Mixed Parentage | | | | | Nonwhite | | | |
| N-W Europe Parentage, living in-- | | Other Parentage, living in-- | | Foreign-Born White | Born in South, living in-- | | Born in North or West, living in-- | |
Region of Birth	Other Region	Region of Birth	Other Region		Region of Birth	Other Region	Region of Birth	Other Region
2,419	574	3,797	895	2,515	2,155	1,672	665	87
1,904	447	3,422	800	1,950	1,085	1,133	518	67
515	128	375	96	565	1,070	539	147	20
3.9	7.2	1.6	4.7	0.3	-19.3	-14.7	-6.2	-2.7
3.2	4.9	1.3	0.6	0.1	-8.6	-6.9	-4.4	-8.8
4.0	8.1	-0.4	2.7	-0.1	-20.4	-17.8	-6.4	-2.5
3.6	6.2	1.3	0.2	-0.2	-9.7	-9.5	-3.5	-8.0
0.1	3.0	-2.7	1.9	-1.3	-11.4	-7.7	-7.7	1.7
0.8	1.6	-2.2	2.8	0.7	-5.9	-4.3	-7.1	1.7
2.3	3.2	1.3	4.0	2.2	-11.6	-7.4	-4.3	2.5
2.2	1.5	1.9	0.8	2.1	-3.8	-1.7	-3.0	4.7
1.9	3.6	-0.5	2.9	2.5	-12.2	-9.1	-5.1	0.3
2.1	2.0	1.8	0.9	2.5	-4.3	-3.0	-2.9	-4.3
0.1	0.4	-1.3	-1.7	-0.8	-5.1	-3.3	-2.7	8.9
1.3	-0.1	-0.7	-1.3	0.5	-2.1	-1.1	-2.5	-1.9
0.04	0.28	0.05	0.49	-0.27	-1.69	-0.92	0.14	0.34
0.01	0.14	0.41	0.67	-0.24	-1.00	-0.47	0.26	0.00
0.00	0.20	-0.17	0.39	-0.23	-1.52	-0.90	-0.03	0.13
0.03	0.07	0.32	0.67	-0.18	-0.81	-0.38	0.19	-0.45
-0.10	0.38	0.05	-0.40	-0.59	-1.34	-0.78	0.42	0.16
-0.11	0.28	0.34	0.09	-0.50	-1.06	-0.56	0.35	0.15

TABLE J6.3. PER CENT OF NATIVE WHITES OF NATIVE PARENTAGE AND NONWHITES CONTINUING THEIR EDUCATION AT SUCCESSIVE LEVELS

Nativity, Color, and Migration Status	Through Eighth Grade (1)	Eighth Grade to Some High School (2)	Some High School to High-School Graduation (3)	High-School Graduation to Some College (4)	Some College to College Graduation (5)	College Graduation to Graduate School (6)
Native whites of native parentage—Northern born,						
Living in region of birth	91.5	85.3	76.7	44.5	51.2	38.8
Living elsewhere	96.3	91.8	79.3	59.0	55.1	42.9
Native whites of native parentage—Southern born,						
Living in region of birth	75.2	85.3	70.5	42.7	46.5	36.5
Living elsewhere	86.0	80.7	72.5	41.3	47.4	31.9
Nonwhites—Northern born,						
Living in region of birth	91.1	90.6	71.5	40.1	27.4	20.9[a]
Living elsewhere	83.9[a]	93.2[a]	89.7[a]	45.9[a]	42.9[a]	41.7[a]
Nonwhites—Southern born,						
Living in region of birth	49.3	79.2	44.0	34.1	44.2	28.1[a]
Living elsewhere	69.5	76.3	55.1	34.4	31.9	46.2[a]
All[b]	84.9	84.0	73.6	45.8	51.2	41.1

[a] Population base less than 100,000.
[b] Includes all men in the sample, not just those covered by the rest of this table.

TABLE J7.1.   INTERGENERATIONAL MOBILITY DISTRIBUTION OF ETHNICITY, NATIVITY, AND WHETHER LIVING IN REGION OF BIRTH, STANDARDIZED FOR FATHER'S OCC. (IN PERCENTAGES)

Color and Migration Status	Moving up 26 to 96 Points	Moving up 6 to 25 Points	Stable (-5 to +5 Points)	Moving down 6 Points or More	Total
Northern white					
Living in region of birth	19.0	28.1	37.8	15.1	100.0
Living elsewhere	17.8	31.6	37.0	13.6	100.0
Southern white,					
Living in region of birth	18.3	27.2	37.5	17.0	100.0
Living elsewhere	20.1	27.6	35.2	17.1	100.0
Second generation of					
North or West European descent					
Living in region of birth	19.8	27.1	36.7	16.4	100.0
Living elsewhere	17.6	28.9	33.8	19.7	100.0
Second generation of other descent,					
Living in region of birth	21.7	28.1	36.3	13.9	100.0
Living elsewhere	17.3	32.5	36.6	13.5	100.0
Foreign-born white	19.7	27.9	36.6	15.9	100.0
Northern nonwhite					
Living in region of birth	21.1	26.7	37.8	14.4	100.0
Living elsewhere	4.2	40.2	46.7	8.9	100.0
Southern nonwhite					
Living in region of birth	24.7	19.7	30.0	25.6	100.0
Living elsewhere	22.8	25.9	32.9	18.4	100.0

TABLE J7.2.   PER CENT DISTRIBUTION BY TYPE OF GEOGRAPHIC MOBILITY FROM AGE 16 TO MARCH 1962, BY AGE

Migration Status and Community of Destination	Total, 20 to 64	Age (Years)				
		20 to 24	25 to 34	35 to 44	45 to 54	55 to 64
Total, number in thousands	44,984	5,015	10,614	11,609	10,162	7,584
Total, per cent	100.0	100.0	100.0	100.0	100.0	100.0
Nonmigrant						
Large city	22.7	33.8	23.3	20.8	22.0	18.6
Small city	6.3	9.6	6.8	5.6	5.9	4.8
Rural nonfarm	6.5	10.7	8.4	6.1	5.0	3.9
Rural farm	7.7	7.5	5.7	7.5	8.8	9.7
Migrant, within same type of community						
Large city	12.4	9.9	11.9	14.5	12.3	11.5
Small city	3.7	4.2	3.6	3.5	3.7	3.5
Rural nonfarm	2.2	2.1	3.0	2.3	2.1	1.4
Rural farm	1.9	0.7	1.1	1.7	2.3	3.4
Migrant, between types of community						
Large to small city	1.5	1.6	1.5	1.9	1.3	0.9
Small to large city	10.5	6.1	11.4	10.7	10.3	12.1
Urban to rural[a]	7.2	4.2	8.6	8.0	6.9	6.2
Rural nonfarm to large city	3.1	2.6	3.0	2.6	3.0	4.5
Rural nonfarm to small city	1.1	1.4	1.1	0.9	0.9	1.3
Rural farm to large city	5.4	1.7	4.4	5.4	6.8	7.1
Rural farm to small city	2.3	1.2	1.7	2.4	2.6	3.5
Rural nonfarm to farm	0.4	0.3	0.3	0.4	0.4	0.6
Rural farm to nonfarm	3.6	1.0	2.7	4.1	4.4	4.7
Migration status unknown	1.6	1.5	1.5	1.4	1.5	2.2

[a]At least 9/10 of the destinations are rural nonfarm.

TABLE J10.1.   HUSBAND'S FATHER'S OCC. BY WIFE'S FATHER'S OCC., FOR OCG MARRIED COUPLES WITH WIFE 22 TO 61 YEARS OLD IN MARCH 1962 (FREQUENCIES IN THOUSANDS)

Husband's Father's Occ.	Wife's Father's Occ. (see stub)												
	(1)	(2)	(3)	(4)	(5)	(6)	(7)	(8)	(9)	(10)	(11)	(12)	Total
(1) Prof., SE	22	40	34	66	35	20	73	30	12	6	57	2	397
(2) Prof., sal.	57	100	82	132	57	39	207	125	42	26	110	6	983
(3) MOP, sal.	51	72	107	122	86	72	200	160	60	35	131	2	1,098
(4) MOP, SE	106	135	102	334	141	85	418	319	108	76	358	11	2,193
(5) Sales	32	69	78	134	128	54	266	151	57	55	130	18	1,172
(6) Clerical	28	53	48	98	62	30	196	129	55	55	142	19	915
(7) Crafts	73	255	223	358	208	207	1,464	1,074	226	377	785	77	5,327
(8) Operatives	44	132	105	244	173	120	997	1,313	183	315	600	75	4,301
(9) Service	22	65	64	96	45	54	343	208	93	100	168	24	1,282
(10) Laborers	24	49	28	72	62	52	273	358	81	297	237	81	1,614
(11) Farmers	59	166	157	323	151	123	894	895	184	392	4,174	219	7,737
(12) Farm laborers	8	18	12	18	20	12	112	102	23	80	161	148	714
Total	526	1,154	1,040	1,997	1,168	868	5,443	4,864	1,124	1,814	7,053	682	27,733[a]

[a]Excludes 5,139 couples with one or both occupations not reported.

TABLE J11.1.   SUMMARY OF GROSS AND NET EFFECTS OF OCC. CLASSIFICATIONS ON FERTILITY OF WIVES 42 TO 61 YEARS OLD, LIVING WITH HUSBANDS, IN OCG SAMPLE

Occupation Status and Type of Effect	Broad Occ. Group					
	White collar		Manual			Not
	Higher	Lower	Higher	Lower	Farm	stated
Number[a] of couples (thousands) by						
(1) Wife's father's occ.	2,081	805	2,273	3,139	4,145	1,312
(2) Husband's father's occ.	2,006	830	2,304	2,924	4,542	1,142
(3) Husband's first job	1,038	2,584	1,184	5,742	2,796	422
(4) Husband's occ., 1962	3,778	1,418	2,894	3,719	1,109	853
Gross effects[b] for						
(1) Wife's father's occ.	-.31	-.32	-.15	-.13	.37	.08
(2) Husband's father's occ.	-.47	-.46	-.06	-.12	.39	.02
(3) Husband's first job	-.49	-.50	-.14	.02	.67	.06
(4) Husband's occ. 1962	-.32	-.53	.12	.17	.74	.26
Net effects[b] for						
(1) net of (3)	-.14	-.17	-.08	-.10	.20	.07
(1) net of (4)	-.19	-.20	-.10	-.13	.27	.05
(2) net of (4)	-.32	-.33	-.01	-.11	.28	.01
(3) net of (1)	-.45	-.45	-.12	.03	.57	.02
(3) net of (4)	-.36	-.38	-.13	.00	.53	.02
(4) net of (1)	-.28	-.49	.12	.15	.57	.25
(4) net of (2)	-.24	-.46	.10	.13	.53	.23
(4) net of (3)	-.17	-.38	.09	.09	.37	.21

[a]Row sum may differ from grand total of 13,736 owing to accumulation of rounding errors in tabulation.
[b]Deviations from grand mean of 2.45 children ever born per wife.

TABLE J11.2.   NUMBER OF COUPLES AND NUMBER OF CHILDREN EVER BORN PER WIFE, BY WIFE'S FATHER'S OCC. AND HUSBAND'S FIRST JOB, FOR MARRIED COUPLES, SPOUSE PRESENT, WIFE 42 TO 61 YEARS OLD, CIVILIAN NONINSTITUTIONAL POPULATION OF THE UNITED STATES, MARCH 1962

Wife's Father's Occ.	All Couples	Husband's First Job					
		White-collar		Manual			Not
		Higher	Lower	Higher	Lower	Farm	Stated
Number of couples (thousands)							
All couples	13,755[a]	1,035	2,581	1,194	5,732	2,793	420
Higher white-collar	2,081	379	606	192	668	191	45
Lower white-collar	805	106	259	76	265	72	27
Higher manual	2,273	137	534	279	1,031	234	58
Lower manual	3,139	136	554	269	1,754	364	62
Farm	4,145	199	412	262	1,453	1,694	125
Not stated	1,312	78	216	116	561	238	103
Children ever born per wife							
All couples	2.45	1.96	1.95	2.29	2.46	3.11	2.53
Higher white-collar	2.14	1.75	1.99	1.87	2.37	2.86	2.20
Lower white-collar	2.13	1.92	1.92	2.78	2.12	2.42	2.48
Higher manual	2.30	2.08	1.84	2.30	2.44	2.93	2.05
Lower manual	2.32	2.01	1.97	2.01	2.41	2.76	2.13
Farm	2.82	2.30	2.04	2.58	2.68	3.24	2.76
Not stated	2.53	1.85	1.92	2.66	2.40	3.38	2.91

[a]Marginal and grand totals are sums of cell frequencies; totals vary between tabulations because of accumulated rounding errors.

Name Index

Subject Index